Modern Imaging Evaluation of the Brain, Body and Spine

Editor

LARA A. BRANDÃO

MAGNETIC RESONANCE IMAGING CLINICS OF NORTH AMERICA

www.mri.theclinics.com

Consulting Editors
SURESH K. MUKHERJI
LYNNE STEINBACH

May 2013 • Volume 21 • Number 2

ELSEVIER

1600 John F. Kennedy Boulevard • Suite 1800 • Philadelphia, Pennsylvania, 19103-2899

http://www.theclinics.com

MRI CLINICS OF NORTH AMERICA Volume 21, Number 2
May 2013 ISSN 1064-9689, ISBN 13: 978-1-4557-7115-8

Editor: Pamela Hetherington

Magnetic Resonance Imaging Clinics of North America (ISSN 1064-9689) is published quarterly by Elsevier Inc., 360 Park Avenue South, New York, NY 10010-1710. Months of issue are February, May, August, and November. Business and Editorial Offices: 1600 John F. Kennedy Blvd., Ste. 1800, Philadelphia, PA 19103-2899. Customer Service Office: 3251 Riverport Lane, Maryland Heights, MO 63043. Periodicals postage paid at New York, NY and additional mailing offices. Subscription prices are $357.00 per year (domestic individuals), $573.00 per year (domestic institutions), $182.00 per year (domestic students/residents), $399.00 per year (Canadian individuals), $716.00 per year (Canadian institutions), $517.00 per year (international individuals), $716.00 per year (international institutions), and $263.00 per year (international and Canadian students/residents). International air speed delivery is included in all *Clinics* subscription prices. All prices are subject to change without notice. **POSTMASTER:** Send address changes to *Magnetic Resonance Imaging Clinics*, Elsevier Health Sciences Division, Subscription Customer Service, 3251 Riverport Lane, Maryland Heights, MO 63043. Customer Service (orders, claims, online, change of address): Elsevier Health Sciences Division, Subscription Customer Service, 3251 Riverport Lane, Maryland Heights, MO 63043. Tel:1-800-654-2452 (U.S. and Canada); 314-447-8871 (outside U.S. and Canada). Fax: 314-447-8029. E-mail: journalscustomerservice-usa@elsevier.com (for print support); journalsonlinesupport-usa@elsevier.com (for online support).

Reprints. For copies of 100 or more of articles in this publication, please contact the Commercial Reprints Department, Elsevier Inc., 360 Park Avenue South, New York, NY 10010-1710. Tel.: 212-633-3812; Fax: 212-462-1935; E-mail: reprints@elsevier.com.

Magnetic Resonance Imaging Clinics of North America is covered in the *RSNA Index of Imaging Literature, MEDLINE/PubMed (Index Medicus),* and *EMBASE/Excerpta Medica.*

Printed and bound by CPI Group (UK) Ltd, Croydon, CR0 4YY

Transferred to digital print 2012

Contributors

CONSULTING EDITOR

SURESH K. MUKHERJI, MD, FACR
Professor and Chief of Neuroradiology,
Department of Radiology, University of
Michigan Health System, Ann Arbor, Michigan

EDITOR

LARA A. BRANDÃO, MD
Chief of Neuroradiology, Radiologic
Department, Clinica Felippe Mattoso,
Barra da Tijuca, Rio de Janeiro, Brazil

AUTHORS

MANYOO AGARWAL, MD
Division of Neuroradiology, Department of
Radiology, Keck School of Medicine,
University of Southern California,
Los Angeles, California

ARTEM S. BELYAEV, BA
Researcher, Functional MRI Laboratory,
Department of Radiology, Memorial
Sloan-Kettering Cancer Center, New York,
New York

MICHAEL T. BOOKER, BS
Division of Neuroradiology, Department of
Radiology, Keck School of Medicine,
University of Southern California,
Los Angeles, California

ALICE C. BRANDÃO, MD
Women's Imaging Radiologist, Clinica Felippe
Mattoso, Barra da Tijuca, Rio de Janeiro, Brazil

LARA A. BRANDÃO, MD
Chief of Neuroradiology, Radiologic
Department, Clinica Felippe Mattoso, Barra da
Tijuca, Rio de Janeiro, Brazil

GINA BROWN, MBBS, MD, MRCP, FRCR
Department of Radiology, Royal Marsden
Hospital, Sutton, United Kingdom

LUCIANA COSTA-SILVA, MD, MSc
Assistant Professor of Radiology and
Medical Faculty, Department of Anatomy
and Imaging, Federal University of Minas
Gerais, Clínica Ecoar Medicina Diagnóstica,
Belo Horizonte, Brazil

ANTONIO LUIS EIRAS DE ARAÚJO, MD
Staff Radiologist, Department of Radiology,
Universidade Federal do Rio de Janeiro, Rua
Rodolpho Paulo Rocco; Staff Radiologist, Labs
D'Or Network – Fleury Group, Rio de Janeiro,
Brazil

DANIEL ANDRADE TINOCO DE SOUZA, MD
Clinical Fellow, PET/CT and Nuclear Medicine,
Dana-Farber Cancer Institute, Harvard Medical
School, Boston, Massachusetts

AARON S. FIELD, MD, PhD
Associate Professor of Radiology and
Biomedical Engineering, Chief of
Neuroradiology, Department of Radiology,
School of Medicine and Public Health,
University of Wisconsin, Madison, Wisconsin

ANDREI I. HOLODNY, MD
Chief of the Neuroradiology Service, Director of
the Functional MRI Laboratory and Professor
of Radiology, Department of Radiology,
Memorial Sloan-Kettering Cancer Center, Weill
Medical College of Cornell University, New
York, New York

JASON M. HUSTON, DO
Neuroradiology Fellow, Department of
Radiology, School of Medicine and Public
Health, University of Wisconsin, Madison,
Wisconsin

PAULA IANEZ, MD
Radiologist, Clinica Felippe Mattoso,
Barra da Tijuca, Rio de Janeiro, Brazil

NIDHI JAIN, MD
Division of Neuroradiology, Department of
Radiology, Keck School of Medicine,
University of Southern California,
Los Angeles, California

MENG LAW, MD
Division of Neuroradiology, Department of
Radiology, Keck School of Medicine,
University of Southern California,
Los Angeles, California

CONSTANCE D. LEHMAN, MD, PhD, FACR
Professor and Vice Chair of Radiology and
Section Head of Breast Imaging, University of
Washington School of Medicine; Director of
Imaging, Seattle Cancer Care Alliance,
Seattle, Washington

ALEXANDER LERNER, MD
Division of Neuroradiology, Department of
Radiology, Keck School of Medicine,
University of Southern California,
Los Angeles, California

KOENRAAD J. MORTELÉ, MD
Director, Division of Clinical MRI; Staff
Radiologist, Abdominal Imaging and
Body MRI, Beth Israel Deaconess Medical
Center; Associate Professor of Radiology,
Harvard Medical School, Boston,
Massachusetts

ILANA NAGHI, MD
Division of Neuroradiology, Department of
Radiology, Keck School of Medicine,
University of Southern California,
Los Angeles, California

JAIME ARAUJO OLIVEIRA NETO, MD
Clinical Researcher, D'Or Institute for
Research and Education; Staff Radiologist,
Labs D'Or Network – Fleury Group and Quinta
D'Or Hospital, Rio de Janeiro, Brazil

DANIELLA BRAZ PARENTE, MD, PhD
Clinical Researcher, D'Or Institute for
Research and Education; Staff Radiologist,
Labs D'Or Network – Fleury Group, Rio de
Janeiro, Brazil

SAVANNAH C. PARTRIDGE, PhD
Research Associate Professor, Department of
Radiology, University of Washington School of
Medicine, Seattle Cancer Care Alliance,
Seattle, Washington

KYUNG K. PECK, PhD
Assistant Attending Physicist, Functional MRI
Laboratory, Department of Radiology and
Medical Physics, Memorial Sloan-Kettering
Cancer Center, New York, New York

NICOLE M. PETROVICH BRENNAN, BA
Neurodiagnostic fMRI Specialist, Functional
MRI Laboratory, Department of Radiology,
Memorial Sloan-Kettering Cancer Center,
New York, New York

MARK S. SHIROISHI, MD
Division of Neuroradiology, Department of
Radiology, Keck School of Medicine,
University of Southern California,
Los Angeles, California

ANELISE OLIVEIRA SILVA, MD
Department of Radiology, Hospital Federal da
Lagoa; IRM, Ressonância Magnética; Clínica
Radiológica Luiz Felippe Mattoso, Rio de
Janeiro, Brazil

LAWRENCE N. TANENBAUM, MD, FACR
Associate Professor and Director of Computed
Tomography and Magnetic Resonance
Imaging, Department of Diagnostic Imaging,
Mount Sinai School of Medicine, New York,
New York

Contents

> This article focuses on advanced magnetic resonance (MR) imaging techniques and
> how they can be used to help diagnose a specific tumor, suggest tumor grade and
> prognosis, follow tumor progression, evaluate tumor extension, suggest the ideal
> site for biopsy, and assess therapeutic response. Advanced MR imaging techniques
> may also help to distinguish between lesions that simulate brain tumors on conven-
> tional MR imaging studies.

> Although conventional contrast-enhanced MR imaging remains the standard-of-
> care imaging method in the posttreatment evaluation of gliomas, recent develop-
> ments in therapeutic options such as chemoradiation and antiangiogenic agents
> have caused the neuro-oncology community to rethink traditional imaging criteria.
> This article highlights the latest recommendations. These recommendations should
> be viewed as works in progress. As more is learned about the pathophysiology of
> glioma treatment response, quantitative imaging biomarkers will be validated within
> this context. There will likely be further refinements to glioma response criteria,
> although the lack of technical standardization in image acquisition, postprocessing,
> and interpretation also need to be addressed.

> Functional magnetic resonance (fMR) imaging for neurosurgical planning has
> become the standard of care in centers where it is available. Although paradigms
> to measure eloquent cortices are not yet standardized, simple tasks elicit reliable
> maps for planning neurosurgical procedures. A patient-specific paradigm design
> will refine the usability of fMR imaging for prognostication and recovery of function.
> Certain pathologic conditions and technical issues limit the interpretation of fMR
> imaging maps in clinical use and should be considered carefully. However, fMR
> imaging for neurosurgical planning continues to provide insights into how the brain
> works and how it responds to pathologic insults.

assessment of disease activity. Knowledge of the location, severity, and presence of complications may assist in providing patients with appropriate treatment options. Other small bowel diseases beyond Crohn disease will also be discussed.

Optimal treatment decisions for patients with rectal cancer are based on knowledge of tumor characteristics and prognostic features and any initial treatment must aim to reduce the risk of both local and distant recurrence. The radiologist has become an increasingly important part of multidisciplinary team managing rectal cancer. The primary goal of MRI staging of rectal tumors is to identify prognostic factors in order to offer patients a tailored treatment based on individual risks. Restaging of rectal tumors using MRI after chemoradiation therapy is becoming more relevant issue, since further tailoring of treatment is increasingly being considered after the treatment.

The multiparametric approach expanded the clinical applications for prostate magnetic resonance (MR) imaging to include not only staging but also a correlation with tumor aggressiveness. It can also help to guide biopsies, to achieve a higher tumor detection rate, and to better reflect the true Gleason grade. The improved accuracy provided by multiparametric MR imaging and a better understanding of the clinical significance of the imaging findings can pave the way to a more direct role of MR imaging in patient management.

Defecography by magnetic resonance (MR) imaging makes it possible to view the multiple compartments of the pelvic floor at one examination, with high-resolution images at rest and dynamic images, providing accurate evaluation of the morphology and function of the anorectal and pelvic organs and muscles, involved in pelvic floor dynamics. MR imaging of the pelvic floor identifies the diseases affecting the evacuation mechanism, providing information essential for surgical planning and choice of treatment approach. This article focuses on the MR details of the pelvic floor anatomy and the most commonly observed anatomic and functional abnormalities.

Magnetic resonance (MR) imaging has been widely accepted as a powerful imaging modality for the evaluation of the pelvis because of its intrinsic superior soft tissue contrast compared with that of computed tomography. In certain cases, however, the morphologic study provided by MR imaging may not be enough. Functional evaluation with perfusion and diffusion, which allow estimation of the microvascular characteristics and cellularity of the lesions, favors the differentiation of benign from malignant lesions. This article focuses on new magnetic resonance techniques and their contribution to the differentiation and characterization of pelvic pathologies.

MAGNETIC RESONANCE IMAGING CLINICS OF NORTH AMERICA

FORTHCOMING ISSUES

August 2013
Breast MR Imaging
Bonnie Joe, MD, *Editor*

November 2013
Pediatric Imaging of the Abdomen
Jonathan Dillman, MD and Ethan Smith, MD, *Editors*

February 2014
Imaging of the Bowel
Jordi Rimola, MD, *Editor*

RECENT ISSUES

February 2013
Imaging of the Hip
Miriam A. Bredella, MD, *Editor*

November 2012
MR Contrast Agents
Marco Essig, MD, and
Juan E. Gutierrez, MD, *Editors*

August 2012
Practical MR Imaging in the Head and Neck
Laurie A. Loevner, MD, *Editor*

RELATED INTEREST

***Neuroimaging Clinics*, February 2013**
Head and Neck Cancer
Patricia A. Hudgins, MD, and Amit M. Saindane, MD, *Editors*

PROGRAM OBJECTIVE
The goal of Magnetic Resonance Imaging Clinics of North America is to keep practicing physicians up to date with current clinical practice by providing timely articles reviewing the state of the art in patient care.

TARGET AUDIENCE
All practicing physicians and healthcare professionals who provide patient care utilizing findings from Magnetic Resonance Imaging.

LEARNING OBJECTIVES
Upon completion of this activity, participants will be able to:
1. Recognize clinical applications of functional MRI.
2. Review MRI of the pelvic floor as well as rectal cancer.
3. Discuss advances in imaging evaluation of female pelvis diseases.
4. Utilize magnetic resonance enterography for the assessment of small bowel disease.

ACCREDITATION
The Elsevier Office of Continuing Medical Education (EOCME) is accredited by the Accreditation Council for Continuing Medical Education (ACCME) to provide continuing medical education for physicians.

The EOCME designates this journal-based CME activity for a maximum of 12 *AMA PRA Category 1 Credit*(s)™. Physicians should claim only the credit commensurate with the extent of their participation in the activity.

All other health care professionals completing continuing education credit for this activity will be issued a certificate of participation.

DISCLOSURE OF CONFLICTS OF INTEREST
The EOCME assesses conflict of interest with its instructors, faculty, planners, and other individuals who are in a position to control the content of CME activities. All relevant conflicts of interest that are identified are thoroughly vetted by EOCME for fair balance, scientific objectivity, and patient care recommendations. EOCME is committed to providing its learners with CME activities that promote improvements or quality in healthcare and not a specific proprietary business or a commercial interest.

The planning committee, staff, authors and editors listed below have identified no financial relationships or relationships to products or devices they or their spouse/life partner have with commercial interest related to the content of this CME activity:
Manyoo Agarwal, MD; Artem S. Belyaev, BA; Michael T. Booker, MD; Lara A. Brandao, MD; Alice C. Brandao, MD; Daniella Braz Parente, MD, PhD; Nicole M. Petrovich Brennan, BA; Gina Brown, MBBS, MD, MRCP, FRCR; Mauricio Castillo, MD; Nicole Congleton; Luciana Costa-Silva, MD, MSc; Antonio Luis Eiras de Araujo, MD; Aaron S. Field, MD, PhD; Pamela Hetherington; Jason M. Huston, DO; Paula Ianez, MD; Nidhi Jain, MD; Sandy Lavery; Alexander Lerner, MD; Jill McNair; Koenraad J. Mortele, MD; Ilana Naghi, MD; Anelise Oliveira Silva, MD; Jaime Araujo Oliveira Neto, MD; Savannah C. Partridge, PhD; Kyung K. Peck, PhD; Daniel Andrade Tinoco de Souza, MD; Karthikeyan Subramaniam; and Tina Young Poussaint, MD.

The planning committee, staff, authors and editors listed below have identified financial relationships or relationships to products or devices they or their spouse/life partner have with commercial interest related to the content of this CME activity:
Andrei I. Holodny, MD has stock ownership in fMRI Consultants.
Meng Law, MD, MBBS, FRACR has stock ownership in Prism Clinical Imaging; has research grants from NIH and Bayer; is a consultant/advisor for Bayer; and is on speaker's bureau for Toshiba America Medical, ICad, Inc. and Bracco.
Constance D. Lehman, MD, PhD, FACR is a consultant/advisor for GE and Bayer.
Suresh K. Mukherji, MD, FACR is a consultant/advisor for Philips.
Mark S. Shiroishi, MD is a consultant/advisor for Bayer.
Lawrence N. Tanenbaum, MD, FACR has a research grant from GE Healthcare and is on speaker's bureau for GE Healthcare and Siemens Medical.

UNAPPROVED/OFF-LABEL USE DISCLOSURE
The EOCME requires CME faculty to disclose to the participants:
1. When products or procedures being discussed are off-label, unlabelled, experimental, and/or investigational (not US Food and Drug Administration [FDA]) approved; and
2. Any limitations on the information presented, such as data that are preliminary or that represent ongoing research, interim analyses, and/or unsupported opinions. Faculty may discuss information about pharmaceutical agents that is outside of FDA-approved labelling. This information is intended solely for CME and is not intended to promote off-label use of these medications. If you have any questions, contact the medical affairs department of the manufacturer for the most recent prescribing information.

TO ENROLL
To enroll in the *Magnetic Resonance Imaging Clinics of North* Continuing Medical Education program, call customer service at 1-800-654-2452 or sign up online at http://www.theclinics.com/home/cme. The CME program is available to subscribers for an additional annual fee of $223 USD.

METHOD OF PARTICIPATION
In order to claim credit, participants must complete the following:
1. Complete enrolment as indicated above.
2. Read the activity.
3. Complete the CME Test and Evaluation. Participants must achieve a score of 70% on the test. All CME Tests and Evaluations must be completed online.

CME INQUIRIES/SPECIAL NEEDS
For all CME inquiries or special needs, please contact elsevierCME@elsevier.com.

Foreword

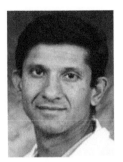

Suresh K. Mukherji, MD, FACR
Consulting Editor

It is my distinct pleasure to thank Lara Brandao for editing this edition of *Magnetic Resonance Imaging Clinics of North America* on MR of the Brain, Body, and Spine. Dr Brandao had focused this edition on advanced MR techniques for imaging various parts of the brain, body, and spine. The techniques she reviews are emerging MR techniques that have direct clinical applications. Some examples include fMRI, diffusion imaging of the spine, diffusion imaging of the breast, multiparametric MR imaging of the prostate, and MR enterography. The authors are recognized experts in the respective specialties and I thank them for their efforts.

This edition also highlights the tremendous talent of individuals outside the usual confines of the United States and Europe. Dr Brandao is from Brazil, which is where the "action" will be over the next few years. Both the Football (Soccer) World Cup and Olympics will be held in Brazil and I encourage all of you to visit this wonderful country. The beauty of the country is only superseded by the warmth and hospitality of its people.

I am not quite sure how Lara was able to edit this edition with 2 young children. However, she is a very special individual and I personally thank her for creating such an outstanding edition.

Suresh K. Mukherji, MD, FACR
Department of Radiology
University of Michigan Health System
1500 East Medical Center
Ann Arbor, MI, 48109-0030, USA

E-mail address:
mukherji@med.umich.edu

Magn Reson Imaging Clin N Am 21 (2013) xi
http://dx.doi.org/10.1016/j.mric.2013.02.001
1064-9689/13/$ – see front matter © 2013 Published by Elsevier Inc.

mri.theclinics.com

Preface

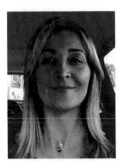

Lara A. Brandão, MD
Editor

This issue of *Magnetic Resonance Imaging Clinics of North America* focuses on modern imaging techniques in the evaluation of the brain, spine, and body.

In the beginning of this issue, the readers are provided with two articles on brain tumors. The first article, entitled "Brain Tumors: A Multimodality Approach with DWI, DTI, MRS, DSC, and DCE MRI," focuses on advanced MR imaging techniques and how they can be used to help diagnose a specific tumor, suggest tumor grade and prognosis, detect tumor progression, evaluate tumor extension, suggest the ideal site for biopsy, and assess therapeutic response.

The next article, entitled "Posttreatment Evaluation of CNS Gliomas," addresses posttreatment evaluation of CNS gliomas. Limitations of the Macdonald criteria and the latest RANO Working group recommendations, with particular attention to pseudoprogression and pseudoresponse, are discussed. In addition, a review of the developing role of advanced MR imaging techniques is provided.

In the article entitled, "Clinical Applications of Functional MRI," basic principles, anatomy of the functional areas, as well as task and paradigm selection are extensively reviewed, with special attention to motor and language pradigms. Issues concerning data acquisition, analysis and interpretation, as well as artifacts and pitfalls are also addressed.

In "Clinical Applications of DTI," the authors discuss the physical principles of DTI, as well as DTI quantification and display. Clinical applications of DTI in the brain, brainstem, and spinal cord are discussed.

The article entitled, "Clinical Applications of Diffusion Imaging in the Spine," in addition to discussing technical issues, demonstrates that diffusion imaging adds sensitivity and specificity in evaluating the osseous and soft tissue structures of the spine for neoplastic involvement as well as in cases of suspected infection. Diffusion-weighted imaging (DWI) can also contribute valuable information to the evaluation of lesions of the spinal cord, offering improved lesion characterization.

The remaining seven articles concern advances in body imaging. "Breast MRI-Diffusion-weighted Imaging" offers a great review of the role of DWI in the evaluation of breast lesions. The principles and the technique of DWI, as well as example protocols, are discussed. Clinical applications of diffusion MRI are reviewed, such as distinguishing malignant from benign lesions as well as a discussion on false-negative and false-positive findings.

Modern MRI evaluation of the liver includes a comprehensive morphologic and functional assessment of the liver parenchyma, hepatic vessels, and biliary tree. The article entitled, "Modern Imaging Evaluation of the Liver: Emerging MRI Techniques," discusses the role of conventional MR imaging in the quantification of liver fat and iron deposition, as well as the role of DWI in the identification and characterization of both focal and diffuse diseases. Potential indications of MR elastrography are also addressed.

The article entitled, "MR Enterography for the Assessment of Small Bowel Diseases," addresses the role of MR enterography in the evaluation of small bowel diseases. The protocol for the examination is discussed, including enteric contrast agents, imaging timing, and sequence selection. Imaging findings in Crohn disease as well as in bowel neoplasms and celiac disease are addressed.

http://dx.doi.org/10.1016/j.mric.2013.02.002
1064-9689/13/$ – see front matter © 2013 Published by Elsevier Inc.

mri.theclinics.com

In "Magnetic Resonance Imaging of Rectal Cancer," the readers are provided with an extensive review of the rectal anatomy as well as important technical issues in the evaluation of the rectum. Risk factors for local recurrence and distant metastatic disease are discussed.

In the article entitled, "Multiparametric MR Imaging of the Prostate," MR imaging techniques in the evaluation of the prostate gland are discussed, including the role of DWI, dynamic contrast-enhanced imaging, and MR spectroscopy. Clinical applications of prostate MRI such as diagnosis and staging of prostate tumors are addressed.

There are two articles concerning the pelvis: one on pelvic floor entitled, "MRI of the Pelvic Floor—Defecography," that discusses normal pelvic floor anatomy, dynamic MR defecography technique, as well as the main imaging findings in diseases of the pelvic floor. The second article on the female pelvis entitled, "Diseases of the Female Pelvis—Advances in Imaging Evaluation," describes how DWI and dynamic contrast-enhanced MRI may help characterize endometrium carcinoma, myometrial focal lesions, as well as adenomyosis and cervical cancer. The role of SWI in endometriomas and of DWI in tubo-ovarian abscesses, adnexial torsion, and adnexial neoplasms is also demonstrated.

In this issue we intend to share author experience as well as to offer the readers an extensive literature review on modern imaging techniques that help us to improve our diagnostic abilities in daily practice. The articles were written by experienced radiologists and address topics relevant to daily practice.

I would like to sincerely and whole-heartedly thank all of the authors of this issue for their invaluable contributions to this work. I wish to express my sincere gratitude to the consulting editor, Dr Suresh Mukherji, MD, for the opportunity and privilege to lead this project. I would also like to thank the series editors, Pamela Hetherington and Nicole Congleton, for their guidance and support during the process of preparation of this work.

I would like to dedicate this issue to my husband, Sergio, and my daughters, Carolina (8 years) and Camila (5 years), for their support, love, and understanding during the process of preparing this work.

To my father, Adelmo, my best friend!

Lara A. Brandão, MD
Radiologic Department, Clinica Felippe Mattoso
Barra da Tijuca, Rio de Janeiro 22640-100, Brazil

E-mail address:
larabrandao.rad@terra.com.br

Brain Tumors
A Multimodality Approach with Diffusion-Weighted Imaging, Diffusion Tensor Imaging, Magnetic Resonance Spectroscopy, Dynamic Susceptibility Contrast and Dynamic Contrast-Enhanced Magnetic Resonance Imaging

Lara A. Brandão, MD[a,b,*], Mark S. Shiroishi, MD[c],
Meng Law, MD[c]

KEYWORDS

- Diffusion • Fractional anisotropy • Magnetic resonance spectroscopy • Perfusion
- Dynamic susceptibility contrast MR imaging • Dynamic contrast-enhanced MR imaging • Permeability
- Brain tumor

KEY POINTS

- High choline levels in the spectrum and high blood volumes in the perfusion study of the peritumoral region favors glioblastoma multiforme (GBM) rather than single brain metastasis with high specificity.
- Low apparent diffusion coefficient (ADC), along with low blood volumes and mild elevation of the permeability, favors lymphoma over GBM.
- Restricted diffusion and prominent choline peak, along with the presence of taurine in the spectrum favors medulloblastoma rather than ependymoma; on the other hand, a high myo-inositol (mI) peak in the spectrum along with high blood volume and low percentage of signal intensity recovery of the time-intensity curve favors ependymoma.
- High-grade gliomas typically present with high choline in the spectrum, high blood volumes, and high permeability. High ADC measurements, discrete or no elevation of the choline peak along with high mI peak, low blood volumes, and no or low elevation of the permeability characterize low-grade (grade II) gliomas. Beware: high blood volumes may be seen in low-grade gliomas, usually in oligodendrogliomas.
- ADC, cerebral blood volume (CBV) and multivoxel ^{1}H magnetic resonance spectroscopy (MV-MRS) may better indicate the ideal site for biopsy in an infiltrative tumor than a conventional magnetic resonance (cMR) imaging study.
- Tumor extension is better estimated by perfusion study and MV-MRS than cMR imaging.
- Elevated ADC and low choline levels along with high lipids, low blood volumes and, probably, lower permeability characterize favorable tumor response to therapy. Beware: elevated choline levels may be seen in radiation necrosis.

Funding Sources: None.
Conflict of Interest: L.A. Brandão: None. M.S. Shiroishi: Bayer Healthcare: Consultant. M. Law: Toshiba America Medical Systems: Speaker Bureau, Bayer Healthcare: Research Grant, Bracco Diagnostics: Honorarium, iCAD Inc: Honorarium; Prism Clinical Imaging: Stock Options, Fuji Inc: Honorarium.
[a] Radiologic Department, Clínica Felippe Mattoso, Fleury Medicina Diagnóstica, Av. Das Américas 700, Sala 320, Barra da Tijuca, Rio de Janeiro 22640-100, Brazil; [b] Clínica IRM, Ressonância Magnética, Rua Capitão Salomão 44-Humaitá, Rio de Janeiro 22271-040, Brazil; [c] Department of Radiology, Keck School of Medicine, University of Southern California, 1520 San Pablo Street, Lower Level Imaging, L1600, Los Angeles, CA 90033, USA
* Corresponding author.
E-mail address: larabrandao.rad@terra.com.br

Magn Reson Imaging Clin N Am 21 (2013) 199–239
http://dx.doi.org/10.1016/j.mric.2013.02.003
1064-9689/13/$ – see front matter © 2013 Published by Elsevier Inc.

INTRODUCTION

In addition to conventional magnetic resonance (MR) imaging techniques, advanced techniques including diffusion-weighted (DW) imaging, proton nuclear magnetic resonance spectroscopy (^{1}H-MRS), perfusion-weighted (PW) imaging, and dynamic contrast-enhanced (DCE) imaging studies can provide information beyond mere anatomy and have been commonly used in clinical practice. Maps of apparent diffusion coefficient (ADC), fractional anisotropy (FA), and relative cerebral blood volume (rCBV), as well as the metabolic abnormalities in the spectrum and the permeability maps and curves generated by advanced imaging techniques, may enable the radiologist to identify tumor tissue, differentiate tumor types, grade tumors, evaluate tumor extent, guide stereotactic biopsy, and determine early response to treatment.[1–19]

Diffusion-Weighted Imaging

DW imaging has been used to grade brain tumors on the basis of cellularity.

Low ADC values have been correlated with increasing cellularity, increasing grade, and increasing Ki-67 cellular proliferation index in cerebral gliomas.[20–33]

Fractional Anisotropy

FA represents the magnitude and directionality of water diffusion. FA measurements may help distinguish glioblastoma multiforme (GBM) from solitary brain metastases.[34,35]

[1]H Magnetic Resonance Spectroscopy

^{1}H-MRS is a noninvasive, in vivo technique that provides additional metabolic diagnostic indices beyond anatomic information, which has been extensively used to evaluate brain tumors. High choline (Cho) and lipids (Lip), along with low N-acetylaspartate (NAA) peaks, are related to tumor aggressiveness.[36]

Dynamic Susceptibility Contrast (Perfusion) MR Imaging

rCBV maps can be generated from dynamic susceptibility contrast (DSC) T2* gradient-echo–echo-planar sequence (GE-EPI), acquired during the first pass of the standard dose of a gadolinium-based contrast agent. Tumor blood volume (TBV) values can be measured from the rCBV map, and TBV has been correlated with tumor grade and vascularity, with higher TBV associated with gliomas of higher grade.[37–39]

Dynamic Contrast-Enhanced (Permeability) MR Imaging

DCE studies allow estimation of brain tumor permeability, and have been used more recently in the characterization of brain tumors.[40] While pharmacokinetic modeling and determination of metrics such as volume transfer constant (K^{trans}), volume of the extravascular-extracellular space (Ve), and blood plasma volume (Vp) have been commonly used in the literature, one of the authors (L.A.B.) has had extensive experience in subjective analysis of dynamic changes in signal enhancement using the Maximum Slope of Increase algorithm with the aid of GE Functool (GE Healthcare, Waukesha, WI). Such changes are likely correlated with microvascular permeability, and the content referred to as "permeability" herein is reflective of that experience, unless otherwise noted.

MAIN CLINICAL APPLICATIONS
Determination of Tumor Type

On contrast-enhanced T1-weighted images (CE-T1WI), high-grade gliomas (HGGs), lymphomas, and metastasis show enhancement, which are sometimes difficult to specify using conventional MR (cMR) images.[5]

The information obtained from advanced MR imaging techniques may help indicate a specific diagnosis.

GBM versus solitary metastasis

It is clinically important to differentiate GBM from a solitary brain metastasis because medical staging, surgical planning, and therapeutic decisions are vastly different for each tumor type.[41–43]

On conventional MR images, HGGs and solitary metastatic brain tumors often display similar signal-intensity characteristics and contrast-enhancement patterns. Advanced MR imaging techniques may help in differentiating solitary brain metastasis from high-grade glial tumors such as GBM.[43]

Peritumoral ADC

GBMs and metastatic tumors often contain heterogeneous signal intensity secondary to necrosis and susceptibility artifacts. As a result of this heterogeneity, DW imaging metrics obtained from the tumor can be imprecise or inaccurate. Lee and colleagues[41] demonstrated that tumoral ADC showed no statistically significant difference between the two groups (GBM and metastasis). On the other hand, the mean minimum ADC value in the peritumoral region of GBMs (1.149 $\pm$ 0.119 [standard deviation]) was significantly lower than that in metastases (1.413 $\pm$ 0.147) ($P<.05$). The mean peritumoral ADC ratio (minimum ADC in the peritumoral edema of the affected hemisphere divided by that from the normal white matter in the contralateral hemisphere) was also significantly lower in GBMs (1.466 ± 0.24) than in metastases (1.829 ± 0.25) (P<.05). These results support the hypothesis that minimum ADC values can detect neoplastic cell infiltration in peritumoral edema in patients with GBM, distinguishing these tumors from solitary brain metastasis.

Differentiation of vasogenic edema from infiltrative edema has been attempted using DW imaging, based on the premise that water diffusivity is facilitated to a greater degree in vasogenic edema surrounding brain metastasis than in infiltrative edema surrounding GBMs, because of a lack of intervening tumor cells in the former.[44–48] However, the authors believe that ADC measurements in the peritumoral areas of GBM and metastasis cannot be used to distinguish between these lesions, as a large overlap is often demonstrated. This finding is in agreement with previous studies, which have shown that peritumoral ADC is not useful for distinguishing between GBMs and metastatic tumors.[21,44,49,50]

Peritumoral diffusion tensor imaging metrics

Areas of extensive edema on T2-weighted imaging surround both GBMs and metastatic tumors. In metastatic tumors, this peritumoral edema is assumed to be composed of pure water, whereas for GBMs the edema is assumed to contain tumor cells that have infiltrated into the tissue.[18,35,51,52]

Diffusion tensor (DT) imaging is an advanced MR technique that describes the movement of water molecules by using 2 metrics, mean diffusivity (MD) and FA, which represent the magnitude and directionality of water diffusion, respectively. DT imaging may be able to detect changes in the white matter surrounding malignant gliomas that are not visible on cMR imaging. In a study by Lu and colleagues[35] the peritumoral MD of metastatic lesions was significantly greater (average 0.798 ± 0.109) than that of gliomas (average 0.622 ± 0.111) (P<.005). The average FA was 0.181 ± 0.049 around metastatic lesions, whereas the average FA around HGGs was 0.248 ± 0.063.

Although peritumoral MD could be used to distinguish HGGs from metastatic tumors, peritumoral FA demonstrated no statistically significant difference.[35]

¹H-MRS

To differentiate a solitary brain metastasis from GBM, the voxel should be placed in the peritumoral area.[52,53] No evidence of tumor infiltration is demonstrated in the peritumoral vasogenic edema surrounding a metastatic brain lesion. No elevation of the Cho, Cho/creatine (Cho/Cr), and Cho/NAA ratios will be demonstrated in the spectrum (Fig. 1A, B). On the other hand, evidence of tumor infiltration outside the tumor nodule may be demonstrated in the peritumoral area surrounding a GBM (see Fig. 1C, D).

Beware that high Cho peak, Cho/Cr ratio, and Cho/NAA ratio in the peritumoral region surrounding a GBM may not be demonstrated in the spectrum, as these changes are related to the number of tumor cells that have infiltrated the peritumoral area (Fig. 2). If no elevation of the Cho peak is seen in the peritumoral area, a high-grade primary tumor cannot be ruled out.

Dynamic susceptibility contrast MR imaging

Tumoral CBV In a retrospective study of 83 tumors, spin-echo echo-planar images (SE-EPI)–derived rCBV maps allowed reliable distinction of brain metastasis from HGGs and were superior to percentage recovery analysis for distinguishing brain metastasis from HGG.[54] In this study, the average normalized CBV (nCBV) obtained from the maximum rCBV within the tumor divided by the rCBV of an equivalent region of interest (ROI) in the contralateral normal-appearing white matter was 1.53 ± 0.79 (0.59–4.05) within HGG compared with 0.82 ± 0.40 for brain metastasis (0.48–2.12), and differences between nCBV averages and ranges for the two groups were significant (P<.05).[54]

The optimal threshold occurred at 1.0, where sensitivity and specificity for detection of brain metastasis were 88% and 72%, respectively. Therefore if the tumoral CBV is less than the CBV measured in the contralateral normal white matter, metastasis should be suggested instead of a HGG.

Peritumoral CBV When a focal brain lesion presents with high blood volume, GBM and metastasis should be both considered in the differential diagnosis. In metastatic brain lesions, the area with high blood volume will correspond exactly to the tumoral-enhancing nodule. On the other hand, GBMs tend to have angiogenesis beyond the contrast-enhancing portion of the tumor, so that high blood volume may be demonstrated outside the tumor nodule (Fig. 3).

In a study of 75 brain tumors, peritumoral CBV values (rCBVp) were more effective than tumoral rCBV (rCBVt) in differentiation of metastasis from both LGG and HGG. rCBVp cutoff values of 1.1 and 1.2 were used for the differentiation.[55]

Percentage of signal-intensity recovery (curve analysis) Percentage recovery analysis of time-intensity curves from GE-EPI DSC PW imaging

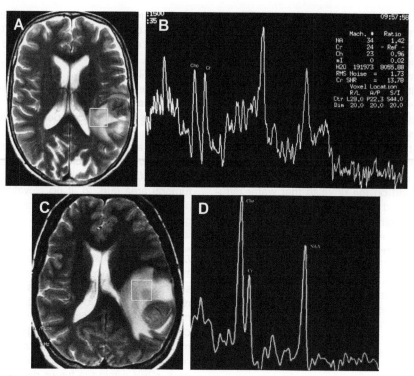

Fig. 1. Magnetic resonance spectroscopy (MRS) of perilesional edema. (*A, B*) A 66-year-old woman diagnosed with breast cancer metastasis. There is a solitary nodular metastatic lesion in the left parietal lobe, surrounded by vasogenic edema (*A*: axial T2). Spectrum from the perilesional edema (*B*) demonstrates no signs of tumor infiltration: there is no elevation of the choline (Cho) peak, Cho/creatine (Cr) ratio, and Cho/N-acetylaspartate (NAA) ratio. (*C, D*) A 39-year-old woman presenting with aphasia. There is a left parietal nodular lesion, isointense on T2 (*C*) surrounded by vasogenic edema. Spectrum from the perilesional "edema" (*D*) demonstrates significant elevation of the Cho peak, Cho/Cr ratio, and Cho/NAA ratio, consistent with tumor infiltration. Final diagnosis: glioblastoma multiforme (GBM).

has been proposed to distinguish GBMs from metastasis by assessing the profound difference in capillary permeability between the 2 tumor types with increased capillary permeability in brain metastasis.[54–59]

The percentage of signal-intensity recovery (PSR) is a hemodynamic variable derived from DSC perfusion MR imaging that provides additional information on tumor vasculature. PSR is defined as the percentage of signal-intensity recovery relative to the precontrast baseline at the end of the first pass, and is influenced by the amount of contrast agent leaked during the first pass, thus reflecting alteration in capillary permeability.

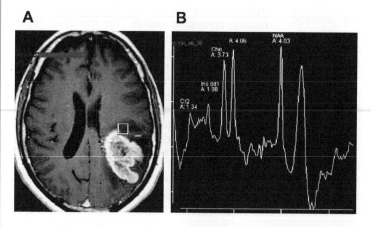

Fig. 2. MRS of the perilesional edema surrounding a GBM. A 50-year-old man presenting with headaches and paresthesia on the right. There is a left frontoparietal GBM presenting with irregular enhancement (*A*: axial T1 with contrast). Spectrum from the perilesional area (*B*) shows no signs of tumor infiltration. The Cho peak is smaller than the Cr peak.

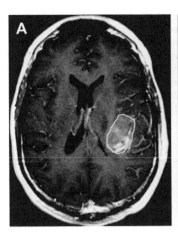
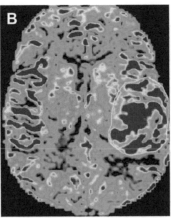

Fig. 3. Peritumoral relative cerebral blood volume (rCBV). A 67-year-old woman presenting with headaches. There is a nodular enhancing lesion close to the posterior margin of the left ventricle (A: axial T1 with contrast) that was diagnosed as a GBM. High blood volume (B) can be seen extending beyond the limits of the enhancing lesion in A, related to vascular proliferation as well as tumor infiltration into the peritumoral tissue.

Cha and colleagues[56] demonstrated that both the minimum and average percentages of signal-intensity recovery were significantly greater for patients with GBM compared with the values for patients with metastasis ($P<.05$). When the average PSR in the contrast-enhancing lesion was more than 82% and less than 66%, the prediction of GBM and single brain metastasis, respectively, had specificity of 100% (**Fig. 4**).

Beware: Some GBMs with significant disruption of the blood-brain barrier (BBB) will demonstrate a very low PSR of the time-intensity curve, resembling metastasis (**Fig. 5**).

Dynamic contrast-enhanced MR imaging
Permeability is typically high in aggressive tumors such as metastasis and GBM, owing to significant disruption of the BBB. There is greater permeability in metastasis than in GBM because metastases have no BBB, whereas GBMs have a "damaged" BBB.

GBM versus lymphoma
Despite some characteristic conventional MR imaging findings, it may be difficult or even impossible to distinguish cerebral lymphomas from GBM.[60]

Accurate preoperative differentiation between these 2 tumors is important for appropriate treatment.

GBMs are usually treated with surgical resection plus radiation therapy and chemotherapy, whereas lymphoma is not treated with surgery.

ADC and FA
Lymphomas demonstrate low ADC values (**Fig. 6A–C**), a finding consistent with restricted water diffusion related to high tumor-cell density.[21,22,49,61] By contrast, HGGs are relatively hyperintense to gray matter on both trace DW imaging and ADC maps (**Fig. 7B**), findings consistent with elevated diffusivity.[49,62,63] Prior studies have shown statistically significant differences in

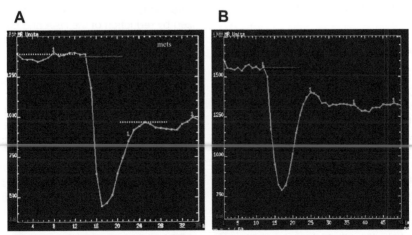

Fig. 4. Percentage of signal intensity recovery: mets × GBM. A low percentage of signal intensity recovery (PSR) of the time-intensity curve is demonstrated in the perfusion study in metastasis (A). In the GBM a greater PSR is usually seen (B).

A **B**

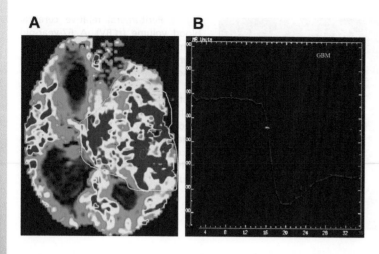

Fig. 5. Percentage of signal intensity recovery: drawback. GBM in the left frontoparietal region presenting with very high blood volume (A: CBV map). The time-intensity curve (B) demonstrates a very low PSR, resembling metastasis (compare with Fig. 4A).

ADC between the cerebral lymphoma and GBM.[22,49] However, GBMs with restricted water diffusion have also been reported.[64–68] Therefore, discrimination of lymphoma from some GBMs may be difficult.

A study by Toh and colleagues[61] demonstrated that the FA and ADC of lymphomas were significantly lower than those of GBMs. Cutoff values to differentiate lymphomas from GBM were 0.192 for FA, 0.33 for FA ratio, 0.818 for ADC, and 1.06 for ADC ratio. Accuracy of 100% was reached in the distinction between lymphoma and GBM using a cutoff value of 1.06 for the ADC ratio (see **Fig. 6**C).

The specificity and accuracy of ADC were higher than those of FA in differentiating the two.

ADC measurements are also useful in the distinction between lymphoma and GBM infiltrating the corpus callosum.[69]

1H-MRS

When lipids are demonstrated in a solid-appearing tumor, lymphoma should be considered (see **Fig. 6**D, E).[36]

Lipids are also typically seen in the spectrum of the GBM (see **Fig. 7**C), related to the presence of necrosis.

DSC and DCE MR imaging

CBV and cerebral blood flow are much lower in lymphomas than in GBMs.[70–72]

Angiogenesis is not a prominent finding in lymphomas, so perfusion may not be elevated (see **Fig. 6**F).[70]

In the authors' experience, despite being an aggressive tumor, lymphomas may present with minimal or mild elevation of the permeability (see **Fig. 6**G). On the other hand, high blood volumes[37,38] and significantly high permeability[73,74] are typically demonstrated in high-grade glial tumors such as GBM (see **Fig. 7**D, E).

Gliomatosis cerebri versus lymphomatosis cerebri

Intracranial gliomas may present as infiltrative lesions known as gliomatosis cerebri. These tumors usually infiltrate at least 2 or 3 lobes, sometimes in a bilateral and fairly symmetric fashion, usually with no or minimum mass effect.

Lymphomas may also present as infiltrative tumors known as lymphomatosis cerebri. This rare presentation of intracranial primary lymphomas may resemble gliomatosis cerebri on cMR imaging. Discrete or no enhancement is demonstrated in both tumors.

ADC measurements are not helpful in the differentiation of these lesions. Restricted diffusion, typically seen in lymphomas, is mild or absent in lymphomatosis cerebri.[75]

1H-MRS may be helpful, and a high mI peak has been described as the most characteristic spectral finding in gliomatosis grade II, especially if the Cho peak is not elevated (**Fig. 8**A, B).[53,76–78] On the other hand, lymphomatosis cerebri is characterized by reduction of the NAA and mI peaks, along with elevation of the Cho and lipid peaks (see **Fig. 8**C, D).[53]

Medulloblastoma versus ependymoma

Medulloblastoma, a highly malignant neoplasm, is the most common neoplasm of the posterior fossa in children.[9,79–84] The tumor usually arises at the midline within the vermis, and exhibits growth into the fourth ventricle.[84–89]

Medulloblastomas and ependymomas may look very similar on cMR imaging. Accurate diagnosis is crucial, as treatment strategies and prognosis are different.

ADC

ADC values are significantly lower in medulloblastomas than in all other posterior fossa tumors

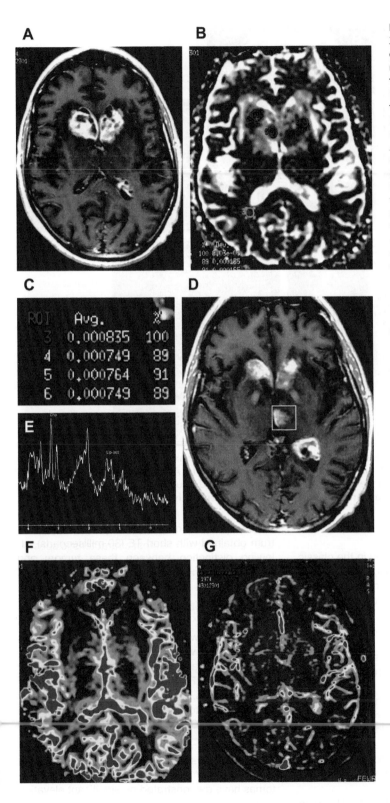

Fig. 6. GBM versus lymphoma. A 37-year-old man, human immuno-deficiency virus (HIV)-positive, diagnosed with lymphoma involving the basal ganglia and periventricular regions (A: axial T1 with contrast). The solid areas present with low apparent diffusion coefficient (ADC) values (B: ADC map). The ADC ratio (ADC from the lesion divided by the ADC from the normal white matter) is less than 1 (C). Spectrum from the solid thalamic lesion on the left (D, E) demonstrates high Cho peak along with high lipid-lactate peaks. There is no elevation of the blood volume (F: CBV map) and only minimal elevation of the permeability (G: permeability map), which favors lymphoma over GBM. The minimal elevation of permeability in this lymphoma could represent a limitation of trying to estimate permeability without pharmacokinetic modeling, and further confirmation is necessary.

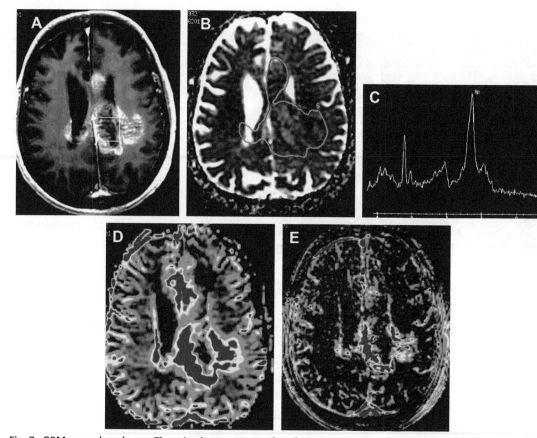

Fig. 7. GBM versus lymphoma. There is a heterogeneously enhancing GBM (*A*: axial T1 with contrast) involving the parietal lobes and the cingulate gyrus bilaterally, presenting with high ADC (*B*: ADC map). A prominent lipid peak is demonstrated in the spectrum from the necrotic area (*C*). Very high blood volume (*D*: CBV map) and significantly high permeability (*E*: permeability map) are demonstrated, very consistent with the diagnosis of GBM.

(*P*<.001) related to high cell density (**Fig. 9A, B**).[8,11,20,49]

Diffusion is not typically restricted in the classic ependymomas (see **Fig. 9C, D**), but may be restricted in the anaplastic ones, making distinction between these tumors and medulloblastomas more difficult.

^{1}H-MRS
Medulloblastomas usually demonstrate a significant elevation of the Cho peak, Cho/Cr ratio, and Cho/NAA ratio in the spectrum, related to the high cell density and reflecting its malignant nature (**Fig. 10A**).[9–11,20,36,49,86–91] Majós and colleagues[92] demonstrated that significantly elevated levels in the Cho peak could be used to distinguish primitive neuroectodermal tumors (PNET) from non-PNET tumors with a high degree of accuracy (94%).

Also, spectrum with a short echo time (TE) show a significantly elevated taurine concentration at 3.3 ppm in patients with medulloblastoma when compared with other tumors (see **Fig. 10A**).[6,10,93–96]

Ependymomas may show very high ml in spectrum obtained with short TE (30 milliseconds), allowing distinction between these tumors and medulloblastomas (see **Fig. 10B**).[9,10,97,98]

Dynamic susceptibility contrast MR imaging
In the authors' experience, some medulloblastomas present with high blood volumes and others with low blood volumes.

Ependymomas generally demonstrate markedly elevated rCBV (**Fig. 11A–C**) and, unlike many other glial neoplasms, a poor return to baseline that may be attributable to fenestrated blood vessels and an incomplete BBB (see **Fig. 11C**).[99–101]

Dynamic contrast-enhanced MR imaging
In the authors' experience, some medulloblastomas have demonstrated no significant elevation of the permeability (**Fig. 12A–C**).

Permeability in ependymomas is highly variable, with some ependymomas presenting with high permeability (**Fig. 13A, B**) and some with no

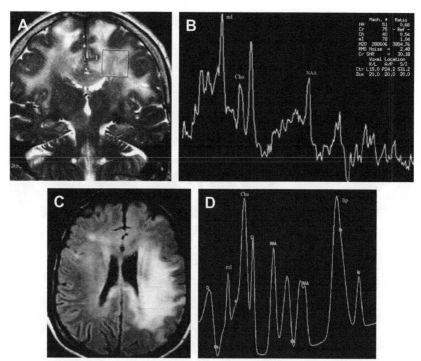

Fig. 8. Lymphomatosis versus gliomatosis cerebri. Gliomatosis cerebri infiltrating the white matter bilaterally (*A*: coronal T2). The spectrum (*B*) demonstrates reduction of the NAA and Cho peaks along with elevation of the *myo*-inositol (mI) peak. Lymphomatosis cerebri infiltrating the frontal and parietal lobes bilaterally, mostly on the left (*C*: axial fluid-attenuated inversion recovery [FLAIR]). A prominent lipid peak, along with elevation of the Cho peak and reduction of the NAA and mI peaks, are demonstrated in the spectrum (*D*). ([*C, D*] *Courtesy of* Leonardo Avanza MD, Vitória ES, Brazil.)

significant elevation of the permeability (see **Fig. 13**C, D) (authors' personal communication).

Hemangioblastoma versus pilocytic astrocytoma

Hemangioblastomas (HGBLs) are the most common primary brain tumors in the posterior fossa of adult patients. The lesion arises in the cerebellar parenchyma, and usually presents with cystic and solid components (**Fig. 14**). HGBL may resemble a pilocytic astrocytoma (PA) on cMR imaging.

Flow voids consistent with prominent blood vessels may be demonstrated in the solid portion of HGBLs (see **Fig. 14**A), suggesting the diagnosis.

ADC ADC is typically elevated not only in the cysts but also in the solid portions of HGBLs, related to the large amount of capillaries in these tumors (see **Fig. 14**B).[102,103]

A PA has greater ADC values than do other cerebellar tumors such as ependymoma and medulloblastoma, and may look similar to an HGBL on diffusion study.[49,91]

^{1}H-MRS Elevation of the Cho peak in the spectrum of HGBLs is usually minimal, as these are low-grade tumors (see **Fig. 14**C). Lipids may be seen, related to the presence of cysts. On the other hand, despite being a grade I tumor, PAs typically demonstrate a prominent Cho peak, along with reduction of the NAA and Cr peaks and the presence of lipids and lactate, simulating a HGG (see **Fig. 14**D).[7,9,36,91,104]

DSC and DCE MR imaging High blood volume and high permeability may be demonstrated in PAs but, in the authors' experience, never as high as in HGBLs. These neoplasms are truly vascular, and behave like vessels in the perfusion and permeability studies. Very high CBV and very high permeability, related to the presence of enlarged vessels, will be demonstrated in this grade I tumor (see **Fig. 14**E–G).

Determination of Tumor Grade

Differentiation between high-grade and low-grade tumors is important for therapeutic planning. The contrast-enhancement pattern of a tumor on cMR imaging is not always reliable enough to obtain precise information about tumor angiogenesis at a capillary level, because tumoral enhancement is mainly due to disruption of the BBB rather than

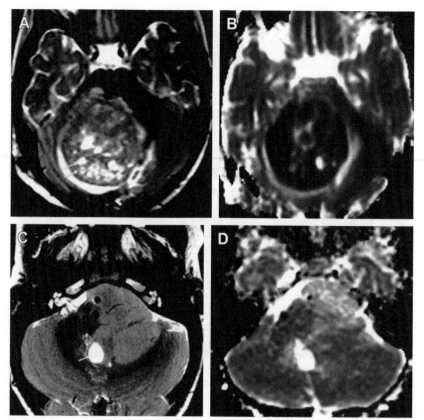

Fig. 9. Medulloblastoma versus ependymoma: ADC map. (*A, B*) Medulloblastoma. (*C, D*) Ependymoma. The solid portions of medulloblastomas and ependymomas may be isointense on the T2 sequence (*A, C*). Cysts may be seen in both tumors (*arrows* in *A, C*). Mass in the cerebellopontine angle is very characteristic of ependymomas (*C*). Restricted diffusion is classically seen in the medulloblastoma (*B*: ADC map) because of high cellularity. There is no restricted diffusion in the classic ependymoma (*D*: ADC map).

the tumoral vascular proliferation itself.[55] Thirty-three percent of high-grade tumors do not enhance, and 20% of low-grade tumors enhance.[105]

Advanced MR imaging techniques such as DW imaging, DT imaging, ^{1}H-MRS, PW imaging, and permeability may better estimate tumor grade than conventional MR imaging studies.

ADC

ADC measurements are related to tumor-cell density and tumor grade.[20,21] Many studies have demonstrated an inverse relationship between ADC values and tumor grade, with lower ADCs found in higher-grade tumors (**Figs. 15** and **16**) in comparison with lower-grade tumors (**Fig. 17**).[20,22–27,29–32]

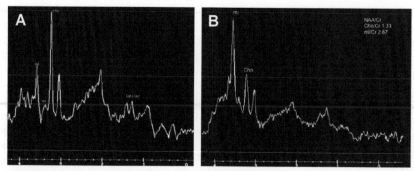

Fig. 10. Medulloblastoma versus ependymoma: ^{1}H-MRS. (*A*) Spectrum from a medulloblastoma demonstrates significant elevation of the Cho peak, along with presence of lipids, lactate, and taurine (tau) peaks. (*B*) Spectrum from the posterior fossa ependymoma shown in **Fig. 9**C demonstrates a very high mI peak.

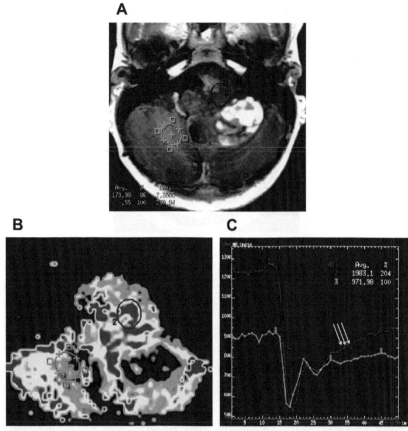

Fig. 11. Ependymoma versus medulloblastoma: dynamic susceptibility contrast (DSC) study. There is a heterogeneously enhancing ependymoma arising from the fourth ventricle extending to the left cerebellopontine angle (CPA) (*A*: axial T1 with contrast). The lesion has very high blood volume (*B*: rCBV map). A very low PSR of the time-intensity curve is demonstrated (*C, arrows*) related to fenestrated blood vessels and an incomplete blood-brain barrier. See also Refs.[99–102]

Recent studies have shown that minimum ADCs may facilitate accurate grading of astrocytic tumors, because regions exhibiting the minimum ADC correspond to the highest-grade glioma foci within heterogeneous tumors.[106–108]

Beware: restricted diffusion may be seen in PA, a grade I tumor (**Fig. 18**).

^{1}H-MRS

^{1}H-MRS may indicate tumor grade with more accuracy when compared with a blind biopsy, because it assesses a larger amount of tissue than is usually excised at biopsy.[36,53]

Tumors are commonly heterogeneous, and their spectrum may vary depending on the region sampled by ^{1}H-MRS.[109,110] Hence, the ROI chosen for analysis will have a large influence on the results, and multivoxel (MV) spectroscopy is generally considered preferable because it allows metabolic heterogeneity to be evaluated. ^{1}H-MRS is considered 96% accurate in differentiating LGGs from HGGs.[111]

There is a high correlation between in vivo concentration of Cho in brain tumors and in vitro tumor proliferation markers. Compared with low-grade gliomas (LGGs) (see **Fig. 17**C, D), statistically significantly higher Cho/Cr, Cho/NAA, and rCBV have been reported in HGGs (see **Fig. 15**D, E).[112] although threshold values of metabolite ratios for grading of gliomas are not well established. Cho/Cr is the most frequently used ratio for grading gliomas.

Although Cho is related to tumor-cell density and tumor grade, grade IV GBM usually presents with lower levels of Cho (see **Fig. 16**C) than gliomas of grades III (see **Fig. 15**D) and II (see **Fig. 17**C).[113] This discrepancy may be due to the presence of necrosis in GBMs, because necrosis is associated with a prominent lipid peak along with reduction of all other metabolites.[114] Lipids may be the only spectral finding in a GBM.

Useful information on tumor grade may be acquired by using a short-TE (30–35 milliseconds) ^{1}H-MRS to assess mI.[115] In low-grade tumors, the

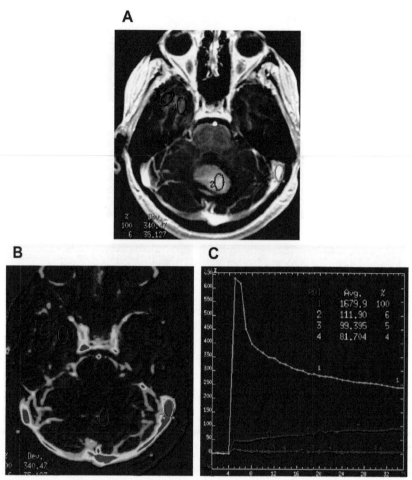

Fig. 12. Medulloblastoma: dynamic contrast-enhanced (DCE) study. Adult patient diagnosed with medulloblastoma. There is a solid enhancing lesion compromising the cerebellar vermis (*A*) presenting with no significant elevation of the permeability (*B*: permeability map; *C*: signal intensity–phase curves). Mild elevation of the permeability in this case could represent a limitation of trying to estimate permeability without pharmacokinetic modeling, and further confirmation is necessary.

ml/Cr ratio is typically higher (see **Fig. 17C**) than in high-grade tumors (see **Fig. 15D**).[113,116] According to Howe and colleagues,[113] high mI is characteristic of grade II astrocytomas. Increased mI levels have been reported to be useful in identifying low-grade astrocytomas in which the Cho/Cr ratio is not altered.[117,118]

In summary
Grade II gliomas The ^{1}H-MRS spectrum in LGGs may look very similar to a normal spectrum, demonstrating a mild reduction of the NAA peak along with a mild elevation of the Cho peak.[105,113,119]

An elevated mI peak may be the only finding in the spectrum of a grade II astrocytoma (see **Fig. 17C**).[113,117,120]

No lipids or lactate are usually demonstrated in the spectrum of a grade II glioma.

Grade III gliomas In grade III gliomas there is a significant elevation of the Cho peak, which correlates well with the high cell density in these tumors.[121] NAA, Cr, and mI peaks are reduced (see **Fig. 15D**). If the lesion does not exhibit mobile lipid signals, anaplastic glioma is more likely than GBM.[122] In the authors' experience, however, some elevation of lipids and lactate may be seen in grade III gliomas.

Grade IV gliomas The spectral pattern of these tumors is characterized by severe reduction of the NAA, Cr, and mI peaks. Cho is elevated, although not as much as in a grade III glioma, because prominent necrosis is usually present in grade IV gliomas. Marked necrosis will result in a prominent lipid peak (see **Fig. 16C**). Typically the higher levels of Cho occur in grade III gliomas, whereas in GBM the Cho levels may be much

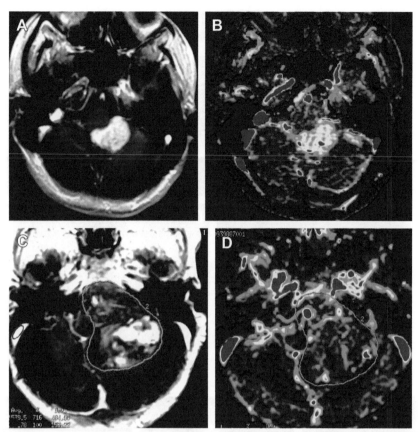

Fig. 13. Ependymoma: DCE study. (*A, B*) Ependymoma in an adult patient. There is a nodular enhancing lesion arising from the fourth ventricle, extending to the left CPA (*A*: axial T1 with contrast), presenting with high permeability (*B*: permeability map). (*C, D*) A 3-year-old boy diagnosed with ependymoma. There is an enhancing lesion (*A*: axial T1 with contrast) extending from the fourth ventricle to the CPA on the left, presenting with much lower permeability (*D*: permeability map) compared with the patient in *A, B*.

lower because of necrosis.[123] In fact, when the voxel is placed within the necrotic area of a GBM, no Cho will be detected and a prominent lipid-lactate peak will be the only spectral abnormality (see **Fig. 16C**).[123]

Key points to remember

1. PAs usually present with a significant elevation of the Cho peak. Some lipids and lactate are also usually seen in these tumors (see **Fig. 18C**).[53]
2. Some overlap between grades II and III gliomas may be seen in the spectrum (**Fig. 19**).
3. Some aggressive tumors, such as metastases and GBM, may present with no elevation of the Cho peak (see **Fig. 16C**).
4. Cho peak and the Cho/Cr and Cho/NAA ratios may be higher in grade III (see **Fig. 15D**) than in grade IV gliomas (see **Fig. 16C**).
5. Lipids do not necessarily represent necrosis. Lipids may be related to the presence of cysts in grade III gliomas (**Fig. 20**).

DSC MR imaging

The rCBV, the most robust and standard hemodynamic variable derived from DSC perfusion MR imaging, has been shown to correlate with grading of pure astrocytomas.[37,53,55,124,125]

CBV is a marker of angiogenesis, tumor grade, and survival.[126–128] CBV is related not only to vascular density but also to tumor-cell density.[129]

Law and colleagues[112] have demonstrated that rCBV is better related to tumor biology than Cho/Cr and Cho/NAA ratios.

Tumor rCBV obtained with GE-EPI is significantly higher than that obtained with the SE-EPI technique in the HGGs. This is probably related to the higher sensitivity of the GE-EPI technique to large vessels, which can be clearly observed in the HGGs. The findings suggest that the GE-EPI technique is more useful for detecting low-versus high-grade gliomas than is the SE-EPI technique.[130] However, SE-EPI may have a better performance than the GE-EPI technique in areas of greater susceptibility, such as close to the bone and surgical cavities.

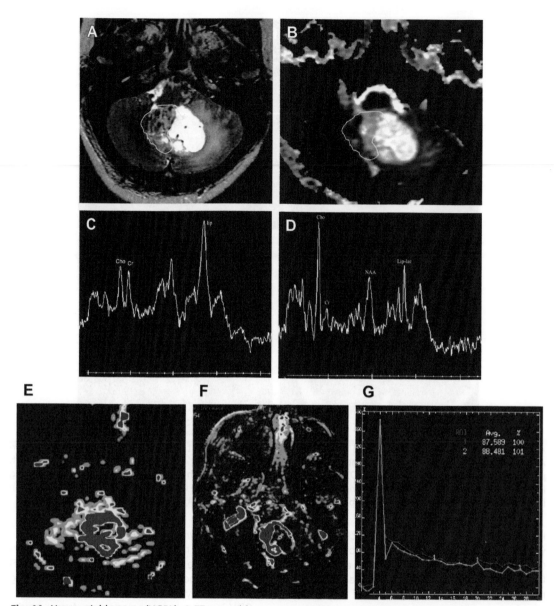

Fig. 14. Hemangioblastoma (HGBL). A 57-year-old woman presenting with vertigo, ataxia, and headaches in the last 2 months. There is a cystic-solid lesion in the cerebellum. Flow voids consistent with prominent vessels are demonstrated within the solid component of the lesion, suggesting the diagnosis of HGBL (*A*: axial T2). There is no restricted diffusion within the cysts as well as in the solid portion of the tumor (*B*: ADC map). There is no significant elevation of the Cho peak in the spectrum (*C*), as this is a low-grade tumor. Lipids are demonstrated, related to the presence of cysts. (*D*) Spectrum from a pilocytic astrocytoma for comparison demonstrates a prominent Cho peak. There is apparent high blood volume (*E*: rCBV map) and significantly high permeability (*F*: permeability map; *G*: signal intensity–phase curves region of interest [ROI] 1, venous sinus and ROI 2, solid lesion), which may both be related to the presence of macrovessels.

Permeability can confound rCBV measurements, and correction for T1 and T2/T2* effects should be done before interpreting the results from the perfusion study.[55,131]

Many different techniques have been advocated, although no standardized methods exist. This ambiguity can result in a wide range of values in the literature, and makes comparison of studies problematic.

Perfusion studies can also be done without gadolinium-based contrast agent (GBCA) injection using the arterial spin-labeling (ASL) technique. The results from this technique are related to the percentage of blood vessels and tumor cellularity,

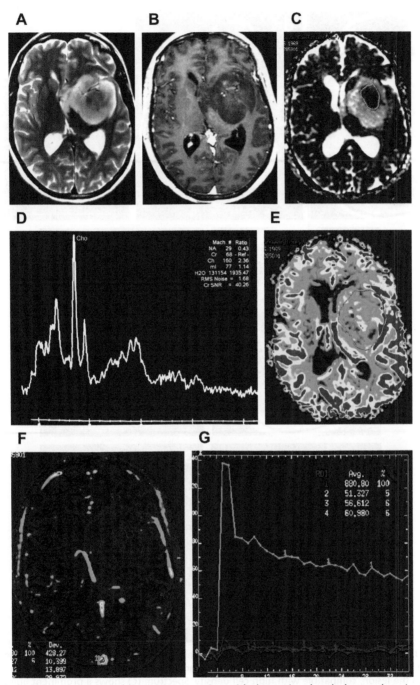

Fig. 15. Grade III glioma. A 41-year-old woman presenting with depression, headaches, and panic attacks. There is a solid mass in the left temporal-frontal region (*A*: axial T2) with a faint nodular enhancement in its anterior portion (*B*: axial T1 with contrast). There is an area of restricted diffusion within the lesion (*circle* in *C*: ADC map) that corresponds to the area of lowest signal intensity on the T2 image (*A*), indicating high cell density. A prominent Cho peak is demonstrated in the spectrum (*D*). There is elevation of the blood volume (*E*: CBV map). No significant elevation of the permeability is demonstrated (*F*: permeability map; *G*: signal intensity–phase curves). Pathology was consistent with grade III (anaplastic) oligoastrocytoma.

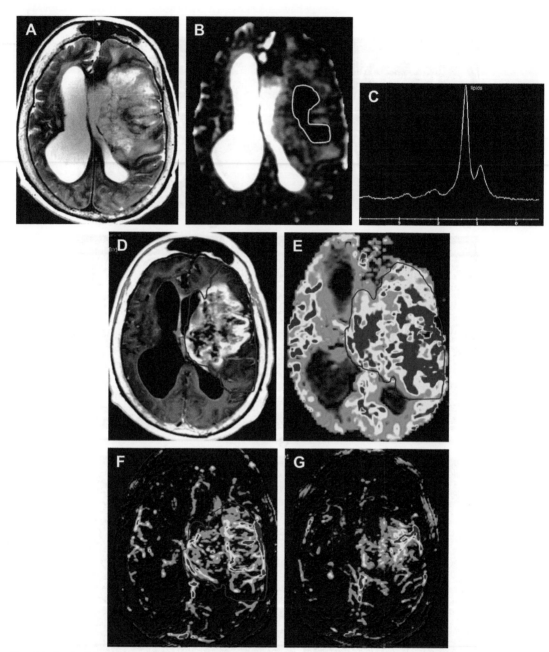

Fig. 16. Grade IV glioma. A 64-year-old woman found unconscious. There is a large heterogeneous lesion involving the left frontal and parietal lobes (*A*: axial T2). An area with restricted diffusion (*B*: ADC map) is demonstrated within the lesion, compatible with high cell density. Spectrum (*C*) shows a prominent lipid peak, due to extensive necrosis. No elevation of the Cho is demonstrated. The lesion presents with heterogeneous enhancement (*D*: axial T1 with contrast). Very high blood volume is demonstrated (*E*: CBV map) extending beyond the limits of the enhancing tumor (*D*), characterizing tumor infiltration beyond the enhancing lesion. Permeability is also very high (*F, G*: permeability maps).

and may be useful in distinguishing between high-grade and LGGs.[132] ASL currently can provide measurements of cerebral blood flow, and absolute quantification is more easily performed in ASL than in DSC MR imaging.

Using the SE-EPI technique, Lev and colleagues[125] found that if the tumoral rCBV was more than 1.5 times the rCBV in the contralateral white matter, a HGG could be suggested with 100% sensitivity and 69% specificity. According

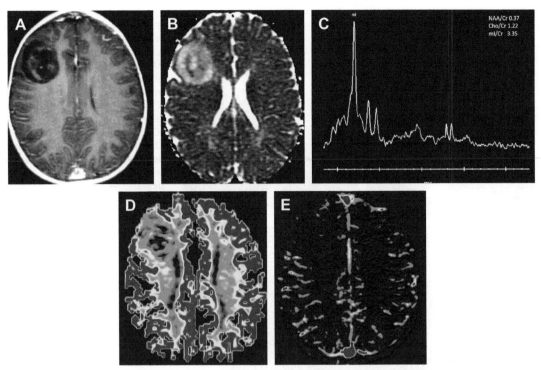

Fig. 17. Low-grade (grade II) astrocytoma. A 5-year-old boy who presented with 1 seizure episode at the age of 7 months. The study was done because of motor delay. A solid lesion is demonstrated in the right frontal lobe, presenting with no significant enhancement (*A*: axial with contrast). There is increased ADC in the mass (*B*: ADC map) suggesting a low-grade tumor. Spectrum (*C*) demonstrates a prominent ml peak, very typical for grade II astrocytomas. Perfusion is low (*D*) and there is no elevation of the permeability (*E*). The findings from the conventional and functional studies were consistent with low-grade tumor (confirmed as grade II astrocytoma).

to this study, none of the HGGs presented with low CBV. On the other hand, using the GE-EPI sequence, Law and colleagues[112] demonstrated that if the measured rCBV in the tumor lesion was more than 1.75 times the rCBV in the contralateral white matter, a HGG could be suggested with 95% sensitivity and 57.5% specificity.

HGGs are characterized by high rCBV (see **Figs. 15E** and **16E; Fig. 21A, B**). However, a high proportion of LGGs can demonstrate foci of high rCBV (**Fig. 22**).

It is important to remember that both low-grade and high-grade oligodendrogliomas may present with high blood volume in the perfusion study, because of their unique "chicken-wire" vascularity. Low-grade oligodendrogliomas with high blood volumes tend to respond better to chemotherapy with procarbazine and vincristine.[55]

Recently, susceptibility-weighted (SW) imaging has been described as a useful tool for the grading of noninvasive glioma. High rCBV values on perfusion imaging in tumors go hand in hand with evidence of blood products detected within the tumor matrix on SW imaging.[133]

Beware: pilocytic astrocytomas may present with high blood volumes.

DCE MR imaging

Like PW MR imaging, permeability MR imaging, also known as DCE MR imaging, is performed through the use of GBCAs. However, it often uses more complex pharmacokinetic models (PKMs) than in PW imaging, and incorporates several assumptions that may potentially result in errors. It is insensitive to magnetic susceptibility and thus has a better performance than perfusion studies in the evaluation of lesions close to the skull base and close to the surgical cavity. The techniques utilized often result in conflicting demands on high temporal resolution, high signal to noise ratio, high spatial resolution, and wide anatomic coverage.[134]

Permeability allows estimation of the BBB integrity through calculation of microvascular permeability.[40,45] The volume-transfer constant between the capillary plasma space and the extravascular-extracellular space (EES), K^{trans}, is the most widely used microvascular permeability metric. It is a potentially intractable combination of flow, permeability, and surface area.[135] Despite the most rapid imaging techniques, it may not be possible to differentiate the contribution of each factor in the resultant K^{trans} and, thus, its physiologic meaning can

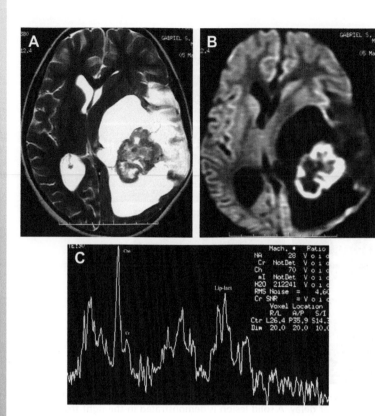

Fig. 18. Pilocytic astrocytoma (PA). A 9-year-old boy presenting with epilepsy and right-side hemiparesis. The solid portion of the PA is isointense on T2 (A) and presents with very high signal intensity on diffusion-weighted (DW) imaging (B) characterizing restricted diffusion. The spectrum (C) demonstrates a prominent Cho peak along with elevation of lipids and lactate (Lip-lact), and reduction of the NAA and Cr peaks.

differ. Furthermore, variations in the DCE technique can also make a comparison of literature values of K^trans difficult.[136–138]

K^trans of the brain parenchyma is insignificant, and consistent with noise.[73]

K^trans and CBV measure different vascular parameters, so areas of high CBV do not necessarily correspond to areas of high permeability.[139] Strong relationships have been demonstrated between both rCBV and K^trans and histologic grade

in gliomas; however, the relationship appears to be stronger with rCBV.[73,140]

More simple methods analysis that do not use PKM, such as qualitative or semiquantitative analysis of signal intensity–time curves, though physiologically less specific, can be beneficial.[141–143] The GE Functool maximum (max) slope of increase is likely correlated with permeability, and subjective dynamic curve analysis can be beneficial.

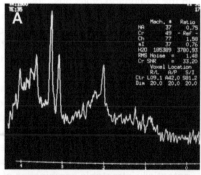
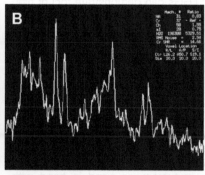

Fig. 19. Overlap in the spectrum between grades II and III gliomas. (A) MRS from a left frontal grade II glioma in a 50-year-old man demonstrates a Cho/Cr ratio of 1.58 and mI/Cr ratio of 0.76. (B) MRS from a left frontal grade III glioma in a 27-year-old man with similar abnormalities: the Cho/Cr ratio is 1.55, a little less than in the grade II glioma (A), and the mI/Cr ratio is about the same (0.75 × 0.76). MRS cannot be used in isolation to differentiate grade II and III gliomas.

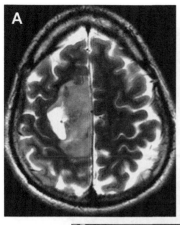
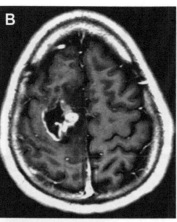
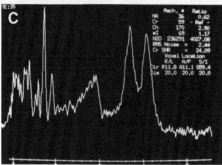

Fig. 20. Grade III glioma misdiagnosed as grade IV glioma. A 24-year-old man presenting with seizures. There is a right fronto-parietal infiltrating tumor, with high signal intensity on the T2 (*A*) and peripheral enhancement (*B*), and a central area that does not enhance, which could represent cystic component or necrosis. There is significant elevation of the Cho peak in the spectrum (*C*), along with a prominent lipid peak. Based on the conventional MR imaging and ¹H-MRS studies, a diagnosis of GBM was suggested. However, the final diagnosis was a grade III anaplastic glioma. The nonenhancing area corresponded to cyst formation. High lipids do not necessarily mean necrosis.

Grade II gliomas Grade II gliomas typically present with no significant elevation of permeability (see **Fig. 17E**).[74]

Grade III gliomas Permeability is variable in grade III gliomas, with some presenting with no significant elevation of the permeability (see **Fig. 15F, G**) and others with high permeability (see **Fig. 21C, D**). Overlap may be seen between grades III and II gliomas in the permeability study.

Grade IV gliomas According to Cha and colleagues,[74] distinction between grade IV gliomas and gliomas of lower grade was only possible using the K^{trans} and not the CBV measurements. K^{trans} was much higher in GBM (see **Fig. 16F, G**) than in lower-grade tumors, and was more predictive of tumor grade than the CBV derived from the perfusion study. Permeability may better distinguish between grades III and IV gliomas than the perfusion study.[74]

A recent study using individual arterial input functions and 5 flip-angle T1 mapping at 1.5 T found that K^{trans} was not only able to distinguish LGGs (grade I and II) from HGGs (grade III and IV) but also grade II from grade III.[144] Nguyen and colleagues[145] used a phase-derived vascular input function (VIP) with the bookend T1 measurement to show that both K^{trans} and plasma volume (Vp)

derived from DCE MR imaging could differentiate LGGs from HGGs. Adoption of a phase-derived VIP may be helpful because changes in the concentration of GBCA are known to vary in a linear fashion with phase changes in vessels that are more or less parallel to the magnetic field.[146,147] This finding is significant because the relationship between MR signal intensity and gadolinium-based contrast agent may not always be linear, and could be complicated by inflow.[73,148]

Special situations

1. Pilocytic astrocytoma may present with high permeability despite being a grade I tumor
2. Steroids and antiangiogenic therapy may reduce the measured K^{trans}

The effects of steroid therapy are predicted to reduce the measured K^{trans}, and reduce or abolish the strength of the relationship between K^{trans} and grade.[73]

Antiangiogenic therapy such as bevacizumab (Avastin) dramatically reduces BBB permeability, and no elevation of the permeability may be seen even if an aggressive tumor is present; this is known as pseudoresponse (see for more detail the article elsewhere in this issue on posttreatment evaluation of central nervous system gliomas).

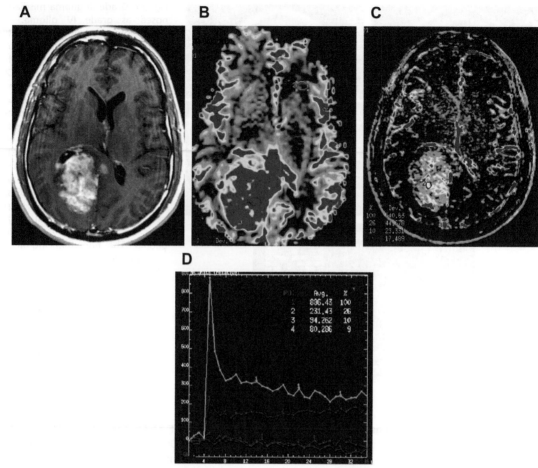

Fig. 21. Grade III glioma. A 28-year-old man presenting with 6-month history of generalized seizures. There is a solid lesion in the right occipital lobe, with heterogeneous enhancement (*A*: axial T1 with contrast). The lesion presents with very high CBV (*B*) and very high permeability (*C*: permeability map; *D*: signal intensity–phase curves). Tumor permeability (ROI 2) is almost 3 times that in the gray matter (ROI 4).

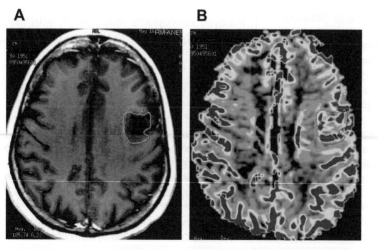

Fig. 22. High rCBV in a grade II glioma. A 60-year-old woman presenting with seizures. There is a solid ill-defined lesion in the left frontal lobe that does not enhance (*A*: axial T1 with contrast). High blood volume is demonstrated in the DSC MR study (*B*: CBV map), a finding that can be seen in low-grade gliomas.

Prediction of Prognosis and Survival

DW imaging, ^{1}H-MRS, and PW imaging yield structural and metabolic information that may provide better insight into tumor functionality and improve the prognostic stratification of brain tumors.[149]

ADC measurements

Some studies have shown that the minimum ADC values of tumors have preoperative prognostic importance in patients with malignant supratentorial astrocytoma.[41,150,151]

ADC values are also predictive of clinical outcome in primary central nervous system lymphoma.[151]

Lymphomas with more restricted diffusion have higher cell density and have a worse prognosis, so these tumors deserve more aggressive treatment.[29]

^{1}H-MRS

Majós and colleagues[149] have demonstrated that a high-intensity value of the peaks at 0.98 and 1.25 ppm, attributed to lipids, correlates with tumoral necrosis and low survival in high-grade astrocytomas. These investigators also found that another region of the short TE spectrum, around 3.67 ppm, likely representing glucose, showed a direct correlation with patient survival. High metabolic activity and, consequently, poor prognosis correlate with depletion of glucose in the extracellular compartment and, accordingly, with low intensity of the resonances that represent this compound in the spectrum, centered at 3.67 ppm. The investigators concluded that ^{1}H-MRS could be used to stratify prognostic groups in HGGs and that this prognostic assessment could be made by evaluating the intensity values of 2 points on the spectrum at short TE (0.98 and 3.67 ppm) and another 2 at long TE (0.98 and 1.25 ppm). Although short-TE ^{1}H-MRS may be considered somewhat superior to long-TE ^{1}H-MRS for prognostic assessment of HGGs, spectrum at both TEs may provide relevant information.[149]

Oh and colleagues[152] found a significantly shorter median survival time for patients with a large volume of metabolic abnormality, measured by ^{1}H-MRS.

In grade IV gliomas, high relative volumes of regions with elevated Cho/NAA index were negatively associated with survival. Survival time was also negatively associated with high lactate and lipid levels and with low ADC within the enhancing volume.[153,154]

DSC MR imaging

The predictive value of perfusion MR imaging for the prognosis of patients with glioma has been well documented.[126,152,155–157] Lev and colleagues[125] reported that in low-grade and HGGs, elevated rCBV was a stronger predictor of survival than the degree of enhancement.

According to Tzika and colleagues,[155] the rCBV value was useful for distinguishing between progressive and stable tumors in pediatric patients with low-grade or high-grade glioma.

Low-grade astrocytomas Law and colleagues[156] suggested that rCBV measurements in LGGs better correlated with time to progression than the initial histopathologic grading of the tumor.

rCBV may be able to distinguish the stable from the rapidly progressing gliomas among patients with the same histopathologic grade (grade II gliomas).[156,158,159] Grade II gliomas that present with high blood volume (see **Fig. 22**B) will probably progress more rapidly than grade II gliomas that present with low blood volume (see **Fig. 17**D). In patients with imaging features of low-grade tumors, high rCBV values suggest a need for a more aggressive approach, with biopsy and treatment and/or MR imaging at closer intervals.[127]

High-grade astrocytomas A long-term follow-up study of patients with high-grade astrocytoma showed that the maximum rCBV value on pretreatment MR imaging scans is useful as a clinical biomarker for predicting the survival of these patients.[159] The presence of an intratumoral area with a high maximum rCBV value ($\geq$2.3) may be predictive of a poor prognosis. The combined assessment of histopathologic and perfusion MR imaging findings obtained before the inception of treatment may be useful in determining optimal management strategies in patients with high-grade astrocytoma.

Anaplastic astrocytomas harboring components manifesting a high maximum rCBV may be associated with a poor prognosis and may require the same aggressive treatment as for GBM. Survival was significantly longer in GBM patients with low rather than high maximum rCBV values.[159]

Determination of Tumor Progression

In patients diagnosed with LGGs, advanced MR imaging techniques may detect malignant transformation earlier than conventional imaging studies.

ADC

Low-grade tumors are typically characterized by relatively higher ADC values related to low cell density. During follow-up, foci of restricted diffusion related to high cellularity and malignant transformation may be demonstrated in these lesions

(Fig. 23). A calculated ADC ratio (tumoral ADC divided by the ADC in the contralateral white matter) of less than 1.0 is related to malignant transformation in LGGs.[30]

¹H-MRS

Malignant degeneration can be demonstrated earlier with ¹H-MRS than with cMR imaging, whereby an increased Cho/Cr or Cho/NAA is suggestive of malignant progression. Tedeschi and colleagues[160] demonstrated that interval percentage change in Cho intensity in stable gliomas and progressive gliomas (malignant degeneration or recurrent disease) is less than 35 and more than 45, respectively (Fig. 24A–D).

DSC MR imaging

An increase in rCBV is likely to provide an early noninvasive indicator of malignant progression and activation of the "angiogenic switch." Increases in rCBV may precede the development of contrast enhancement by at least 12 months in transforming LGGs (see Fig. 24E–G).[161] This finding indicates that high capillary density can be demonstrated well before the appearance of contrast enhancement secondary to disruption of the BBB. It is recommended that MR perfusion imaging be used routinely in the initial assessment and subsequent evaluation of patients with LGGs who are treated conservatively.[161]

DCE MR imaging

During the follow-up of a grade II glioma, appearance of foci of high permeability in the permeability study within the tumor should raise concern for malignant transformation (authors' personal communication).

Determining the Ideal Site for Biopsy

Although histopathology is primarily used to determine the WHO tumor grade, there is the possibility of histopathologic misdiagnosis attributable to sampling error at pathologic examination. When only a few small tissue samples are assessed, particularly from stereotactic biopsy, suboptimal sampling may result in inaccurate glioma grading because of the histologic heterogeneity of tumor tissues.[162,163]

It is estimated that up to 25% of brain tumors are undergraded because the most malignant portion of a neoplasm may not enhance.[164,165]

Advanced imaging techniques can help to indicate the ideal site for biopsy.[36,53]

ADC

Because studies[106–108] have shown that regions of minimum ADC in glial tumors correspond to the highest-grade foci, measuring the lowest ADC within a tumor might aid in selecting an appropriate site for biopsy.[41]

MRS

The role of ¹H-MRS in biopsy guidance is to recognize regions of high metabolic activity: regions of elevated Cho levels (and low NAA levels) indicating tumor tissue represent a good target for biopsy (Fig. 25).[166–171]

DSC MR imaging

Because perfusion MR imaging facilitates assessment of the entire tumor and identification of the

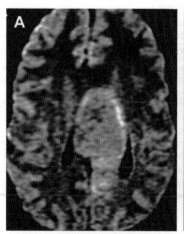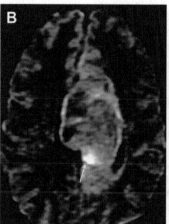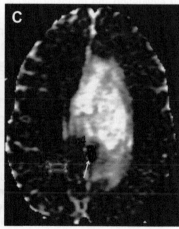

Fig. 23. Tumor progression: ADC. A 22-year-old woman presenting with headaches and seizures. There is a lesion of high signal intensity infiltrating the left frontoparietal lobes, extending to the contralateral hemisphere (A: DW imaging). No areas of restricted diffusion are demonstrated. Nine months later (B, C) a follow-up MR study demonstrates a small area of restricted diffusion (high signal intensity on the DW image, *arrow* in B) and low signal intensity on the ADC map (ROI indicated by *arrow* in C), suggesting anaplastic transformation.

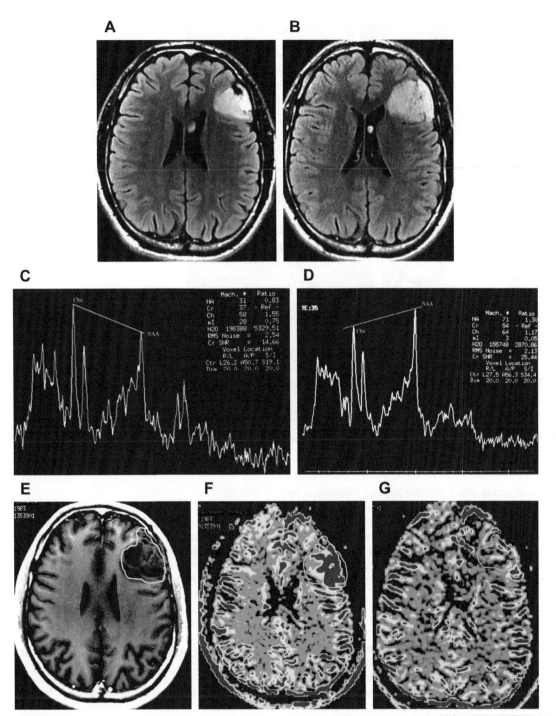

Fig. 24. Tumor progression: MRS and DSC MR imaging. A 27-year-old man presenting with seizures. There is a solid hyperintense lesion in the left inferior frontal gyrus (A: FLAIR). Biopsy was compatible with a grade II glioma. The patient was monitored with follow-up imaging. (B) Follow-up 9 months later demonstrates tumor growth. Spectrum from the lesion (C) shows elevation of the Cho/Cr and Cho/NAA ratios, suggesting high cell density. Compare with the spectrum obtained 9 months before (D) where the NAA is the highest peak. Malignant transformation was suggested based on interval elevation of the Cho/Cr and Cho/NAA ratios. There is subtle enhancement (E: axial T1 with contrast). CBV is very high (F), also suggesting malignant transformation. Compare with the perfusion study from 9 months before (G). Based on the results from the ^{1}H-MRS and perfusion-weighted imaging studies, a diagnosis of anaplastic transformation was suggested and surgical resection was performed. The lesion diagnosed as a grade II glioma 9 months ago was now confirmed as a grade III anaplastic oligoastrocytoma with high cell density and significant vascular proliferation.

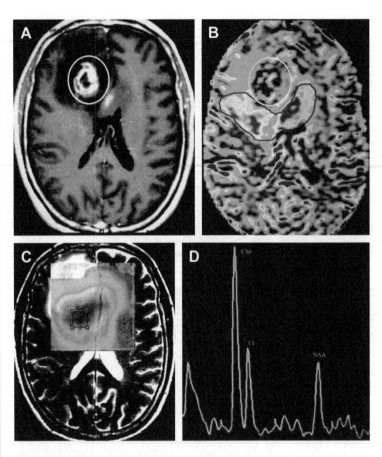

Fig. 25. Determining the ideal site for biopsy. A 47-year-old man status post surgical resection of a right frontal lesion 3 months ago; pathology was negative. The area that enhances (*circle* in *A*) presents with low capillary density (*B*: DSC) and is not the ideal site for biopsy. Surrounding the area of enhancement posteriorly there is an area of high capillary density (*area bordered by red* in *B*) and high cell density (*C, D*: multivoxel MRS) presenting with high Cho peak and high Cho/Cr and Cho/NAA ratios. This area is probably the best site for biopsy.

intratumoral areas with the highest microvascular density, it may be helpful for selection of the biopsy targets. The area with maximum rCBV value in a high-grade glial tumor will be the best site for biopsy (see **Fig. 25**). This technique may prevent undergrading (eg, sampling error) and may demonstrate biologic differences (eg, genetic change) in the tumor.[159]

DCE MR imaging

The permeability map may indicate the more malignant area in a heterogeneous brain tumor, suggesting the ideal site for biopsy.

The best place for biopsy is likely the area of highest permeability, which corresponds to the presence of leaky vessels derived from angiogenesis, known to occur in more malignant tumors/areas.

Assessment of Tumor Extension

ADC

In the authors' experience, ADC cannot demonstrate tumor extension. Some studies also have demonstrated that ADC cannot depict peritumoral neoplastic cell infiltration.[28,60,171–174]

¹H-MRS

In high-grade infiltrative tumors, tumor activity can be demonstrated by MRS imaging beyond the enhanced area identified on gadolinium-enhanced cMR imaging (**Fig. 26A–C**). Comparison of the extent (and location) of active tumor as defined by MR imaging and MRS imaging demonstrates differences between the two techniques.[175] The area of metabolic abnormality as defined by MRS imaging may exceed the area of abnormal T2-weighted signal.[91,175–177] ¹H-MRS may better define tumor extension than cMR imaging.[53]

Special consideration If no elevation of the Cho/NAA ratio is demonstrated beyond the enhancing lesion, tumor infiltration cannot be ruled out. The reason for this is probably the fact that elevation of the Cho/Cr and Cho/NAA ratio is related to the number of neoplastic cells that have infiltrated outside the enhancing lesion.[53]

DSC MR imaging

High-grade tumors tend to infiltrate the parenchyma around the enhancing tumor nodule.

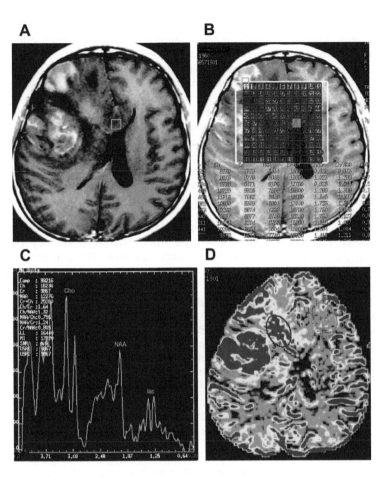

Fig. 26. Evaluation of tumor extension. A 48-year-old woman diagnosed with GBM. There is a large infiltrative lesion in the right frontal lobe, crossing the midline and presenting with some areas of enhancement (*A*: axial T1 with contrast). Multivoxel ¹H-MRS (*B*, *C*) demonstrates significant elevation of the Cho peak and Cho/Cr and Cho/NAA ratios in the corpus callosum, along with the presence of lactate peak, compatible with tumor infiltration beyond the areas of enhancement. There is also elevation of the blood volume in the same area (*D*: rCBV map).

Perfusion alone or in combination with MRS imaging may better define tumor borders than cMR imaging (see **Fig. 26**D).[72,178]

Assessment of Therapeutic Response

An important issue in patients with brain tumors is the differentiation between recurrent brain tumor and radiation injury/change, particularly when new contrast-enhancing lesions are seen in previously operated and/or irradiated regions.[179–183] At present, the 2-dimensional measurements of contrast enhancement on MR imaging along with clinical status and corticosteroid dosage (collectively referred to as the Macdonald criteria) are the methods most widely used to assess therapeutic response in patients with HGG.[184] However, a well-known pitfall of this approach is that contrast enhancement is a result of nonspecific BBB damage and can be due to many causes including, but not limited to, tumor progression, postoperative changes, ischemia, and treatment-related effects.[185–189]

Differentiating residual or recurrent tumors from treatment-related changes is limited on cMR imaging as well as on histologic examination; areas of T1 contrast enhancement after radiation treatment often contain both residual and recurrent tumor and tissue affected by therapy-related changes. Furthermore, the heterogeneity of gliomas before and after therapy and the inaccuracy of biopsy sampling pose another challenge in the histologic separation of tumors from necrosis.[45] On cMR imaging, the evaluation of treatment response and categorization as stable disease, responder (partial remission), and nonresponder (progression) are based predominantly on changes in tumor volumes, which can take some time.[190]

Since the introduction of combined chemoradiation with temozolamide as the current standard of care for HGGs, the phenomenon of pseudoprogression (PsP) has been increasingly recognized. Although the exact definition of PsP is still debated, it most often refers to a new or increased contrast enhancement on MR imaging within the first 3 to 6 months of chemoradiation, earlier than occurs with radiation therapy alone. This enhancement is due to treatment-related changes rather than to true early progression (TEP) and, if therapy is unchanged, will stabilize or improve over time.[191,192]

Advanced imaging methods may show some promise in the distinction between TEP and PsP. Perfusion studies, for example, have demonstrated that rCBV is higher in TEP than in PsP.[193–195] However, there are still currently no validated advanced imaging methods to distinguish TEP from PsP, so follow-up cMR imaging is still considered the gold-standard imaging technique.[196]

In response to the possibility of PsP, the Response Assessment in Neuro-Oncology (RANO) Working Group recently recommended that for patients within 3 months of completion of chemoradiation, the diagnosis of disease progression could be made only if there is new enhancement beyond the radiation field or if there is unequivocal histopathologic evidence of tumor.[197] However, there is some concern that this recommendation could exclude the rapidly progressing, malignant tumors and that, because these types of patients were not prevented from enrolling in prior clinical trials, a new bias could be encountered when trying to determine the efficacy of a new drug on comparison with historical controls.[198]

Advanced MR imaging techniques and their role in the evaluation of treated gliomas

ADC
Diffusion can be used to assess tumor response to therapy.[28,199–202]

Successful radiation and/or chemotherapy will result in tumor cell necrosis; as a result, restricted diffusion related to high cell density will be converted to high diffusivity, characterized by increased ADC values.

Postresection injury Diffusion may help to distinguish tumor recurrence from postresection injury.[203] Infarcts occur in up to two-thirds of surgically treated gliomas in the immediate postsurgery period, and enhancement will be demonstrated in the follow-up studies in this area. Enhancement may persist for up to 2 to 3 months, simulating residual/recurrent tumor. Evaluation of the immediate postsurgery MR imaging may demonstrate restricted diffusion within the surgical margins corresponding to the area of enhancement in the follow-up MR imaging, compatible with postresection injury (**Fig. 27**).[45]

TEP versus pseudoprogression Some studies demonstrate that ADC measurements may be used in the distinction between TEP and pseudprogression.[204] According to Matsusue and colleagues,[204] restricted diffusion would indicate TEP, and high signal intensity on the ADC maps would represent inflammatory abnormalities related to PsP. However, the authors of this chapter have experienced a large overlap when ADC measurements are used in the distinction between TEP and PsP. The heterogeneity of both TEP and PsP lesions limits the use of ADC in this setting, and currently there is insufficient evidence from either DW imaging or DT imaging to be able to differentiate TEP from PsP.[192,196]

Antiangiogenic-related changes Antiangiogenic drugs such as Avastin (bevacizumab) have been used as a treatment option for recurrent GBMs. Antiangiogenic agents are thought to result in "vascular normalization," a rapid but transient effect on GBM vasculature whereby there is a decrease in vascular permeability and vessel diameter, improved tumor oxygenation and thinning of the abnormally thick basement membrane.[205,206] The often reversible marked

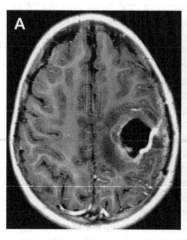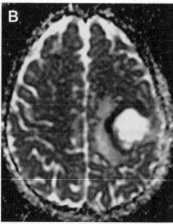

Fig. 27. Postresection injury. A 7-year-old boy presenting with paresthesia and paresis in the right hand. He was previously diagnosed with high-grade glioma in the left frontal-parietal region and underwent resection. Enhancement is demonstrated in the surgical borders (*A*: axial T1 with contrast) that could represent residual tumor versus ischemic changes. Corresponding to the area that enhances, diffusion restriction is demonstrated on the ADC map (*B*), characterizing postsurgical ischemic changes. In the follow-up study (not shown), enhancement and restricted diffusion had resolved.

decrease in contrast enhancement and impressive 6-month progression-free survival, but with modest effect on overall survival, support the notion that these changes are more attributable to changes in vascular permeability rather than to a true antitumoral response.[207,208] Angiogenesis inhibition may result in alternative routes of nonenhancing tumor progression, likely through vessel co-option.[209] As a result, reliance on changes in contrast enhancement on cMR imaging may not be appropriate for the assessment of response to antiangiogenic agents. The term pseudoresponse has been applied to this dramatic decrease in contrast enhancement seen with antiangiogenic agents, and some patients may develop nonenhancing evidence of disease progression such as regions of diffusion restriction and increased fluid-attenuated inversion recovery (FLAIR) signal.[200,201,210–215]

Restricted diffusion may be demonstrated before the appearance of enhancement in progressive tumors during bevacizumab therapy.[200,214] These restricted-diffusion abnormalities may develop both in and outside the setting of bevacizumab treatment.[32]

There is still some debate as to whether these restricted-diffusion lesions represent aggressive tumor or ischemic changes. Mong and colleagues[216] have demonstrated that regions of persistent diffusion restriction after bevacizumab treatment in patients with malignant gliomas are not associated with growing tumor, but rather may be related to atypical necrosis in many patients. These investigators have demonstrated that these areas of restricted diffusion tend to be stable within 6 months, present with low rCBV and reduced metabolism in positron emission tomography (PET) studies and, moreover, that these patients live longer, which all are very suggestive of a benign process rather than aggressive tumor growth (Fig. 28). High signal intensity on the T1 within the margins of these lesions is commonly seen, and is usually associated with necrosis.

The decreased vasogenic edema from vascular normalization can result in decreased morbidity, improved clinical status, and reduced steroid dosing, regardless of whether a patient is experiencing a pseudoresponse or true response to antiangiogenic agents.[207,217]

At present there are no validated biomarkers with which to appropriately select patients with cancer for antiangiogenic therapy. Contrast-enhanced cMR imaging studies, as well as permeability study, may fail to demonstrate tumor progression during bevacizumab therapy.

Enlargement of the T2 and FLAIR abnormalities on cMR imaging in patients undergoing bevacizumab therapy may be suggestive of tumor progression, although demyelination secondary to radiation therapy and chemotherapy cannot be ruled out.

¹H-MRS

¹H-MRS has been applied to differentiate between radiation-induced tissue injury and tumor recurrence in adult and pediatric patients with brain tumor following external beam radiation, gamma-knife radiosurgery, and brachytherapy.[218–224] Significantly reduced Cho and Cr levels are suggestive of radiation necrosis.[32,207,215–220,225,226] Necrotic regions may also show elevated lipid and lactate signals (Fig. 29A, B).[221,222] On the other hand, increased Cho (evaluated as Cho levels relative to Cho signal in normal-appearing tissue, Cho/Cr or Cho/NAA ratios) is suggestive of recurrence (see Fig. 29D).[219,220,225] Many studies have found that Cho/Cr and/or Cho/NAA ratios are significantly higher in recurrent tumor (or predominantly tumor) than in radiation injury.[180–183] In a retrospective MRS imaging study of 33 tumors using an intermediate TE of 144 milliseconds, Smith and colleagues[181] demonstrated that higher Cho/Cr and Cho/NAA ratios and a lower NAA/Cr ratio suggest tumor recurrence rather than radiation change. According to this study, the Cho/NAA ratio demonstrated the best confidence interval to distinguish between tumor recurrence and radiation change. The distinction between recurrent tumor and radiation necrosis using the Cho/NAA ratio could be made with 85% sensitivity and 69% specificity.[181]

According to Elias and colleagues,[223] Cho/NAA and NAA/Cr were the 2 ratios with the best discriminating ability to differentiate recurrent brain tumor from radiation change.

Tumor recurrence may be detected by ¹H-MRS in a site remote from the irradiated area. In some cases, elevation of the Cho may precede a coincident increase in contrast enhancement by 1 to 2 months.[226]

Some overlap may be seen in the ¹H-MRS of tumors and radiation change. An increase in Cho-containing compounds after radiation therapy as a result of cell damage and astrogliosis may be seen in radiation necrosis misclassified as tumors.[224] In addition, both tumors and necrotic tissue have low levels of NAA, consistent with neuronal damage. Also, residual tumor may be present along with some radiation changes in the same patient. If the spectrum is indeterminate (ie, indicating the presence of both residual tumor and radiation change), repeated examination is suggested after an interval of 6 to 8 weeks.[221] If

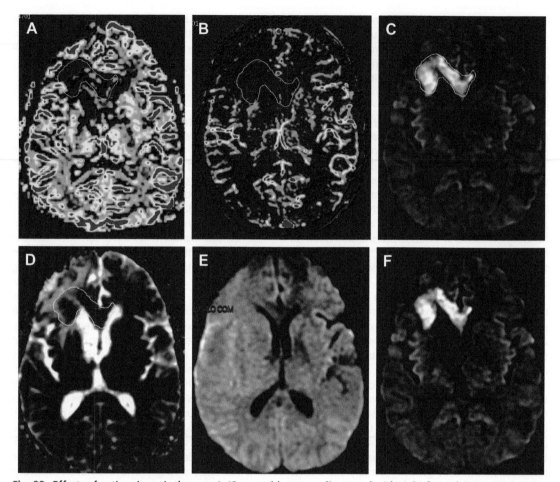

Fig. 28. Effects of antiangiogenic therapy. A 48-year-old woman diagnosed with right frontal GBM. MR imaging after surgical resection + radiation therapy + chemotherapy demonstrates no elevation of the blood volume (*A*: rCBV map) and no elevation of the permeability (*B*: permeability map) in the right frontal lobe. Restricted diffusion (high signal intensity on DW imaging [*C*] and low signal intensity on the ADC map [*D*])is demonstrated in the right frontal region, which could be related to tumor growth or hypoxic changes/atypical necrosis. Compare with the DW image at the time of diagnosis (*E*). Follow-up 1 year later demonstrates that the area of restricted diffusion is exactly the same (*F*), which rules out aggressive tumor and suggests chronic hypoxic changes.

the elevation of Cho is related to radiation change, it will normalize with time.

Finally, a discrete and isolated elevation of Cho in serial examinations should not be considered evidence of tumor recurrence. Interval increased Cho/Cr or Cho/NAA is suggestive of malignant progression/tumor recurrence if the percentage change in Cho is more than 45%,[155] and/or is associated with elevation of the blood volume and permeability indicating vascular proliferation and significant compromise of the BBB, respectively.

DSC and DCE MR imaging

Additional information from the perfusion and permeability studies may also help in the correct distinction between tumors (see **Fig. 29**E–G) and radiation necrosis (see **Fig. 29**C).

In recurrent tumor, vascular proliferation results in elevated rCBV, whereas in delayed radiation necrosis (DRN), lower rCBV is seen because it is the result of extensive fibrinoid necrosis, vascular dilation, and endothelial injury.[227–230]

The use of other PW MR imaging parameters such as increased peak height (PH) and lower relative PSR has been reported in recurrent glioblastoma in comparison with DRN.[227]

The use of DCE MR imaging to diagnose DRN is much more limited than with the use of rCBV. However, there is some evidence to indicate that there is lower permeability in DRN compared with recurrent tumor.[143,231] A recent study of 18 patients with HGG showed that a K^{trans} threshold of greater than 0.19 produced 100% sensitivity and 83% specificity for detecting recurrent glioma versus DRN.[232]

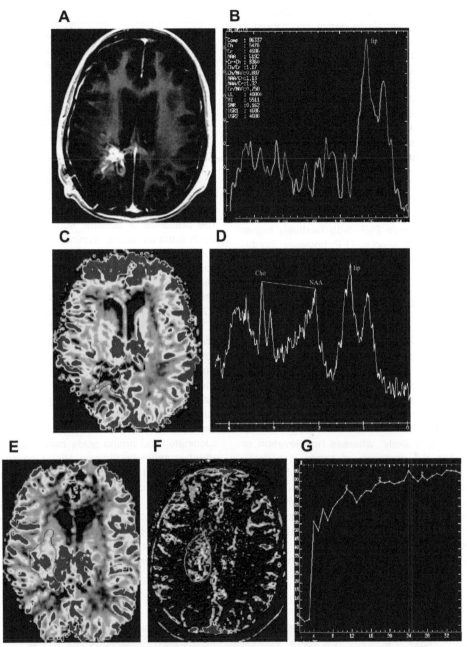

Fig. 29. Radiation necrosis versus tumor recurrence. A 24-year-old woman diagnosed with GBM who underwent surgery, chemoradiation therapy, and steroid administration. There is irregular enhancement in the surgical bed (A). The spectrum (B) demonstrates significant reduction of the NAA, Cho, and Cr peaks, along with a prominent lipid peak, consistent with radiation necrosis. Perfusion is reduced (C: CBV map) and there is mildly increased permeability also indicating therapeutic response. Four months later the spectroscopy demonstrates elevation of the Cho peak and Cho/NAA ratio indicating tumor-cell proliferation (D). The perfusion study (E) demonstrates high capillary density, and there is also significant elevation of the permeability (F, G) in the same area. The results from the MRS, DSC, MR imaging, and DCE MR imaging are now compatible with tumor recurrence.

Another recent study used a nonmodel-based semiquantitative permeability MR imaging technique to differentiate recurrent/progressive brain tumor from treatment-induced necrosis.[141] In this study, recurrent/progressive tumor demonstrated greater maximum slope of enhancement in the initial vascular phase of signal intensity–time curves. This study seemed to indicate that although semiquantitative metrics are less physiologically specific, they are simple to derive and robust in differentiating between the two conditions.

Besides antiangiogenic therapy, steroids may also affect the perfusion and permeability of brain tumors. Steroid therapy is intended to stabilize the endothelium and, consequently, is expected to reduce measured values of K^{trans}.[73]

Concerning the distinction between tumor progression and pseudoprogression, some studies have demonstrated that an increase in the relative CBV value favors TEP and a decrease indicates PsP, but there is still some degree of overlap.[193–195,233]

DCE MR imaging may potentially be useful to distinguish TEP from PsP, with relatively higher permeability to be seen in TEP; however, confirmatory studies are currently lacking.

DIFFERENTIAL DIAGNOSIS FOR FOCAL BRAIN TUMORS
Tumor Versus Infarct

Differentiation between a glioma and an infarct may be difficult or even impossible using cMR imaging. Restricted diffusion may be demonstrated in high-grade tumors as well as in acute and subacute infarcts.

Increased Cho makes the diagnosis of neoplasm more likely, whereas no elevation of Cho makes the diagnosis of tumor less likely. Elevation of lipids along with reduction of all other metabolites is characteristic of infarcts, but this finding may also be present in tumors with extensive necrosis. Moreover, elevation of Cho may be seen in infarction especially in the subacute stage, mimicking tumor (**Fig. 30**).

High blood volume, along with high permeability, favors neoplasm over infarct.

Tumor Versus Abscess

The differential diagnosis between brain abscess and neoplasms (primary and secondary) is a challenge. Both may appear as cystic lesions with rim enhancement on cMR imaging. Pyogenic abscesses typically demonstrate diffusion restriction (**Fig. 31A, B**), which is usually not seen in tumors. Nevertheless, some neoplasms may occasionally have restricted diffusion, and biopsy is inevitable.

^{1}H-MRS may help establish a diagnosis. In the case of a rim-enhancing lesion, to differentiate between a necrotic tumor and an abscess the voxel should be placed within the cystic-necrotic area.[234] The presence of acetate, succinate, and amino acids such as valine, alanine, and leucine in the core of the lesion has high sensitivity for pyogenic abscess (see **Fig. 31C**).[116,234,235] To demonstrate the typical spectral abnormalities in the abscess cavity, an intermediate (144 milliseconds) or high (270 milliseconds) TE should be used.[234]

Typical spectrum of anaerobic bacterial abscesses (acetate, succinate, and amino acids) do not exist in *Staphylococcal aureus* abscesses, which are one of the aerobic bacterial abscesses.[234] In this situation, lipids and lactate may be the only spectral findings, and the spectrum will be similar to that of a necrotic brain tumor. Moreover, the resonances of acetate, succinate, and amino acids may disappear with effective antibiotic therapy. High Cho peak, Cho/NAA ratio, and Cho/Cr ratio may be seen in infection and should not be considered as evidence of tumor.

A thin rim of high CBV may be seen in the subacute and chronic abscesses (see **Fig. 31D**).

In the authors' experience, no significant elevation of the permeability has been demonstrated (see **Fig. 31E**).

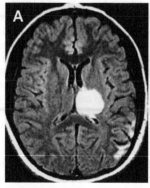
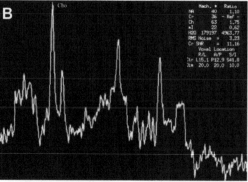

Fig. 30. Infarct with high choline. Significant elevation of the Cho peak is demonstrated in the spectrum from the left thalamic infarct (*A*: axial T2 FLAIR; *B*: spectroscopy). The spectral pattern resembles that of a brain tumor.

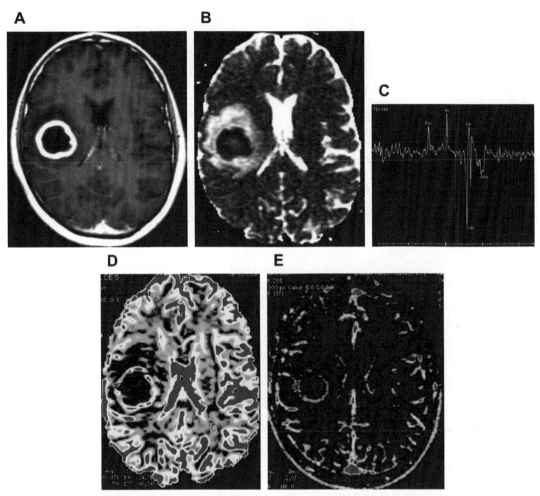

Fig. 31. Tumor versus abscess. A 39-year-old man, HIV-positive, presenting with a ring-enhancing lesion in the right frontal lobe (*A*). There is restricted diffusion (low signal intensity on the ADC map, *B*) compatible with the diagnosis of pyogenic abscess. Spectrum from the abscess cavity (*C*) performed with intermediate echo time (TE; 144 milliseconds) demonstrates lipids (Lip) and lactate (Lac), which are also seen in the GBM. However, amino acids (Aas; 0.9 ppm), acetate (Ac; 1.9 ppm), and succinate (Suc; 2.4 ppm) are also demonstrated. These findings have high sensitivity for the diagnosis of pyogenic abscesses. A thin rim of high blood volume may be demonstrated in subacute and chronic abscesses (*D*) and should not be confused with tumors. Mildly increased permeability is typically seen (*E*).

Tumor Versus Tumefactive Demyelinating Lesions

Restricted diffusion is typically demonstrated in high-grade glial tumors and lymphomas, and is related to high cell density. While acute demyelinating plaques may demonstrate restricted diffusion within its margins (**Fig. 32**A, B), a rim of restricted diffusion is not a characteristic finding in lymphomas.[236]

Differentiation between HGGs and some acute demyelinating lesions based on ^{1}H-MRS alone may be difficult because of histopathologic similarities, which include hypercellularity, reactive astrocytes, mitotic figures, and areas of necrosis.[45,237,238]

Aggressive tumors and acute demyelinating plaques typically present with elevated Cho and decreased NAA, as well as often-increased lactate and lipids (see **Fig. 32**C).[239,240]

In the acute stage of a demyelinating disease, increased lactate is reflective of the metabolism of inflammatory cells.[239–242]

Majós and colleagues[120] found that the increased Cho and decreased NAA at long TE were even higher in tumors and that these metabolites could discriminate between tumors and pseudotumoral lesions. However, in the authors' experience, a significant elevation of Cho along with significant reduction of NAA may be demonstrated in acute demyelinating plaques (see

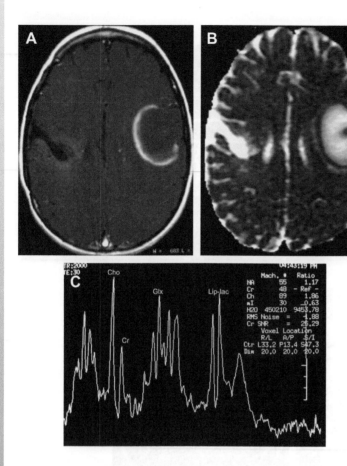

Fig. 32. Tumor versus tumefactive demyelinating lesion. An 11-year-old boy presenting with right-side hemiparesis. Two years ago he underwent surgical resection of an acute demyelinating plaque in the right frontal lobe, which was diagnosed as a brain glioma. Now there is a new acute demyelinating plaque in the left frontal lobe, presenting with a peripheral incomplete rim of enhancement (A: axial T1 with contrast) and a rim of restricted diffusion (B: ADC map). Spectrum from the lesion (C) demonstrates reduction of the NAA peak along with high Cho, and lipids and lactate (Lip-lac) peaks. The spectral findings resemble those of brain gliomas, except for the high glutamate and glutamine (Glx) peak.

Fig. 32C). According to Cianfoni and colleagues,[240] elevation of glutamine and glutamate helps differentiate tumefactive demyelinating lesions from neoplastic masses, avoiding unnecessary biopsy and potentially harmful surgery, as well as providing a more specific diagnosis during the initial MR examination, thus allowing earlier institution of appropriate therapy.

Low CBV values and no significant elevation of the permeability are more consistent with acute demyelinating plaque than aggressive tumor.

SUMMARY

Advanced MR imaging techniques can provide additional diagnostic indices beyond anatomic information that is typically generated with cMR imaging. Indeed, with the introduction of DW imaging, advanced MRS, DSC MR imaging, and DCE MR imaging studies, the neuroradiologist now has the tools needed to exploit a body of imaging information, including the likely histology of a lesion, cellularity, capillary density, and metabolic profiles—information that is essential to understanding tumor characteristics and to developing appropriate differential diagnoses.

The primary objective of this article is to demonstrate how different MR techniques can be used to suggest tumor type and tumor grade, indicate the ideal site for biopsy, assess tumor extension, and follow tumor progression.

Advanced MR imaging techniques may also provide prognostic information and may be used to guide therapy early on in the patient's treatment, effectively improving outcomes and minimizing side effects, both in the short and long term. Therapeutic response to therapy may be better estimated by use of advanced MR imaging techniques than simply through cMR imaging.

REFERENCES

1. Al-Okaili RN, Krejza J, Wang S, et al. Advanced MR imaging techniques in the diagnosis of intraaxial brain tumors in adults. Radiographics 2006; 26(Suppl 1):S173–89.
2. Al-Okaili RN, Krejza J, Woo JH, et al. Intraaxial brain masses: MR imaging-based diagnostic strategy-initial experience. Radiology 2007;243:539–50.
3. Catalaa I, Henry R, Dillon WP, et al. Perfusion, diffusion and spectroscopy values in newly diagnosed cerebral gliomas. NMR Biomed 2006;19:463–75.

4. Fayed N, Dávila J, Medrano J, et al. Malignancy assessment of brain tumors with magnetic resonance spectroscopy and dynamic susceptibility contrast MRI. Eur J Radiol 2008;67:427–33.

5. Morita N, Harada M, Otsuka H, et al. Clinical application of MR spectroscopy and imaging of brain tumor. Magn Reson Med Sci 2010;9(4):167–75.

6. Tong Z, Yamaki T, Harada K, et al. In vivo quantification of the metabolites in normal brain and brain tumors by proton MR spectroscopy using water as an internal standard. Magn Reson Imaging 2004; 22:1017–24.

7. Hwang JH, Egnaczyk GF, Ballard E, et al. Proton MR spectroscopic characteristics of pediatric pilocytic astrocytomas. AJNR Am J Neuroradiol 1998; 19:535–40.

8. Poussaint TY, Rodriguez D. Advanced neuroimaging of pediatric brain tumors: MR diffusion, MR perfusion, and MR spectroscopy. Neuroimaging Clin N Am 2006;16:169–92.

9. Barkovich AJ, Raybaud C. Intracranial, orbital and neck masses of childhood. In: Pediatric neuroimaging. 5th edition. Philadelphia: Lippincott Williams & Wilkins and Wolters Kluwer; 2012. p. 637–711.

10. Panigrahy A, Krieger I, Gonzalez G, et al. Quantitative short echo time ^{1}H-MR spectroscopy of untreated pediatric brain tumors: preoperative diagnosis and characterization. AJNR Am J Neuroradiol 2006;27:560–72.

11. Wang Z, Sutton LN, Cnaan A, et al. Proton MR spectroscopy of pediatric cerebellar tumors. AJNR Am J Neuroradiol 1995;16:1821–33.

12. Sutton LN, Wang Z, Gusnard D, et al. Proton magnetic resonance spectroscopy of pediatric brain tumors. Neurosurgery 1992;31:195–202.

13. Lazareff JA, Bockhorst KH, Curran J, et al. Pediatric low-grade gliomas: prognosis with proton magnetic resonance spectroscopic imaging. Neurosurgery 1998;43:809–17.

14. Lazareff JA, Olmstead C, Bockhorst KH, et al. Proton magnetic resonance spectroscopic imaging of pediatric low-grade astrocytomas. Childs Nerv Syst 1996;12:130–5.

15. Horska A, Ulug AM, Melhem ER, et al. Proton magnetic resonance spectroscopy of choroid plexus tumors in children. J Magn Reson Imaging 2001;14:78–82.

16. Tzika AA, Vigneron DB, Dunn RS, et al. Intracranial tumors in children: small single-voxel proton MR spectroscopy using short and long-echo sequences. Neuroradiology 1996;38:254–6.

17. Girard N, Wang ZJ, Erbetta A, et al. Prognostic value of proton MR spectroscopy of cerebral hemisphere tumors in children. Neuroradiology 1998; 40:121–5.

18. Arle JE, Morriss C, Wang ZJ, et al. Prediction of posterior fossa tumor type in children by means of magnetic resonance image properties, spectroscopy, and neural networks. J Neurosurg 1997; 86:755–61.

19. Dezortova M, Hajek M, Cap F, et al. Comparison of MR spectroscopy and MR imaging with contrast agent in children with cerebral astrocytomas. Childs Nerv Syst 1999;15(8):408–12.

20. Rumboldt A, Camacho DL, Lake CT, et al. Apparent diffusion coefficients for differentiation of cerebellar tumors in children. AJNR Am J Neuroradiol 2006;27:1362–9.

21. Stadnik TW, Chaskis C, Michotte A, et al. Diffusion-weighted MR imaging of intracerebral masses: comparison with conventional MR imaging and histologic findings. AJNR Am J Neuroradiol 2001; 22:969–76.

22. Guo AC, Cummings TJ, Dash RC, et al. Lymphomas and high-grade astrocytomas: comparison of water diffusibility and histologic characteristics. Radiology 2002;224(1):177–83.

23. Herneth AM, Guccione S, Bednarski M. Apparent diffusion coefficient: a quantitative parameter for in-vivo tumor characterization. Eur J Radiol 2003; 45(3):208–13.

24. Yamashita Y, Kumabe T, Higano S. Minimum apparent diffusion coefficient is significantly correlated with cellularity in medulloblastomas. J Neuroradiol 2004;31(3):234–7.

25. Khayal IS, Crawford FW, Saraswathy MS, et al. Relationship between choline and apparent diffusion coefficient in patients with gliomas. J Comput Assist Tomogr 2004;28:735–46.

26. Hayashida Y, Hirai T, Morishita S, et al. Diffusion-weighted imaging of metastatic brain tumors: comparison with histologic type and tumor cellularity. AJNR Am J Neuroradiol 2006;27(7):1419–25.

27. Kim HS, Kim SY. A prospective study on the added value of pulsed arterial spin-labeling and apparent diffusion coefficients in the grading of gliomas. AJNR Am J Neuroradiol 2007;28:1693–9.

28. Cruz LC, Domingues R, Sorensen GH. Diffusion magnetic resonance imaging in brain tumors. In: Newton HB, Jolesz FA, editors. Handbook of neuro-oncology neuroimaging. New York: Elsevier; 2008. p. 215–38.

29. Barajas RF, Rubenstein JL, Chang JS, et al. Diffusion-weighted MR imaging derived apparent diffusion coefficient is predictive of clinical outcome in primary central nervous system lymphoma. AJNR Am J Neuroradiol 2010;31:60–6.

30. Holodny AI, Makeyev S, Beattie BJ, et al. Apparent diffusion coefficient of glial neoplasms: correlation with fluorodeoxyglucose–positron-emission tomography and gadolinium-enhanced MR imaging. AJNR Am J Neuroradiol 2010;31:1042–8.

31. Mills SJ, Soh C, Rose CJ, et al. Candidate biomarkers of extravascular extracellular space: a

direct comparison of apparent diffusion coefficient and dynamic contrast-enhanced MR imaging-derived measurement of the volume of the extravascular extracellular space in glioblastoma multiforme. AJNR Am J Neuroradiol 2010;31: 549–53.

32. Gupta A, Young RJ, Karimi A, et al. Isolated diffusion restriction precedes the development of enhancing tumor in a subset of patients with glioblastoma. AJNR Am J Neuroradiol 2011;32: 1301–6.

33. Cruz LC, Vieira IG, Domingues R. Diffusion MR imaging: an important tool in the assessment of brain tumors. Neuroimaging Clin N Am 2011; 21(1):27–49.

34. Wang W, Steward CE, Desmond PM. Diffusion tensor imaging in glioblastoma multiforme and brain metastases: the role of p, q, L, and fractional anisotropy. AJNR Am J Neuroradiol 2009;30:203–8.

35. Lu S, Ahn D, Johnson G, et al. Peritumoral diffusion tensor imaging of high-grade gliomas and metastatic brain tumors. AJNR Am J Neuroradiol 2003; 24:937–41.

36. Brandão L, Domingues R. Intracranial neoplasms. In: MR spectroscopy of the brain. Philadelphia: Lippincott Williams & Wilkins; 2003. p. 130–67.

37. Aronen HJ, Gazit IE, Lous DN, et al. Cerebral blood volume maps of gliomas: comparison with tumor grade and histologic findings. Radiology 1994; 191:41–51.

38. Young R, Babb J, Law M, et al. Comparison of region-of-interest analysis with three different histogram analysis methods in the determination of perfusion metrics in patients with brain gliomas. J Magn Reson Imaging 2007;26:1053–63.

39. Emblem KE, Nedregaard B, Nome T, et al. Glioma grading by using histogram analysis of blood volume maps. Radiology 2008;247:808–17.

40. Roberts HC, Roberts TP, Brasch RC, et al. Quantitative measurement of microvascular permeability in human brain tumors achieved using dynamic contrast-enhanced MR imaging: correlation with histologic grade. AJNR Am J Neuroradiol 2000; 21:891–9.

41. Lee EJ, Brugge K, Mikulis D, et al. Diagnostic value of peritumoral minimum apparent diffusion coefficient for differentiation of glioblastoma multiforme from solitary metastatic lesions. AJR Am J Roentgenol 2011;196:71–6.

42. Tsuchiya K, Fujikawa A, Nakajima M, et al. Differentiation between solitary brain metastasis and high-grade glioma by diffusion tensor imaging. Br J Radiol 2005;78:533–7.

43. Law M, Cha S, Knopp EA, et al. High-grade gliomas and solitary metastases: differentiation by using perfusion and proton spectroscopic MR imaging. Radiology 2002;222:715–21.

44. Oh J, Cha S, Aiken AH, et al. Quantitative apparent diffusion coefficients and T2 relaxation times in characterizing contrast enhancing brain tumors and regions of peritumoral edema. J Magn Reson Imaging 2005;21:701–8.

45. Cha S. Update on brain tumor imaging: from anatomy to physiology. AJNR Am J Neuroradiol 2006;27:475–87.

46. Chiang IC, Kuo YT, Lu CY, et al. Distinction between high-grade gliomas and solitary metastases using peritumoral 3-T magnetic resonance spectroscopy, diffusion, and perfusion imaging. Neuroradiology 2004;46:619–27.

47. Krabbe K, Gideon P, Wagn P, et al. MR diffusion imaging of human intracranial tumors. Neuroradiology 1997;39:483–9.

48. Rollin N, Guyotat J, Streichenberger N, et al. Clinical relevance of diffusion and perfusion magnetic resonance imaging in assessing intra-axial brain tumors. Neuroradiology 2006;48:150–9.

49. Yamasaki F, Kurisu K, Satoh K, et al. Apparent diffusion coefficient of human brain tumors at MR imaging. Radiology 2005;235:985–91.

50. Bulakbasi N, Kocaoglu M, Ors F, et al. Combination of single-voxel proton MR spectroscopy and apparent diffusion coefficient calculation in the evaluation of common brain tumors. AJNR Am J Neuroradiol 2003;24:225–33.

51. Kelly P, Daumas-Duport C, Kispert D, et al. Imaging-based stereotaxic serial biopsies in untreated intracranial glial neoplasms. J Neurosurg 1987;66:865–74.

52. Ricci R, Bacci A, Tugnoli V, et al. Metabolic findings on 3T ^{1}H-MR spectroscopy in peritumoral brain edema. AJNR Am J Neuroradiol 2007;28:1287–91.

53. Brandão L, Castillo M. MR spectroscopy in adult brain tumors. Neuroimaging Clinics of North America. Elsevier, in press.

54. Young GS, Setayesh K. Spin-echo echo-planar perfusion MR imaging in the differential diagnosis of solitary enhancing brain lesions: distinguishing solitary metastases from primary glioma. AJNR Am J Neuroradiol 2009;30:575–7.

55. Bulakbasi N, Kocaoglu M, Farzaliyev A, et al. Assessment of diagnostic accuracy of perfusion MR imaging in primary and metastatic solitary malignant brain tumors. AJNR Am J Neuroradiol 2005;26:2187–99.

56. Cha S, Lupo JM, Chen MH. Differentiation of glioblastoma multiforme and single brain metastasis by peak height and percentage of signal intensity recovery derived from dynamic susceptibility-weighted contrast-enhanced perfusion MR imaging. AJNR Am J Neuroradiol 2007;28:1078–84.

57. Wesseling P, Ruiter DJ, Burger PC. Angiogenesis in brain tumors; pathobiological and clinical aspects. J Neurooncol 1997;32:253–65.

58. Jinnouchi T, Shibata S, Fukushima M, et al. Ultrastructure of capillary permeability in human brain tumor—part 6: metastatic brain tumor with brain edema. No Shinkei Geka 1988;16:563–8 [in Japanese].

59. Long DM. Capillary ultrastructure in human metastatic brain tumors. J Neurosurg 1979;51:53–8.

60. Stadnik TW, Demaerel P, Luypaert RR, et al. Imaging tutorial: differential diagnosis of bright lesions on diffusion-weighted MR images. Radiographics 2003;23:e7.

61. Toh CH, Castillo M, Wong AC, et al. Primary cerebral lymphoma and glioblastoma multiforme: differences in diffusion characteristics evaluated with diffusion tensor imaging. AJNR Am J Neuroradiol 2008;29:471–5.

62. Sugahara T, Korogi Y, Kochi M, et al. Usefulness of diffusion-weighted MRI with echo-planar technique in the evaluation of cellularity in gliomas. J Magn Reson Imaging 1999;9:53–60.

63. Kono K, Inoue Y, Nakayama K, et al. The role of diffusion-weighted imaging in patients with brain tumors. AJNR Am J Neuroradiol 2001;22:1081–8.

64. Chang YW, Yoon HK, Shin HJ, et al. MR imaging of glioblastoma in children: usefulness of diffusion/perfusion-weighted MRI and MR spectroscopy. Pediatr Radiol 2003;33:836–42.

65. Batra A, Tripathi RP. Atypical diffusion-weighted magnetic resonance findings in glioblastoma multiforme. Australas Radiol 2004;48:388–91.

66. Hakyemez B, Erdogan C, Yildirim N, et al. Glioblastoma multiforme with atypical diffusion-weighted MR findings. Br J Radiol 2005;78:989–92.

67. Toh CH, Chen YL, Hsieh TC, et al. Glioblastoma multiforme with diffusion-weighted magnetic resonance imaging characteristics mimicking primary brain lymphoma. Case report. J Neurosurg 2006;105:132–5.

68. Baehring JM, Bi WL, Bannykh S, et al. Diffusion MRI in the early diagnosis of malignant glioma. J Neurooncol 2007;82:221–5.

69. Horger M, Fenchel M, Nägele T, et al. Water diffusivity: comparison of primary CNS lymphoma and astrocytic tumor infiltrating the corpus callosum. AJR Am J Roentgenol 2009;193:1384–7.

70. Cha S, Knopp EA, Johnson G, et al. Intracranial mass lesions: dynamic contrast-enhanced susceptibility-weighted echo-planar perfusion MR imaging. Radiology 2002;223:11–29.

71. Rowland LA, Pedley TA, Merritt HH. Distinguishing of primary cerebral lymphoma from high-grade glioma with perfusion-weighted magnetic resonance imaging. Neurosci Lett 2003;338:119–22.

72. Weber MA, Zoubaa S, Schlieter M, et al. Diagnostic performance of spectroscopic and perfusion MRI for distinction of brain tumors. Neurology 2006;66:1899–906.

73. Patankar TF, Haroon HA, Mills SJ, et al. Is volume transfer coefficient (Ktrans) related to histologic grade in human gliomas? AJNR Am J Neuroradiol 2005;26:2455–65.

74. Cha S, Yang L, Johnson G, et al. Comparison of microvascular permeability measurements, k trans, determined with conventional steady-state T1-weighted and first-pass T2*-weighted MR imaging methods in gliomas and meningiomas. AJNR Am J Neuroradiol 2006;27:409–17.

75. Raz E, Tinelli E, Antonelli M, et al. MRI findings in lymphomatosis cerebri: description of a case and revision of the literature. J Neuroimaging 2011;21(2):e183–6.

76. Mohana-Borges AV, Imbesi SG, Dietrich R, et al. Role of proton magnetic resonance spectroscopy in the diagnosis of gliomatosis cerebri. J Comput Assist Tomogr 2004;28(1):103–5.

77. Sarafi-Lavi E, Bowen BC, Pattany PM, et al. Proton MR spectroscopy of gliomatosis cerebri: case report of elevated myoinositol with normal choline levels. AJNR Am J Neuroradiol 2003;24:946–51.

78. Guzmán-de-Villoria JA, Sánchez-González J, Muñoz L, et al. 1H MR spectroscopy in the assessment of gliomatosis cerebri. AJR Am J Roentgenol 2007;188:710–4.

79. Barkovich A. Posterior fossa tumors. In: Pediatric neuroimaging. 3rd edition. Philadelphia: Lippincott Williams & Wilkins; 2005. p. 446–72.

80. Nagel BJ, Palmer LS, Reddick WE, et al. Abnormal hippocampal development in children with medulloblastoma treated with risk-adapted irradiation. AJNR Am J Neuroradiol 2004;25:1575–82.

81. Khong P, Kwong DL, Chan GC, et al. Diffusion-tensor imaging for the detection and quantification of treatment-induced white matter injury in children with medulloblastoma: a pilot study. AJNR Am J Neuroradiol 2003;24:734–40.

82. Kovantikaya A, Panigrahy A, Krieger MD, et al. Untreated pediatric primitive neuroectodermal tumor in vivo: quantification of taurine with MR spectroscopy. Radiology 2005;236:1020–5.

83. Annette C, Akinwandea D, Paynerb TD, et al. Medulloblastoma mimicking Lhermitte-Duclos disease on MRI and CT. Clin Neurol Neurosurg 2009;111:536–53.

84. Bourgouin PM, Tampieri D, Grahovac SZ, et al. CT and MR imaging findings in adults with cerebellar medulloblastoma: comparison with findings in children. AJR Am J Roentgenol 1992;159:609–12.

85. Koci TM, Chiang F, Mehringer CM, et al. Adult cerebellar medulloblastoma: imaging features with emphasis on MR findings. AJNR Am J Neuroradiol 1993;14:929–39.

86. Meyers SP, Kemp SS, Tarr RW. MR imaging features of medulloblastomas. AJR Am J Roentgenol 1992;158:859–65.

87. Rollins N, Mendelshon D, Mulne A, et al. Recurrent medulloblastoma: frequency of tumor enhancement on Gd-DTPA MR imaging. AJNR Am J Neuroradiol 1990;11:583–7.

88. Zerbini C, Gelber RD, Weinberg D, et al. Prognostic factors in medulloblastoma, including DNA ploidy. J Clin Oncol 1993;11:616–22.

89. Kuhl J. Modern treatment strategies in medulloblastoma. Childs Nerv Syst 1998;14:2–5.

90. Jaremko JL, Jans LB, Coleman LT, et al. Value and limitations of diffusion-weighted imaging in grading and diagnosis of pediatric posterior fossa tumors. AJNR Am J Neuroradiol 2010;31:1613–6.

91. Poussaint TY. Pediatric brain tumors. In: Newton HB, Jolesz FA, editors. Handbook of neuro-oncology neuroimaging. New York: Elsevier; 2008. p. 469–84.

92. Majós C, Alonso J, Aguilera C, et al. Adult primitive neuroectodemal tumor: proton MR spectroscopic findings with possible application for differential diagnosis. Radiology 2002;225:556–66.

93. Schneider JF, Gouny C, Viola A, et al. Multiparametric differentiation of posterior fossa tumors in children using diffusion-weighted imaging and short echo-time ^{1}H-MR spectroscopy. J Magn Reson Imaging 2007;26:1390–8.

94. Panigrahy A, Nelson M, Blúml S. Magnetic resonance spectroscopy in pediatric neuroradiology: clinical and research applications. Pediatr Radiol 2010;40:3–30.

95. Majós C, Aguilera C, Cós M, et al. In vivo proton magnetic resonance spectroscopy of intraventricular tumors of the brain. Eur Radiol 2009;19: 2049–59.

96. Jouanneau E, Tovar RA, Desuzinges C. Very late frontal relapse of medulloblastoma mimicking a meningioma in an adult. Usefulness of ^{1}H magnetic resonance spectroscopy and diffusion-perfusion magnetic resonance imaging for preoperative diagnosis: case report. Neurosurgery 2006;58:E789–90.

97. Harris L, Davies N, MacPherson L, et al. The use of short-echo time ^{1}H MRS for childhood with cerebellar tumors prior to histopathological diagnosis. Pediatr Radiol 2007;37:1101–9.

98. Schneider JF, Viola A, Confort-Gouny S, et al. Infratentorial pediatric brain tumors: the value of new imaging modalities. J Neuroradiol 2007;34:49–58.

99. Yuh EL, Barkovich AJ, Gupta N. Imaging of ependymomas: MRI and CT. Childs Nerv Syst 2009; 25:1203–13.

100. Uematsu Y, Hirano A, Llena JF. Electron microscopic observations of blood vessels in ependymoma. No Shinkei Geka 1988;16:1235–42 [in Japanese].

101. Chen CJ, Tseng YC, Hsu HL, et al. Imaging predictors' intracranial ependymomas. J Comput Assist Tomogr 2004;28:407–13.

102. Quadery FA, Okamoto K. Diffusion-weighted MRI of haemangioblastomas and other cerebellar tumours. Neuroradiology 2003;45(4):212–9.

103. Barboriak DP. Imaging of brain tumors with diffusion-weighted and diffusion tensor MR imaging. Magn Reson Imaging Clin N Am 2003; 11:379–401.

104. Porto L, Kieslich M, Franz K, et al. Spectroscopy of untreated pilocytic astrocytomas: do children and adults share some metabolic features in addition to their morphologic similarities? Childs Nerv Syst 2010;26:801–6.

105. Maia AC Jr, Malheiros SM, Rocha AJ, et al. MR cerebral blood volume maps correlated with vascular endothelial growth factor expression and tumor grade in nonenhancing gliomas. AJNR Am J Neuroradiol 2005;26:777–83.

106. Kitis O, Altay H, Calli C, et al. Minimum apparent diffusion coefficients in the evaluation of brain tumors. Eur J Radiol 2005;55:393–400.

107. Murakami R, Hirai T, Sugahara T, et al. Grading astrocytic tumors by using apparent diffusion coefficient parameters: superiority of a one- versus two-parameter pilot method. Radiology 2009;251: 838–45.

108. Lee EJ, Lee SK, Agid R, et al. Preoperative grading of presumptive low-grade astrocytomas on MR imaging: diagnostic value of minimum apparent diffusion coefficient. AJNR Am J Neuroradiol 2008;29:1872–7.

109. Movsas B, Li BS, Babb JS. Quantifying radiation therapy-induced brain injury with whole-brain proton MR spectroscopy: initial observations. Radiology 2001;221:327–31.

110. Ricci PE, Pitt A, Keller PJ, et al. Effect of voxel position on single-voxel MR spectroscopy findings. AJNR Am J Neuroradiol 2000;21:367–74.

111. Hollingworth W, Medina LS, Lenkinski RE, et al. A systematic literature review of magnetic resonance spectroscopy for the characterization of brain tumors. AJNR Am J Neuroradiol 2006;27: 1404–11.

112. Law M, Yang S, Wang H, et al. Glioma grading: sensitivity, specificity, and predictive values of perfusion MR imaging and proton MR spectroscopic imaging compared with conventional MR imaging. AJNR Am J Neuroradiol 2003;24: 1989–98.

113. Howe FA, Barton SJ, Cudlip SA, et al. Metabolic profiles of human brain tumors using quantitative in vivo ^{1}H magnetic resonance spectroscopy. Magn Reson Med 2003;49:223–32.

114. Preul MC, Leblanc R, Caramanos Z, et al. Magnetic resonance spectroscopy guided brain tumor resection: differentiation between recurrent glioma and radiation change in two diagnostically difficult cases. Can J Neurol Sci 1998;25:13–22.

115. Palasis S. Utility of short TE MR spectroscopy in determination of histology, grade and behavior of pediatric brain tumors. Presented at the 39th Annual Meeting of the American Society of Neuroradiology, Boston, April, 2001.

116. Castillo M, Smith JK, Kwock L. Correlation of myoinositol levels and grading of cerebral astrocytomas. AJNR Am J Neuroradiol 2000;21:1645–9.

117. Rock JP, Hearshen D, Scarpace L, et al. Correlations between magnetic resonance spectroscopy and image-guided histopathology, with special attention to radiation necrosis. Neurosurgery 2002;51:912–9.

118. Covarrubias DJ, Rosen BR, Lev MH. Dynamic magnetic resonance perfusion imaging of brain tumors. Oncologist 2004;9:528–37.

119. Isobe T, Matsumura A, Anno I, et al. Quantification of cerebral metabolites in glioma patients with proton MR spectroscopy using T2 relaxation time correction. Magn Reson Imaging 2002;20: 343–9.

120. Majós C, Aguilera C, Alonso J, et al. Proton MR spectroscopy improves discrimination between tumor and pseudotumoral lesion in solid brain masses. AJNR Am J Neuroradiol 2009;30:544–51.

121. Gupta RK, Cloughesy TF, Sinha U, et al. Relationships between choline magnetic resonance spectroscopy, apparent diffusion coefficient and quantitative histopathology in human glioma. J Neurooncol 2000;50:215–26.

122. Ishimaru H, Morikawa M, Iwanaga S, et al. Differentiation between high-grade glioma and metastatic brain tumor using single-voxel proton MR spectroscopy. Eur Radiol 2001;11:1784–91.

123. Grand S, Passaro C, Ziegler A, et al. Necrotic tumor versus brain abscess: importance of aminoacids detected at ^{1}H MR spectroscopy-initial results. Radiology 1999;213:785–93.

124. Knopp EA, Cha S, Johnson G, et al. Glial neoplasms: dynamic contrast-enhanced T2*-weighted MR imaging. Radiology 1999;211:791–8.

125. Lev MH, Ozsunar Y, Henson JW, et al. Glial tumor grading and outcome prediction using dynamic spin-echo MR susceptibility mapping compared with conventional contrast-enhanced MR: confounding effect of elevated rCBV of oligodendrogliomas. AJNR Am J Neuroradiol 2004;25:214–21.

126. Barajas RF, Chang JS, Sneed PK, et al. Distinguishing recurrent intra-axial metastatic tumor from radiation necrosis following gamma knife radiosurgery using dynamic susceptibility-weighted contrast-enhanced perfusion MR imaging. AJNR Am J Neuroradiol 2009;30:367–72.

127. Bisdas S, Kirkpatrick M, Giglio P, et al. Cerebral blood volume measurements by perfusion-weighted MR imaging in gliomas: ready for prime time in predicting short-term outcome and recurrent disease? AJNR Am J Neuroradiol 2009; 30:681–8.

128. Cha S. Dynamic susceptibility-weighted contrast-enhanced perfusion MR imaging in pediatric patients. Neuroimaging Clin N Am 2006;16(1): 137–47.

129. Sadeghi N, D'Haene N, Decaestecker C, et al. Apparent diffusion coefficient and cerebral blood volume in brain gliomas: relation to tumor cell density and tumor microvessel density based on stereotactic biopsies. AJNR Am J Neuroradiol 2008;29:476–82.

130. Sugahara T, Korogi Y, Kochi M, et al. Perfusion-sensitive MR Imaging of gliomas: comparison between gradient-echo and spin-echo echo-planar imaging techniques. AJNR Am J Neuroradiol 2001; 22:1306–15.

131. Hu LS, Baxter LC, Pinnaduwage DS, et al. Optimized preload leakage-correction methods to improve the diagnostic accuracy of dynamic susceptibility-weighted contrast-enhanced perfusion MR imaging in posttreatment gliomas. AJNR Am J Neuroradiol 2010;31:40–8.

132. Noguchi T, Yoshiura T, Hiwatashi A, et al. Perfusion imaging of brain tumors using arterial spin-labeling: correlation with histopathologic vascular density. AJNR Am J Neuroradiol 2008;29:688–93.

133. Park MJ, Kim HS, Jahng GH, et al. Semiquantitative assessment of intratumoral susceptibility signals using non-contrast-enhanced high-field high-resolution susceptibility-weighted imaging in patients with gliomas: comparison with MR perfusion imaging. AJNR Am J Neuroradiol 2009;30: 1402–8.

134. Parker GJ, Padhani AR. T1-weighted dynamic contrast-enhanced MRI. In: Tofts PS, editor. Quantitative MRI of the brain. Chichester (England): John Wiley & Sons; 2003. p. 341–64.

135. Parker GJ, Tofts PS. Pharmacokinetic analysis of neoplasms using contrast-enhanced dynamic magnetic resonance imaging. Top Magn Reson Imaging 1999;10:130–42.

136. Paldino MJ. Fundamentals of quantitative dynamic contrast-enhanced MR imaging. Magn Reson Imaging Clin N Am 2009;17:277–89.

137. O'Connor JP, Jackson A, Asselin MC, et al. Quantitative imaging biomarkers in the clinical development of targeted therapeutics: current and future perspectives. Lancet Oncol 2008;9:766–76.

138. O'Connor JP, Jackson A, Parker GJ, et al. DCE-MRI biomarkers in the clinical evaluation of antiangiogenic and vascular disrupting agents. Br J Cancer 2007;96:189–95.

139. Provenzale JM, York G, Moya MG, et al. Correlation of relative permeability and relative cerebral blood volume in high-grade cerebral neoplasms. AJR Am J Roentgenol 2006;187:1036–42.

140. Law M, Yang S, Babb JS, et al. Comparison of cerebral blood volume and vascular permeability from dynamic susceptibility contrast-enhanced perfusion MR imaging with glioma grade. AJNR Am J Neuroradiol 2004;25:746–55.

141. Narang J, Jain R, Arbab AS, et al. Differentiating treatment-induced necrosis from recurrent/progressive brain tumor using nonmodel-based semiquantitative indices derived from dynamic contrast-enhanced T1-weighted MR perfusion. Neuro Oncol 2011;13(9):1037–46.

142. Thompson G, Mills SJ, Stivaros SM, et al. Imaging of brain tumors: perfusion/permeability. Neuroimaging Clin N Am 2010;20:337–53.

143. Lacerda S, Law M. Magnetic resonance perfusion and permeability imaging in brain tumors. Neuroimaging Clin N Am 2009;19:527–57.

144. Zhang N, Zhang L, Qiu B, et al. Correlation of volume transfer coefficient K(trans) with histopathologic grades of gliomas. J Magn Reson Imaging 2012;36(2):355–63. http://dx.doi.org/10.1002/jmri.23675.

145. Nguyen TB, Cron GO, Mercier JF, et al. Diagnostic accuracy of dynamic contrast-enhanced MR imaging using a phase-derived vascular input function in the preoperative grading of gliomas. AJNR Am J Neuroradiol 2012;33(8):1539–45.

146. Foottit C, Cron GO, Hogan MJ, et al. Determination of the venous output function from MR signal phase: feasibility for quantitative DCE-MRI in human brain. Magn Reson Med 2010;63:772–82.

147. Cron GO, Foottit C, Yankeelov TE, et al. Arterial input functions determined from MR signal magnitude and phase for quantitative dynamic contrast-enhanced MRI in the human pelvis. Magn Reson Med 2011;66:498–504.

148. Donahue KM, Weissokoff RM, Burstein D, et al. Water diffusion and exchange as they influence contrast enhancement. J Magn Reson Imaging 1997;7:102–10.

149. Majós C, Bruna J, Julià-Sapé M, et al. Proton MR spectroscopy provides relevant prognostic information in high-grade astrocytomas. AJNR Am J Neuroradiol 2011;32:74–80.

150. Higano S, Yun X, Kumabe T, et al. Malignant astrocytic tumors: clinical importance of apparent diffusion coefficient in prediction of grade and prognosis. Radiology 2006;241:839–46.

151. Murakami R, Sugahara T, Nakamura H, et al. Malignant supratentorial astrocytoma treated with postoperative radiation therapy: prognostic value of pretreatment quantitative diffusion-weighted MR imaging. Radiology 2007;243:493–9.

152. Oh J, Henry RG, Pirzkall A, et al. Survival analysis in patients with glioblastoma multiforme: predictive value of choline-to-N-acetylaspartate index, apparent diffusion coefficient, and relative cerebral blood volume. J Magn Reson Imaging 2004;19:546–54.

153. Kuztnesov YE, Caramanos MA, Antel SB, et al. Proton magnetic resonance spectroscopic imaging can predict length of survival in patients with supra-tentorial gliomas. Neurosurgery 2003;53:565–76.

154. Li X, Jin H, Lu Y, et al. Identification of MRI and ^{1}H MRSI parameters that may predict survival for patients with malignant gliomas. NMR Biomed 2004;17:10–20.

155. Tzika AA, Astrakas LG, Zarifi MK, et al. Spectroscopic and perfusion magnetic resonance imaging predictors of progression in pediatric brain tumors. Cancer 2004;100:1246–56.

156. Law M, Oh S, Babb JS, et al. Low-grade gliomas: dynamic susceptibility-weighted contrast-enhanced perfusion MR imaging—prediction of patient clinical response. Radiology 2006;238:658–71.

157. Mills SJ, Patankar TA, Haroon HA, et al. Do cerebral blood volume and contrast transfer coefficient predict prognosis in human glioma? AJNR Am J Neuroradiol 2006;27:853–8.

158. Law M, Young RJ, Babb JS, et al. Gliomas: predicting time to progression or survival with cerebral blood volume measurements at dynamic susceptibility-weighted contrast-enhanced perfusion MR imaging. Radiology 2008;247:490–8.

159. Hirai T, Murakami R, Nakamura H, et al. Prognostic value of perfusion MR imaging of high-grade astrocytomas: long-term follow-up study. AJNR Am J Neuroradiol 2008;29:1505–10.

160. Tedeschi G, Lundbom N, Ramon R, et al. Increased choline signal coinciding with malignant degeneration of cerebral gliomas: a serial proton magnetic resonance spectroscopy imaging study. J Neurosurg 1997;87:516–24.

161. Danchaivijitr N, Waldman AD, Tozer DJ, et al. Low-grade gliomas: do changes in RCBV measurements at longitudinal perfusion-weighted MR imaging predict malignant transformation? Radiology 2008;247:170–8.

162. Jackson RJ, Fuller GN, Abi-Said D, et al. Limitations of stereotactic biopsy in the initial management of gliomas. Neuro Oncol 2001;3:193–200.

163. Gilles FH, Brown WD, Leviton A, et al. Limitations of the world health organization classification of childhood supratentorial astrocytic tumors: children brain tumor consortium. Cancer 2000;88:1477–83.

164. Earnest FT 4th, Kelly PJ, Scheithauer BW, et al. Cerebral astrocytomas: histopathologic correlation of MR and CT contrast enhancement with stereotactic biopsy. Radiology 1988;166:823–7.

165. Lev MH, Rosen BR. Clinical applications of intracranial perfusion MR imaging. Neuroimaging Clin N Am 1999;9:309–31.

166. Martin AJ, Liu H, Hall WA, et al. Preliminary assessment of turbo spectroscopic imaging for targeting in brain biopsy. AJNR Am J Neuroradiol 2001;22: 959–68.

167. Dowling C, Bollen AW, Noworolski SM, et al. Preoperative proton MR spectroscopic imaging of brain tumors: correlation with histopathologic analysis of resection specimens. AJNR Am J Neuroradiol 2001;22:604–12.

168. Hall WA, Martin A, Liu H, et al. Improving diagnostic yield in brain biopsy: coupling spectroscopic targeting with real-time needle placement. J Magn Reson Imaging 2001;13:12–5.

169. Hall WA, Galicich W, Bergman T, et al. 3-Tesla intraoperative MR imaging for neurosurgery. J Neurooncol 2006;77:297–303.

170. Hermann EJ, Hattingen E, Krauss JK, et al. Stereotactic biopsy in gliomas guided by 3-Tesla ^{1}H chemical-shift imaging of choline. Stereotact Funct Neurosurg 2008;86:300–7.

171. Moritani T, Ekholm S, Westesson PL. Diffusion-weighted MR imaging of the brain. Springer; 2005.

172. Sagar P, Grant E. Diffusion-weighted MR imaging: pediatric clinical applications. Neuroimaging Clin N Am 2006;16(1):45–74.

173. Eis M, Els T, Hoehn-Berlage M, et al. Quantitative diffusion MR imaging of cerebral tumor and edema. Acta Neurochir Suppl (Wien) 1994;60: 344–6.

174. Xu M, See SJ, Wh Ng, et al. Comparison of magnetic resonance spectroscopy and perfusion-weighted imaging in presurgical grading of oligodendroglial tumors. Neurosurgery 2005;56:919–26.

175. Pirzkall A, McKnight TR, Graves EE, et al. MR-spectroscopy guided target delineation for high-grade gliomas. Int J Radiat Oncol Biol Phys 2001; 50:915–28.

176. Ganslandt O, Stadlbauer A, Fahlbusch R, et al. Proton magnetic resonance spectroscopic imaging integrated into image-guided surgery: correlation to standard magnetic resonance imaging and tumor cell density. Neurosurgery 2005;56:291–8.

177. McKnight TR, Von Dem Bussche MH, Vigneron DB, et al. Histopathological validation of a three-dimensional magnetic resonance spectroscopy index as a predictor of tumor presence. J Neurosurg 2002;97:794–802.

178. Provenzale JM, Schmainda K. Perfusion imaging for brain tumor characterization and assessment of treatment response. In: Newton HB, Jolesz FA, editors. Handbook of neuro-oncology neuroimaging. New York: Elsevier; 2008. p. 264–77.

179. Yang I, Aghi MK. New advances that enable identification of glioblastoma recurrence. Nat Rev Clin Oncol 2009;6:648–57.

180. Rabinov JD, Lee PL, Barker FG, et al. In vivo 3-T MR spectroscopy in the distinction of recurrent glioma versus radiation effects: initial experience. Radiology 2002;225:871–9.

181. Smith EA, Carlos RC, Junck LR, et al. Developing a clinical decision model: MR spectroscopy to differentiate between recurrent tumor and radiation change in Patients with new contrast-enhancing lesions. AJR Am J Roentgenol 2009;192:W45–52.

182. Weybright P, Sundgren PC, Maly P, et al. Differentiation between brain tumor recurrence and radiation injury using MR spectroscopy. AJR Am J Roentgenol 2005;185:1471–6.

183. Zeng QS, Li CF, Liu H, et al. Distinction between recurrent glioma and radiation injury using magnetic resonance spectroscopy in combination with diffusion-weighted imaging. Int J Radiat Oncol Biol Phys 2007;68:151.

184. Macdonald DR, Cascino T, Schold SJ, et al. Response criteria for phase II studies of supratentorial malignant glioma. J Clin Oncol 1990;8:1277–80.

185. Henegar MM, Moran CJ, Silbergeld DL. Early postoperative magnetic resonance imaging following nonneoplastic cortical resection. J Neurosurg 1996;84(2):174–9.

186. Kumar AJ, Leeds NE, Fuller GN, et al. Malignant gliomas: MR imaging spectrum of radiation therapy- and chemotherapy-induced necrosis of the brain after treatment. Radiology 2000;217: 377–84.

187. Ulmer S, Braga TA, Baker FG 2nd, et al. Clinical and radiographic features of peritumoral infarction following resection of glioblastoma. Neurology 2006;67:1668–70.

188. Finn MA, Blumenthal DT, Salzman KL, et al. Transient postictal MRI changes in patients with brain tumors may mimic disease progression. Surg Neurol 2007;67:246–50.

189. Hattingen E, Raab P, Franz K, et al. Prognostic value of choline and creatine in WHO grade II gliomas. Neuroradiology 2008;50:759–67.

190. Weber MA, Giesel FL, Stieltjes B. MRI for identification of progression in brain tumors: from morphology to function. Expert Rev Neurother 2008;8:1507–25.

191. Clarke JL, Chang S. Pseudoprogression and pseudoresponse: challenges in brain tumor imaging. Curr Neurol Neurosci Rep 2009;9:241–6.

192. Brandes AA, Franceschi E, Tosoni A, et al. MGMT promoter methylation status can predict the incidence and outcome of pseudoprogression after concomitant radiochemotherapy in newly diagnosed glioblastoma patients. J Clin Oncol 2008; 26:2192–7.

193. Mangla R, Singh G, Ziegelitz D, et al. Changes in relative cerebral blood volume 1 month after radiation-temozolomide therapy can help predict overall survival in patients with glioblastoma. Radiology 2010;256:575–84.

194. Tsien C, Galbán CJ, Chenevert TL, et al. Parametric response map as an imaging biomarker to distinguish progression from pseudoprogression in high-grade glioma. J Clin Oncol 2010;28:2293–9.

195. Hu LS, Eschbacher JM, Heiserman JE, et al. Reevaluating the imaging definition of tumor progression: perfusion MRI quantifies recurrent glioblastoma tumor fraction, pseudoprogression, and radiation necrosis to predict survival. Neuro Oncol 2012;14(7):919–30.

196. Hygino da Cruz LC Jr, Rodriguez I, Domingues RC, et al. Pseudoprogression and pseudoresponse: imaging challenges in the assessment of posttreatment glioma. AJNR Am J Neuroradiol 2011;32: 1978–85.

197. Wen PY, Macdonald DR, Reardon DA, et al. Updated response assessment criteria for high-grade gliomas: response assessment in neuro-oncology working group. J Clin Oncol 2010;28:1963–72.

198. Pope WB, Hessel C. Response assessment in neuro-oncology criteria: implementation challenges in multicenter neuro-oncology trials. AJNR Am J Neuroradiol 2011;32:794–7.

199. Mardor Y, Pfeffer R, Spiegelmann R, et al. Early detection of response to radiation therapy in patients with brain malignancies using conventional and high b-value diffusion-weighted magnetic resonance imaging. J Clin Oncol 2003;21:1094–100.

200. Galbán S, Brisset JC, Rehemtulla A, et al. Diffusion-weighted MRI for assessment of early cancer treatment response. Curr Pharm Biotechnol 2010;11(6): 701–8.

201. Pope WB, Kim HJ, Huo J, et al. Recurrent glioblastoma multiforme: ADC histogram analysis predicts response to bevacizumab treatment. Radiology 2009;252:182–9.

202. Al Sayyari A, Buckley R, McHenery C, et al. Distinguishing recurrent primary brain tumor from radiation injury: a preliminary study using a susceptibility-weighted MR imaging-guided apparent diffusion coefficient analysis strategy. AJNR Am J Neuroradiol 2010;31:1049–54.

203. Henson JW, Ulmer S, Harris GJ. Brain tumor imaging in clinical trials. AJNR Am J Neuroradiol 2008;29:419–24.

204. Matsusue E, Fink JR, Rockhill JK, et al. Distinction between glioma progression and post-radiation change by combined physiologic MR imaging. Neuroradiology 2010;52(4):297–306.

205. Jain RK. Normalization of tumor vasculature: an emerging concept in antiangiogenic therapy. Science 2005;307:58–62.

206. Winkler F, Kozin SV, Tong RT, et al. Kinetics of vascular normalization by VEGFR2 blockade governs brain tumor response to radiation: role of oxygenation, angiopoietin-1, and matrix metalloproteinases. Cancer Cell 2004;6:553–63.

207. Batchelor TT, Sorensen AG, di Tomaso E, et al. AZD2171, a pan-VEGF receptor tyrosine kinase inhibitor, normalizes tumor vasculature and alleviates edema in glioblastoma patients. Cancer Cell 2007;11:83–95.

208. Pope WB, Lai A, Nghiemphu P, et al. MRI in patients with high-grade gliomas treated with bevacizumab and chemotherapy. Neurology 2006;66: 1258–60.

209. Jain RK, Duda DG, Willett CG, et al. Biomarkers of response and resistance to antiangiogenic therapy. Nat Rev Clin Oncol 2009;6:327–38.

210. Norden AD, Young GS, Setayesh K, et al. Bevacizumab for recurrent malignant gliomas: efficacy, toxicity, and patterns of recurrence. Neurology 2008;70:779–87.

211. Gerstner ER, Chen PJ, Wen PY, et al. Infiltrative patterns of glioblastoma spread detected via diffusion MRI after treatment with cediranib. Neuro Oncol 2010;12:466–72.

212. Maier R, Eiter H, Burger R. Bevacizumab in recurrence or progress of high-grade gliomas. Lancet Neurol 2009;7:1152–60.

213. Quinn JA, Jiang SX, Reardon DA, et al. Phase II trial of temozolamide (TMZ) plus irinotecan (CPT-11) in adults with newly diagnosed glioblastoma multiforme before radiotherapy. J Neurooncol 2009; 95(3):393–400.

214. Gerstner ER, Frosch MP, Batchelor TT. Diffusion magnetic resonance imaging detects pathologically confirmed, nonenhancing tumor progression in a patient with recurrent glioblastoma receiving bevacizumab. J Clin Oncol 2010;28:e91–3.

215. Sundgren PC. MR spectroscopy in radiation injury. AJNR Am J Neuroradiol 2009;30:1469–76.

216. Mong S, Ellingson BM, Nghiemphu PL, et al. Persistent diffusion-restricted lesions in bevacizumab-treated malignant gliomas are associated with improved survival compared with matched controls. AJNR Am J Neuroradiol 2012; 33:1763–70.

217. Brandsma D, van de Bent MJ. Pseudoprogression and pseudoresponse in the treatment of gliomas. Curr Opin Neurol 2009;22:633–8.

218. Lichy MP, Plathow C, Schulz-Ertner D, et al. Follow-up gliomas after radiotherapy: 1H MR spectroscopic imaging for increasing diagnostic accuracy. Neuroradiology 2005;47:826–34.

219. Wald LL, Nelson SJ, Day MR, et al. Serial proton magnetic resonance spectroscopy imaging of glioblastoma multiforme after brachytherapy. J Neurosurg 1997;87:525–34.

220. Chernov MF, Hayashi M, Izawa M, et al. Multivoxel proton MRS for differentiation of radiation-induced necrosis and tumor recurrence after gamma knife radiosurgery for brain metastases. Brain Tumor Pathol 2006;23:19–27.

221. Law M. MR spectroscopy of brain tumors. Top Magn Reson Imaging 2004;15:291–313.

222. Li X, Vigneron DB, Cha S, et al. Relationship of MR-derived lactate, mobile lipids, and relative blood volume for gliomas in vivo. AJNR Am J Neuroradiol 2005;26:760–9.

223. Elias AE, Carlos RC, Smith EA, et al. MR spectroscopy using normalized and non-normalized metabolite ratios for differentiating recurrent brain tumor from radiation injury. Acad Radiol 2011;18:1101–8.

224. Hourani R, Brant LS, Rizk T, et al. Can proton MR spectroscopic and perfusion imaging differentiate between neoplastic and non neoplastic brain lesions in adults? AJNR Am J Neuroradiol 2008;29:366–72.

225. Taylor JS, Langston JW, Reddick WE, et al. Clinical value of proton magnetic resonance spectroscopy for differentiating recurrent or residual brain tumor from delayed cerebral necrosis. Int J Radiat Oncol Biol Phys 1996;36:1251–61.

226. Graves EE, Nelson SJ, Vigneron DB, et al. Serial proton MR spectroscopic imaging of recurrent malignant gliomas after gamma knife radiosurgery. AJNR Am J Neuroradiol 2001;22:613–24.

227. Barajas RF, Chang JS, Segal MR, et al. Differentiation of recurrent glioblastoma from radiation necrosis after external beam radiation therapy with dynamic susceptibility-weighted contrast-enhanced perfusion MR imaging. Radiology 2009;253:486–96.

228. Hu LS, Baxter LC, Smith KA, et al. Relative cerebral blood volume values to differentiate high-grade glioma recurrence from posttreatment radiation effect: direct correlation between image-guided tissue histopathology and localized dynamic susceptibility-weighted contrast-enhanced perfusion MR imaging measurements. AJNR Am J Neuroradiol 2009;30:552–8.

229. Hopewell JW, Calvo W, Jaenke R, et al. Microvasculature and radiation damage. Recent Results Cancer Res 1993;130:1–16.

230. Oh BC, Pagnini PG, Wang MY, et al. Stereotactic radiosurgery: adjacent tissue injury and response after high-dose single fraction radiation: part I—histology, imaging, and molecular events. Neurosurgery 2007;60:31–44.

231. Hazle JD, Jackson EF, Schomer DF, et al. Dynamic imaging of intracranial lesions using fast spin-echo imaging: differentiation of brain tumors and treatment effects. J Magn Reson Imaging 1997;7(6):1084–93.

232. Bisdas SS, Naegele TT, Ritz RR, et al. Distinguishing recurrent high-grade gliomas from radiation injury. Acad Radiol 2011;18:575–83.

233. Fatterpekar GM, Galheigo D, Narayana A, et al. Treatment-related change versus tumor recurrence in high-grade gliomas: a diagnostic conundrum—use of dynamic susceptibility contrast-enhanced (DSC) perfusion MRI. AJR Am J Roentgenol 2012;198(1):19–26.

234. Pal D, Bhattacharyya A, Husain M, et al. In vivo proton MR spectroscopy evaluation of pyogenic brain abscesses: a report of 194 cases. AJNR Am J Neuroradiol 2010;31:360–6.

235. Lai PH, Ho JT, Chen WL, et al. Brain abscess and necrotic brain tumor: discrimination with proton MR spectroscopy and diffusion-weighted imaging. AJNR Am J Neuroradiol 2002;23(8):1369–77.

236. Cohen B, Valles FE, Rubenstein JL, et al. Differentiating tumefactive demyelinating lesions and primary CNS lymphoma using quantitative apparent diffusion coefficient analysis. Presented at the ASNR 2011. Seattle.ePoster 058.

237. Rand SD, Prost R, Haughton V, et al. Accuracy of single-voxel proton MR spectroscopy in distinguishing neoplastic from non neoplastic brain lesions. AJNR Am J Neuroradiol 1997;18:1695–704.

238. Saindane AM, Cha S, Law M, et al. Proton MR spectroscopy of tumefactive demyelinating lesions. AJNR Am J Neuroradiol 2002;23:1378–86.

239. De Stefano N, Caramanos Z, Preul MC, et al. In vivo differentiation of astrocytic brain tumors and isolated demyelinating lesions of the type seen in multiple sclerosis using ^1H magnetic resonance spectroscopic imaging. Ann Neurol 1998;44:273–8.

240. Cianfoni A, Niku S, Imbesi SG, et al. Metabolite findings in tumefactive demyelinating lesions utilizing short echo time proton magnetic resonance spectroscopy. AJNR Am J Neuroradiol 2007;28:272–7.

241. Srinivasan R, Sailasuta N, Hurd R, et al. Evidence of elevated glutamate in multiple sclerosis using magnetic resonance spectroscopy at 3 T. Brain 2005;128:1016–25.

242. Bitsch A, Bruhn H, Vougioukas V, et al. Inflammatory CNS demyelination: histopathologic correlation with in vivo quantitative proton MR spectroscopy. AJNR Am J Neuroradiol 1999;20:1619–27.

Posttreatment Evaluation of Central Nervous System Gliomas

Mark S. Shiroishi, MD*, Michael T. Booker, BS,
Manyoo Agarwal, MD, Nidhi Jain, MD, Ilana Naghi, MD,
Alexander Lerner, MD, Meng Law, MD

KEYWORDS

- Glioma • Glioblastoma • MacDonald criteria • Response assessment • Radiation necrosis
- Pseudoresponse • MR imaging • Imaging biomarkers

KEY POINTS

- Use of the MacDonald criteria has been the most widely used method to assess therapeutic response in high-grade gliomas and involves examining changes in contrast-enhancing area, typically on conventional contrast-enhanced magnetic resonance (MR) imaging.
- Several limitations of the MacDonald criteria have been identified since their introduction in 1990. The most critical limitation rests on its reliance on contrast enhancement as a criterion of therapeutic response. Although contrast enhancement is a sensitive marker of blood-brain barrier disruption, it is not a specific finding of active tumor, and can be the result of many other processes including treatment-related effect, ischemia, seizure, inflammation, and postoperative changes.
- With the recent recognition of the entities of pseudoprogression and pseudoresponse associated with chemoradiation with temozolomide and antiangiogenic agents, respectively, the neuro-oncology community has been forced to reevaluate traditional imaging criteria of treatment response.
- The latest Response Assessment in Neuro-Oncology Working Group recommendations to address limitations in the MacDonald criteria are reviewed. In addition, the most recent advances in quantitative biomarker development using advanced imaging modalities are highlighted. However, until these techniques are thoroughly validated, conventional contrast-enhanced MR imaging follow-up should remain the standard of care.

INTRODUCTION

Gliomas represent the most common adult primary brain malignancy with an annual incidence of about 4 to 5 per 100,000.[1] The prognosis for glioblastoma in particular remains dismal. Postoperative radiation therapy has been an integral part of the treatment of high-grade gliomas (HGGs) since the 1970s.[2] Over the next 2 decades, innovations in computed tomography (CT) and magnetic resonance (MR) imaging improved both brain tumor characterization and radiotherapy techniques.[3] However, further attempts using

Funding Sources: None.
Conflicts of Interest: Bayer Healthcare, consultant (M.S.S.). None (M.T.B., M.A., N.J., I.N., A.L.). Toshiba America Medical Systems, Speaker Bureau; Bayer Healthcare, research grant; Bracco Diagnostics, honorarium; iCADInc, honorarium; Prism Clinical Imaging, stock options; Fuji Inc, honorarium (M.L.).
Division of Neuroradiology, Department of Radiology, Keck School of Medicine, University of Southern California, Los Angeles, CA 90033, USA
* Corresponding author. Department of Radiology, Keck School of Medicine, University of Southern California, 1520 San Pablo Street, Lower Level Imaging, L1600, Los Angeles, CA 90033.
E-mail address: mark.shiroishi@med.usc.edu

Magn Reson Imaging Clin N Am 21 (2013) 241–268
http://dx.doi.org/10.1016/j.mric.2013.02.004
1064-9689/13/$ – see front matter © 2013 Elsevier Inc. All rights reserved.

alternative methods of radiotherapy failed to improve outcomes.[4] In 2005, Stupp and colleagues[5] showed improved survival with the addition of concurrent and adjuvant temozolomide (TMZ) to radiotherapy and this regimen, combined with maximal surgical resection, has since become the current standard of care for newly diagnosed glioblastoma. In 2009, the antiangiogenic agent bevacizumab received US Food and Drug Administration approval for the treatment of recurrent/progressive glioblastoma. Therapeutic assessment of high-grade gliomas (HGGs) relies on patient survival or, in cases of recurrent tumor, often the radiographic response rate or progression-free survival (PFS).[6,7] The adoption of chemoradiation with TMZ and antiangiogenic agents into the therapeutic armamentarium has resulted in a reevaluation of conventional contrast-enhanced MR imaging and response criteria.

The most widely used method to assess therapeutic response in HGGs has been to examine changes in contrast-enhancing area, typically on conventional contrast-enhanced MR imaging.[8] Progression on imaging is defined as either a 25% increase in the size of enhancement or new foci of enhancement (Table 1).[8] In addition, corticosteroids and neurologic status are also taken into consideration. Taken together, this schema is known as the MacDonald criteria.

When proposed in 1990, these criteria represented a shift from a subjective evaluation of clinical and radiologic data toward a more objective, image-based methodology.[9]

LIMITATIONS OF THE MACDONALD CRITERIA

Since their introduction, several limitations of the MacDonald criteria have been identified.[10,11] These limitations include interobserver variability, failure to measure nonenhancing portions of tumor (particularly significant for evaluation of low-grade gliomas [LGGs]), difficulty in measuring tumors with irregular shapes, lack of guidance in the evaluation of multifocal tumors, assessment of progression after gross total resection of all enhancing tumor, and difficulties with measuring enhancing lesions in the walls of cysts/surgical cavities because the cysts/cavities may be incorporated into the tumor size measurement.

The most critical limitation rests on the MacDonald criteria's reliance on contrast enhancement as a criterion of therapeutic response. Although contrast enhancement is a sensitive marker of blood-brain barrier (BBB) disruption, it is not a specific finding of active tumor, and can be the result of many other processes including treatment-related effect, ischemia, seizure, inflammation, and postoperative changes.[12–16] In

Table 1
MacDonald criteria

Response	Criteria
Complete response	All of the following are required: Complete disappearance of all enhancing measurable and nonmeasurable disease that is sustained for a minimum of 4 wk No new lesions No use of corticosteroids Stable or improved clinically
Partial response	All of the following are required: ≥50% decrease compared with baseline in the sum of products of perpendicular diameters of all measurable enhancing lesions sustained for a minimum of 4 wk No new lesion Stable or reduced corticosteroid dose Stable or improved clinically
Stable disease	All of the following are required: Does not qualify for complete response, partial response, or progression Stable clinically
Progression	Any of the following: ≥25% increase in sum of the products of perpendicular diameters of enhancing lesions Any new lesion Clinical deterioration

Adapted from Macdonald DR, et al. Response criteria for phase II studies of supratentorial malignant glioma. J Clin Oncol 1990;8(7):1277–80.

addition, corticosteroid dosage can complicate assessment in that this can physiologically decrease the amount of contrast enhancement.[17,18] In particular, the recent recognition of the entities of pseudoprogression (PsP) and pseudoresponse (PsR) associated with chemoradiation with temozolomide and antiangiogenic agents, respectively, has emphasized the need to reevaluate traditional imaging criteria of treatment response.

THERAPEUTIC EVALUATION AFTER CHEMORADIATION WITH TMZ IN HGG-RADIATION NECROSIS AND PSP

Radiation necrosis (RN), and the recently recognized PsP, are forms of treatment-related enhancement mimicking tumor progression that can occur following chemoradiation with TMZ. They pose significant problems for treating physicians because they are essentially indistinguishable from tumor progression using conventional MR imaging methods (Fig. 1).[12,16,19,20] Further complicating matters is the possibility to have both coexisting tumor and therapy-induced necrosis in the same enhancing lesion.[21]

RN

Radiation-induced injury represents not a single instantaneous event but a dynamic, complex process that develops over time, with a significant amount of tissue damage occurring hours to days after the initial injury.[22] These processes can include vascular injury with vasogenic edema, glial and white matter damage, effects on the fibrinolytic enzyme system, and immune mechanisms.[12] Radiation effects are usually divided into acute, subacute, and late effects. Vasodilatation, damage

to the BBB, and edema are thought to underlie both acute and subacute types of radiation injury.[23]

Late radiation effects include RN as well as other processes such as leukoencephalopathy, vascular lesions such as moyamoya syndrome and lacunar infarcts, parenchymal calcifications, and enhancing white matter lesions.[24] RN typically occurs months to years following therapy and may be progressive and irreversible.[12,25–27] The incidence of RN is unclear, but may be as high as 24%.[28] Both the volume of brain irradiated as well as the radiation dose delivered are important factors, particularly when doses are higher than 65 Gy in fractions of 1.8 to 2.0 Gy.[24] In RN, blood vessels show fibrinoid necrosis with surrounding perivascular parenchymal coagulative necrosis.[12,25,26] Endothelial injury from radiation results in fibrinoid necrosis of small vessels, endothelial thickening, hyalinization, and vascular thrombosis. In contrast, recurrent tumor shows vascular proliferation and angiogenesis without vascular luminal obliteration.[21] Patterns described as "soap bubble" or "Swiss cheese" have been described on conventional contrast-enhanced MR imaging in RN; however, these appearances cannot reliably differentiate between tumor recurrence and RN.[12,29,30] Advanced MR imaging techniques (discussed later) have been examined to better characterize RN. However, no technique is widely accepted and this remains an active area of research.

The treatment of RN ranges from observation to medical and surgical therapy. Medical treatment incorporates corticosteroids because of their ability to counteract BBB disruption from radiation-induced vascular endothelial injury.[29] Because there seems to be increased vascular endothelial growth factor (VEGF) and microvascular permeability in RN, there is some evidence

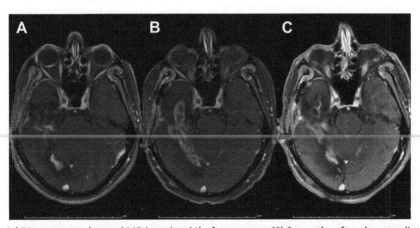

Fig. 1. PsP. Axial T1 contrast-enhanced MR imaging (A) after surgery, (B) 2 months after chemoradiation showing increased enhancement in the right temporo-occipital region, and (C) a significant decrease in enhancement is seen 2 months later without a change in therapy.

to suggest that RN may be responsive to bevacizumab treatment. Hyperbaric oxygen treatment has also been explored as a treatment option because it may stimulate angiogenesis and restore the vascular supply injured by radiation.[29] Medically intractable cases may require surgical resection if the lesion is surgically accessible and will not result in significantly increased morbidity.

PsP

While PsP may occur following radiotherapy alone, there has been a greater focus on PsP since the recent adoption of chemoradiation with TMZ as the standard of care for glioblastoma.[9] Although PsP currently lacks a strict definition, in general it refers to an increase in contrast enhancement within the first 3 to 6 months after chemoradiation that is the result of treatment-induced changes rather than true early progression (TEP).[19,27] The time period of its occurrence is earlier than after radiotherapy alone and, as such, it may represent a mild, self-limiting variant of RN.[19] However, there is evidence to suggest that PsP and RN are distinct entities with PsP representing a combination of treatment effect on residual tumor cells and disruption of the BBB, whereas RN represents radiation damage to the peritumoral white matter.[29] As such, some have argued that the term PsP should replace the outdated term early radionecrosis.[31,32]

Without a change in therapy, PsP may improve or disappear, although in some cases it may remain persistent. Although most patients with PsP are asymptomatic, as many as one-third may need surgery, increased steroids, or possibly antiangiogenic therapy because of symptoms from mass effect.[33]

PsP seems to be a common occurrence, with incidence estimates of approximately 20% to 30% and seems to be more frequent in patients with a methylated O^6-methylguanine–DNA methyltransferase (MGMT) promoter.[11,19,34] More recent analyses seem to support this incidence estimate.[35,36] However, because of varying definitions, uncertainties in image interpretation, as well as variations in the quality and design of studies, the true incidence of PsP is still not clear.[32,37] Clarke and Chang[27] estimate that about half of all patients with glioblastoma develop worrisome contrast-enhancing lesions on follow-up MR imaging after chemoradiation and that many are the result of PsP rather than TEP. In 2011, a retrospective study of the first postradiotherapy scans in 321 patients with glioblastoma treated with chemoradiation with TMZ was reported from a major brain tumor referral center.[20] The investigators reported that

this was, to date, the largest cohort of patients examined to determine whether conventional MR imaging could distinguish PsP from TEP. Suspicious new or enlarging enhancing lesions were found in 93 patients. Of these, 30 patients (32.3%) were determined to have PsP (confirmed pathologically in 6 cases). This incidence is consistent with several prior reports.[24,38–40] Eleven conventional MR imaging signs were evaluated and only subependymal enhancement could predict TEP with 38.1% sensitivity, 93.3% specificity, and 41.8% negative predictive value. The remaining 10 signs were not predictive and there was not a sign with a sufficiently high negative predictive value for PsP. As such, the investigators concluded that conventional MR imaging signs have limited usefulness to diagnose PsP and that an alternative imaging biomarker is needed.

PsP and MGMT promoter methylation status

The MGMT enzyme is a DNA repair protein that provides resistance to the alkylating drug TMZ by removing alkyl groups (such as those placed by chemotherapeutic alkylating agents) from the O^6 position of guanine.[41] Epigenetic silencing of the MGMT gene by promoter methylation causes a loss of its expression, thus inhibiting the DNA repair mechanism and resulting in chemotherapy-induced cytotoxicity and apoptosis.[41–43] The status of the MGMT promoter represents a potentially useful marker to complement imaging because PsP is more frequently seen in cases with a methylated promoter than in those with an unmethylated promoter.[34] Numerous studies have also shown that methylated MGMT promoter status is associated with improved survival with TMZ treatment.[24,34,41,44]

Clinical implications of PsP

The inability of conventional MR imaging methods to differentiate PsP from TEP limits the validity of PFS as a primary end point (unless pathologic confirmation of TEP is made) and confounds the design of salvage clinical trials.[9,11,27] If a patient does not respond to initial therapy with TMZ then treatment should be changed quickly, often into a clinical trial. However, if a patient has developed PsP, then altering management prematurely terminates an effective therapy, and, because PsP tends to improve on its own, can result in a falsely high response rate and PFS as well as lending a false attribution of efficacy to the new agent.

ANTIANGIOGENIC THERAPY AND PSR

Cancers grow beyond their initial local blood supply by developing deregulated angiogenesis, which allows tumors to acquire an abnormal vasculature composed of dilated, tortuous, and hyperpermeable vessels.[45] This results in irregular, inefficient perfusion of tumors, and ultimately hypoxia and necrosis.[46] At first, the mechanism of antiangiogenic agents against tumors was thought to be via reduction or elimination of tumor vasculature, effectively starving the tumor.[45,47–49] However, clinical studies have shown an absence of a clear dose-response relationship as well as a lack of benefit without concomitant cytotoxic therapy. In addition, the resulting hypoxia caused by elimination of blood vessels should result in decreased effectiveness of chemotherapy. However, this has also not been seen in clinical studies.[45,47] As a result, an alternative mechanism termed vascular normalization has been proposed. In vascular normalization, antiangiogenic agents cause a decrease in vessel diameter and permeability as well as thinning of the abnormally thick basement membrane.[50,51]

Treatment with antiangiogenic agents directed against VEGF, such as bevacizumab, can cause a rapid decrease in enhancement caused, at least in part, by a decrease in microvascular permeability secondary to vascular normalization, rather than a true antitumoral effect.[52] This process has become known as PsR.[19] A decrease in contrast enhancement has been documented as early as 24 hours following a single dose of the pan-VEGF tyrosine kinase inhibitor cediranib, and discontinuing the drug leads to a rapid reversal in enhancement, which lends credence to this notion.[48]

Some patients treated with angiangiogenic agents may also experience nonenhancing tumor progression manifesting as increasing T2/fluid-attenuated inversion recovery (FLAIR) signal abnormality (**Fig. 2**).[53,54] Antiangiogenesis therapy may stimulate tumor progression through vascular cooption and develop an invasive, nonenhancing phenotype.[55–57] This process could help explain the large disparity between high response rates in recurrent glioblastoma and modest, if any, survival benefit.[48,53]

Regardless of whether there is a PsR or true antitumoral response, vascular normalization with an associated decrease in vasogenic edema may result in decreased morbidity and steroid usage.[19,48]

Clinical Implications of PsR

There are currently no validated predictive biomarkers for any antiangiogenic agent in cancer.[58] Radiologic responses in patients being treated with antiangiogenic agents must be viewed with skepticism. As with PsP, the possibility of PsR limits the usefulness of PFS as a primary end point in clinical trials.[6] Furthermore, changes in T2/FLAIR signal abnormality have not been explicitly addressed by the traditional MacDonald criteria and should be addressed in updated criteria.

RANO CRITERIA

The Response Assessment in Neuro-Oncology (RANO) Working Group is a multidisciplinary, international collaborative effort whose goal is to provide expert consensus opinion regarding the development of new standardized response criteria for brain tumor clinical trials.[10] In 2010, given concerns raised by PsP and PsR, the RANO Working Group attempted to address some of the limitations of the MacDonald criteria.[11]

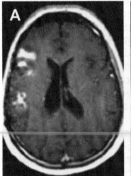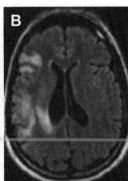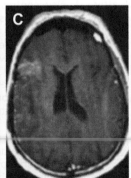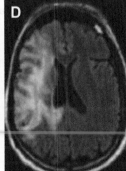

Fig. 2. PsR. Recurrent HGG on axial T1 contrast-enhanced MR imaging (*A*) and axial FLAIR (*B*). The patient was treated with a combination of bevacizumab and VP-16, but clinically worsened significantly despite treatment. Follow-up imaging 2 months later: axial T1 contrast-enhanced MR imaging (*C*) and axial FLAIR (*D*) show decreased enhancement but marked progression of infiltrative FLAIR abnormalities, suggesting nonenhancing tumor progression. (*Reproduced from* Clarke JL, Chang S. Pseudoprogression and pseudoresponse: challenges in brain tumor imaging. Curr Neurol Neurosci Rep 2009;9(3):241–6; with permission.)

Despite many advances in functional MR imaging techniques (discussed later), there is currently insufficient evidence to incorporate them into routine response criteria for use in clinical trials/practice and, therefore, conventional follow-up contrast-enhanced MR imaging remains the standard-of-practice imaging technique.[11,24,32,34] As a result, the determination of PsP by MR imaging alone is inherently a retrospective process.[33] Furthermore, other end points such as quality-of-life measures and neuropsychological testing may be incorporated into response criteria as these metrics are developed and validated.[11]

A summary of the proposed RANO response criteria is given in **Tables 2–4**.

PsP

Because of the possibility of PsP, the RANO recommendations state that patients within 12 weeks of the completion of chemoradiation should be excluded from clinical trials for recurrent glioma unless TEP is shown as new enhancement outside of the radiation field or there is unequivocal evidence of tumor at tissue sampling (see **Table 2**).[11] If patients remain clinically stable and/or are thought to have PsP based on functional imaging, then therapy should remain unchanged. Pope and Hessel[59] raised concern that these new recommendations may exclude the most malignant tumors that progress rapidly, and that, because these patients were not excluded from many prior clinical trials, a bias may be introduced when the therapeutic efficacy of a new drug is compared with historical controls.[59] Furthermore, the RANO guidelines do not account for the possibility of PsP occurring at time later than 3 months. The risk of excluding TEP must be considered against the risk of including PsP in clinical trials.

Table 2
RANO criteria for determining first progression based on time from initial chemoradiation

First Progression	Criteria
Progressive disease <12 wk after completion of chemoradiation	Progression can only be defined using imaging if: There is new enhancement outside the radiation field (beyond the high-dose region or 80% isodose line) or if there is unequivocal evidence of viable tumor on histopathologic sampling (eg, solid tumor areas, ie, greater than 70% tumor cell nuclei in areas; high or progressive increase in MIB-1 proliferation index compared with prior biopsy; or evidence for histologic progression or increased anaplasia in tumor) Because of the difficulty of differentiating TEP from PsP, clinical deterioration alone, in the absence of histologic or radiographic confirmation of progression, is not sufficient for definition of progressive disease in the first 12 wk after completion of concurrent chemoradiation
Progressive disease ≥12 wk after completion of chemoradiation	1. New contrast-enhancing lesion outside radiation field on decreasing, stable, or increasing corticosteroid doses 2. Increase by ≥25% in the sum of the products of perpendicular diameters between the first postradiotherapy scan, or a subsequent scan with smaller tumor size, and the scan at 12 wk or later on stable or increasing corticosteroid doses 3. Clinical deterioration not caused by concurrent medication or comorbid conditions is sufficient to declare progression on current treatment but not for entry onto a clinical trial for tumor recurrence 4. For patients receiving antiangiogenic therapy, significant increase in nonenhancing T2/FLAIR lesion may also be considered progressive disease. The increase must have occurred while on stable or increasing corticosteroid doses compared with baseline scan or best response following initiation of therapy and not be a result of comorbid events (such as radiation therapy effects, demyelination, ischemic injury, infection, seizures, postoperative changes, or other treatment effects)

Adapted from Wen PY, et al. Updated response assessment criteria for high-grade gliomas: Response Assessment in Neuro-Oncology Working Group. J Clin Oncol 2010;28(11):1963–72.

Table 3
RANO criteria for assessment of response using MR imaging and clinical factors

Response	Criteria
Complete response	All of the following are required: Complete disappearance of all enhancing measurable and nonmeasurable disease sustained for a minimum of 4 wk No new lesions Nonenhancing (T2/FLAIR) lesions stable or improved No use of corticosteroids (or on physiologic replacement doses only) Clinically stable or improved Those with nonmeasurable disease only cannot have a complete response. The best possible response is stable disease
Partial response	All of the following are required: ≥50% decrease compared with baseline in the sum of products of perpendicular diameters of all measurable enhancing lesions sustained for a minimum of 4 wk No progression of nonmeasurable disease No new lesions Nonenhancing (T2/FLAIR) lesions stable or improved on same or lower dose of corticosteroids compared with baseline scan Corticosteroid dose at the time of the scan evaluation should be no greater than the dose at time of baseline scan Clinically stable or improved. Those with nonmeasurable disease only cannot have a partial response. The best possible response is stable disease
Stable disease	All of the following are required: Does not qualify for complete response, partial response, or progression Nonenhancing (T2/FLAIR) lesions stable on same or lower dose of corticosteroids compared with baseline scan If the corticosteroid dose was increased for new symptoms and signs without confirmation of disease progression on imaging, and subsequent imaging follow-up shows that this increase in corticosteroid dose was needed because of disease progression, the last scan thought to show stable disease is the scan obtained when the corticosteroid dose was equivalent to the baseline dose
Progression	Any of the following: ≥25% increase in sum of the products of perpendicular diameters of enhancing lesions compared with the smallest tumor measurement obtained either at baseline (if no decrease) or best response Stable or increasing corticosteroids doses[a] Significant increase in nonenhancing T2/FLAIR lesion on stable or increasing corticosteroids doses[a] compared with baseline scan or best response after initiation of therapy[a] that is not the result of comorbid events such as radiation therapy, demyelination, ischemic injury, infection, seizures, postoperative changes, or other treatment effects Any new lesion Obvious clinical deterioration with no causes other than the tumor (such as seizures, adverse effects of medications, therapeutic complications, cerebrovascular events, infection), or corticosteroid dose changes Failure to return for follow-up evaluation because of deteriorating condition or death Obvious progression of nonmeasurable disease

All nonmeasurable and measurable lesions must be assessed using the same techniques as at baseline.
[a] Stable corticosteroid doses include patients not taking corticosteroids.
Adapted from Wen PY, et al. Updated response assessment criteria for high-grade gliomas: Response Assessment in Neuro-Oncology Working Group. J Clin Oncol 2010;28(11):1963–72.

PsR

Given the possibility of PsR, the RANO Working Group has issued new recommendations for patients with recurrent glioblastoma on antiangiogenic therapy (see **Tables 2–4**). These recommendations now state that disease progression can be manifested by a significant increase in the amount

Table 4
Summary of proposed RANO response criteria

Criteria	CR	PR	SD	PD
Enhancing disease	None	≥50% ↓	<50% ↓ but <25% ↑	≥25% ↑[a]
T2/FLAIR	Stable or ↓	Stable or ↓	Stable or ↓	↑[a]
New lesion	None	None	None	Present[a]
Corticosteroids	None	Stable or ↓	Stable or ↓	NA[b]
Clinical status	Stable or ↑	Stable or ↑	Stable or ↑	↓[a]
Requirement for response	All	All	All	Any[a]

Abbreviations: CR, complete response; NA, not applicable; PD, progressive disease; PR, partial response; SD, stable disease.
  [a] Progression occurs when criterion present.
  [b] Corticosteroid dose increase alone is not considered in determining disease progression when there is no persistent clinical deterioration.
  Adapted from Wen PY, et al. Updated response assessment criteria for high-grade gliomas: Response Assessment in Neuro-Oncology Working Group. J Clin Oncol 2010;28(11):1963–72.

of nonenhancing T2W/FLAIR signal while the patient is on stable/increasing corticosteroid dose compared with the baseline scan or best response after the start of therapy.[11] For this reason, the RANO criteria have been referred to as MacDonald plus FLAIR.[59] However, these criteria contain some ambiguity because the definition of a significant increase in T2W/FLAIR signal was not explicitly defined.[59] Another difficulty rests in the recommendation that nonenhancing T2/FLAIR tumor progression must be differentiated from radiation effects, demyelination, infection, decreased corticosteroid dosing, ischemic injury, other treatment effects, and seizures. Imaging findings that would suggest nonenhancing tumor include mass effect, infiltration of the cortical ribbon, and location beyond the radiation field. The RANO criteria also recommend retrospective backdating of the time when nonenhancing progression was first suspected, and although this could increase sensitivity for progression, there is concern that comparison with historical controls could again be difficult.[59] Discordant interpretations can be common in antiangiogenic therapy drug trials and inconsistent progression dating is an issue. Pope and Hessel[59] advocate that making note of suspicious regions of possible nonenhancing progression that are retrospectively confirmed as tumor progression could decrease the discrepancy or adjudication rate.

Other concerns regarding the RANO criteria include issues relating to corticosteroid dosage and lack of validated measures of neurologic function.[11,59] Regarding corticosteroid dosing, what qualifies as a significant change in steroid dose, over what time period before imaging should steroid status be considered relevant, and whether total daily dose or average daily dose should be

considered are also unclear. Both the MacDonald and RANO criteria also consider neurologic function in their assessment criteria. However, a precise definition currently cannot be provided given the lack of validated measures of neurologic function. In RANO, whether a patient is suffering from neurologic deterioration is left to the discretion of the treating physician. They do recommend consideration of a decrease in Karnofsky performance score, Eastern Cooperative Oncology Group performance status or World Health Organization performance score to determine clinical decline.

SURGICALLY DELIVERED THERAPIES

The Surgery Working Group of RANO recently proposed new guidelines regarding response/progression measures following surgically delivered therapies.[10] A summary of their recommendations is given in **Box 1**.

1. *Imaging after surgery for both HGG and LGG.* Because improved outcomes are seen following maximal resection of tumor, recommendations have been set forth regarding the timing of baseline postoperative contrast-enhanced MR imaging to better assess completeness of resection. As was stated by Wen and colleagues,[11] the recent guidelines stressed that, for HGGs, baseline postoperative MR imaging should occur ideally within 24 to 48 hours after surgery, and no later than 72 hours after surgery, because increased enhancement can develop in the wall of the resection cavity 48 to 72 hours after surgery. This postsurgical enhancement can be mistaken for residual or new enhancing tumor. LGGs typically do not

---

Box 1
Summary of RANO surgery task force recommendations

1. Imaging after surgery for HGG and LGG

   a. Should be performed within 72 hours after surgery to determine extent of resection of enhancing tumors (eg, HGG)

   b. For nonenhancing tumors (eg, LGGs), final determination of extent of resection may require a delay of up to 12 weeks to allow for edema resolution

   c. Diffusion-weighted imaging (DWI) should be used to determine regions of perioperative ischemia that could subsequently develop nonspecific areas of enhancement

2. Updated terminology for completeness of surgical resection

   a. When enhancing tumor is present, removal of all enhancing tissue should be called complete resection of enhancing tumor rather than gross total resection

   b. Resection of all enhancing tumor (if present) and all nonenhancing tumor tissue (ie, T2/FLAIR hyperintensity) should be called complete resection of detectable tumor

   c. Partial resections can also be referred to as partial resection of enhancing tumor or partial resection of detectable tumor

3. To determine disease progression, completeness of surgical resection and use of local therapies, if applicable, should be taken into consideration

4. Clinical trials should allow retrospective evaluation of disease progression

5. Blinded central review should be considered for use in clinical trials

6. Volumetric assessment of tumor size and response should be used as these techniques become more widely available

Adapted from Vogelbaum MA, et al. Application of novel response/progression measures for surgically delivered therapies for gliomas: Response Assessment in Neuro-Oncology (RANO) Working Group. Neurosurgery 2012;70(1):234–43. [discussion: 243–4].

---

show significant contrast enhancement and so a delay of up to 12 weeks for postoperative MR imaging may be needed to differentiate nonenhancing tumor from edema. This study should be compared with the appearance of T2/FLAIR hyperintensity on the preoperative MR imaging. For both HGG and LGGs, intraoperative assessment of completeness of resection is thought to be an unreliable measure compared with postoperative MR imaging. The importance of DWI to document possible perioperative ischemia caused by microvascular compromise at the surgical resection margins was emphasized. These regions may go on to show contrast enhancement on follow-up imaging that could be misinterpreted as recurrent tumor, and so comparison with the postoperative DWI images may be critical.

2. *Updated terminology for completeness of surgical resection.* Traditional terminology to describe completeness of surgical resection included descriptors such as gross total resection, near-total resection, subtotal resection, and partial resection. These terms were thought to be subjectively determined and inconsistently used depending on glioma grade, so a set of alternative terms has been suggested. This updated terminology may allow improved design of prospective clinical trials that use a specific extent of tumor debulking for entry and for retrospective studies examining impacts of surgical resection on clinical outcome (see **Box 1**).

3. *To determine disease progression, completeness of surgical resection and use of local therapies, if applicable, should be taken into consideration.* Certain local therapies such as chemotherapy wafers, immunotoxins, or gene therapies given by direct brain delivery, focal irradiation with brachytherapy and stereotactic radiosurgery, and immunotherapies can result in increased contrast enhancement and may simulate recurrent tumor on conventional MR imaging. Because of the nonspecific findings that local therapies can produce, radiographic progression is discouraged as a primary end point in trials using these agents. Although functional imaging techniques may hold promise to distinguish treatment effects from recurrent tumor, none are yet clinically validated so follow-up conventional imaging and clinical evaluation are recommended. Although

biopsy remains an option, there is a concern regarding its ability to determine prognosis in treated glioblastoma.[60,61] However, tissue sampling may be needed if a clinical trial uses an entry criterion or end point of tumor progression.

4. *Clinical trials should allow retrospective evaluation of disease progression.* Given that there are no validated imaging methods to distinguish tumor progression from treatment effects (ie, PsP), serial follow-up conventional MR imaging should be allowed to determine whether there is disease progression. An indeterminate designation may be used if tumor progression is suspected but treatment effects still cannot be excluded. If it is borne out that the patient does have tumor progression, then the date of an indeterminate designation is deemed to be the time of true progression.

5. *Use of blinded central review in clinical trials. PFS is often used as a surrogate for overall survival (OS) in clinical trials.* PFS has the advantage that it can shorten trial duration and is not affected by subsequent salvage treatment. However, its reliance on subjective interpretation of MR imaging studies can be problematic, whereas OS can be assessed objectively. The incorporation of a blinded central review of MR imaging studies into the design of a clinical trial should be considered to address this issue.

6. *Volumetric assessment of tumor size and response.* Given concerns about current nonvolumetric measuring techniques such as poor accuracy and reliability, lack of comparability between studies given different slice positioning, and difficulty in documenting how measurements were made, consideration should be given to the use of volumetric analysis of whole tumor volumes. There is preliminary evidence to suggest that volumetric analysis is effective and this may become realized as the requisite software becomes more widely available. Volumetric techniques may then be applied toward routine assessment of residual enhancing or nonenhancing tumor volume.

LGGs

Although HGGs are the primary focus of this article, a brief overview of response criteria for LGGs is also given. Recent RANO guidelines have also been published regarding assessment criteria in trials of LGG (**Table 5**).[62] The MacDonald criteria are not well suited for use with LGGs because these tumors generally show little to no enhancement.[8,63,64] Although LGGs show a less

aggressive clinical course than HGGs, most ultimately relapse as HGG, with poor outcome. Conventional contrast-enhanced CT or MR imaging seems to be insensitive to detect early malignant degeneration.[65] Low or even absent radiographic responses have been seen in several LGG trials despite clinical benefit, including a reduction in seizures and prolonged disease control.[62] The posttherapeutic imaging evaluation of LGG is difficult because T2-weighted signal abnormalities following successful therapy cannot be differentiated from tumor. As a result, the category of minor response has been created.[66] Further confusing evaluation is the possibility of radiation-induced leukoencephalopathy, which also shows T2-weighted signal abnormalities. The use of PFS as primary end point in clinical trials is problematic in LGG because of the slow growth rate of LGG and the rare radiological true responses despite favorable response to therapy.[62] At the same time, the use of OS as an end point presents logistical challenges and is also prone to the effect of other noninvestigational salvage treatment at recurrence. Regardless of whether PFS or OS is used as a primary end point, RANO also recommends that ancillary measures such as measures of cognition, seizure activity, symptom severity and burden, quality of life, and neurologic deterioration be considered. Response to radiotherapy should be performed with MR imaging 3 to 4 months following the end of radiotherapy given the possibility of PsP in LGG.[62]

ADVANCED IMAGING TECHNIQUES IN THE POSTTREATMENT SETTING

Advanced imaging techniques such as perfusion (dynamic susceptibility contrast and arterial spin labeling [ASL]) MR imaging, permeability (dynamic contrast-enhanced) MR imaging, diffusion MR imaging, MR spectroscopy, and positron emission tomography (PET) are active areas of clinical research and have shown promise when used to assess therapy, predict survival time, and differentiate tumor recurrence from treatment-induced changes. However, these methods require further rigorous clinical validation before they can be incorporated into routine imaging assessment of gliomas.[11] An overview of some recent developments is provided.

Perfusion MR Imaging

Dynamic susceptibility contrast-enhanced (DSC) MR perfusion, sometimes called perfusion-weighted or bolus tracking MR imaging, is a technique in which the first-pass of a bolus of a gadolinium-based contrast agent (GBCA)

Table 5
RANO response criteria for LGG

Response	Criteria
Complete response	All of the following are required compared with the baseline scan: Complete disappearance of the lesion on T2/FLAIR imaging (if enhancement had been present, it must have completely resolved) No new lesions, no new T2 or FLAIR abnormalities apart from those consistent with radiation effects, and no new or increased enhancement Patients must not be taking corticosteroids or only on physiologic replacement doses Patients should be stable or improved clinically
Partial response	All of the following are required compared with the baseline scan: ≥50% decrease in the product of perpendicular diameters of the lesion on T2/FLAIR imaging sustained for a minimum of 4 wk compared with baseline No new lesions, no new T2 or FLAIR abnormalities apart from those consistent with radiation effects, and no new or increased enhancement Patients should be on a corticosteroid dose that is not greater than the dose at time of baseline scan, and should be stable or improved clinically
Minor response	Requires the following criteria compared with baseline: Decrease of the area of nonenhancing lesion on T2/FLAIR imaging between 25% and 50% compared with baseline No new lesions, no new T2/FLAIR abnormalities apart from those consistent with radiation effect, and no new or increased enhancement Patients should be on a corticosteroid dose that should not be greater than the dose at time of baseline scan, and should be stable or improved clinically
Stable disease	If the criteria do not qualify for complete, partial, or minor response or progression, then stable disease is present. It requires: Stable area of nonenhancing abnormalities on T2/FLAIR imaging No new lesions, no new T2/FLAIR abnormalities apart from those consistent with radiation effect, and no new or increased enhancement Patients should be on a corticosteroid dose that should not be greater than the dose at time of baseline scan, and should be stable or improved clinically
Progression	Defined by any of the following: Development of new lesions or increased enhancement (imaging evidence of malignant transformation) A 25% increase of the T2/FLAIR nonenhancing lesion on stable or increasing doses of corticosteroids compared with baseline scan or best response after initiation of therapy, not caused by radiation effect or comorbid events Clear clinical deterioration not from causes other than the tumor, or decrease in corticosteroid dose Failure to return for follow-up evaluation because of deteriorating condition or death, unless caused by documented nonrelated causes

Adapted from van den Bent MJ, et al. Response assessment in neuro-oncology (a report of the RANO group): assessment of outcome in trials of diffuse low-grade gliomas. Lancet Oncol 2011;12(6):583–93.

through the brain parenchyma is monitored by a series of T2-weighted or T2*-weighted MR images.[67] Relative cerebral blood volume (rCBV) is the most robust and commonly used perfusion metric derived from DSC MR imaging and seems to be the most useful parameter in patients with brain tumors.[68,69]

rCBV seems to be increased in tumor progression secondary to increased vascular proliferation, whereas, in RN, rCBV seems to be decreased because of extensive fibrinoid necrosis, vascular dilatation, and endothelial injury (**Fig. 3**).[21,68,70–76]

In addition to finding higher rCBV in recurrent glioblastoma compared with RN, Barajas and colleagues[70] also found that peak height (PH), defined as difference in precontrast T2*-weighted signal intensity and minimum T2*-weighted signal intensity, was also higher in recurrent glioblastoma than RN. Furthermore, recurrent glioblastoma also showed lower relative percentage signal recovery (PSR), a reflection of increased vascular permeability, although a large degree of overlap was seen between the 2 groups, making this a less robust predictor of progression of tumor. A recent

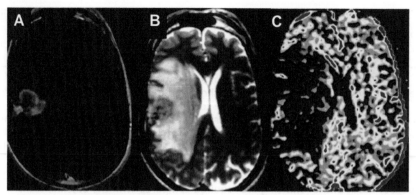

Fig. 3. RN. (*A*) Axial postcontrast T1 MR imaging shows an enhancing mass adjacent to the surgical bed and an axial T2-weighted image (*B*) shows a significant amount of edema with mass effect. (*C*) Gradient-echo axial DSC MR imaging with rCBV color overlay map shows reduced perfusion throughout the lesion. Surgical resection showed this lesion to be RN. (*Reproduced from* Lacerda S, Law M. Magnetic resonance perfusion and permeability imaging in brain tumors. Neuroimaging Clin N Am 2009;19(4):527–57; with permission.)

study addressed the confounding effects of GBCA leakage in rCBV determination and found that a 0.1 mmol/kg preload dose of GBCA with 6 minutes of incubation time along with baseline subtraction techniques seemed to improve the diagnostic accuracy of rCBV to differentiate recurrent glioma from radiation effect.[77] The use of ASL perfusion MR imaging in the posttherapeutic setting is emerging and a recent pilot study using ASL found that it may be more accurate than DSC MR imaging to distinguish RN from progressive HGG, especially in areas of mixed radiation necrosis in which leakage of GBCA could result in underestimation of rCBV.[78]

Like in the case of RN, DSC MR imaging seems to be a promising technique to distinguish PsP from TEP, with several recent studies showing lower rCBV in PsP compared with TEP.[79–81] A recent prospective study by Kong and colleagues[80] examined 90 patients with glioblastoma who were treated with chemoradiation. They found new or enlarging contrast-enhancing lesions in 59 of these patients, with 26 and 33 patients subsequently being classified as PsP and TEP, respectively (based on either imaging follow-up or histopathology). Using the maximum rCBV ratio based on color overlay maps, there was a significantly lower mean rCBV in patients with PsP versus TEP with an rCBV ratio greater than 1.47 demonstrating a sensitivity of 81.5% and specificity of 77.8%. The MGMT promoter methylation was also examined and the unmethylated group had a significant difference in the mean rCBV between PsP and TEP, whereas those with a methylated promoter did not. The investigators postulated that this difference could be a reflection of a higher probability of TEP in tumors

with an unmethylated promoter and, if a patient has an unmethylated promoter, that rCBV may be more useful to determine TEP, which suggests that correlation with MGMT promoter status could improve the validity of the rCBV value. A retrospective study in 36 patients with glioblastoma by Mangla and colleagues[79] reported that, at 1 month after chemoradiation with TMZ, a greater than 5% increase in rCBV seemed to be a strong predictor of less than 1-year survival. In 53% of their patients, an increase in contrast enhancement was noted on posttreatment MR imaging and 37% of these patients were determined to have PsP based on follow-up imaging. The patients with PsP had a mean decrease in rCBV of 41%, whereas those with TEP had a mean increase in rCBV of 12%. To differentiate TEP from PsP, receiver operating characteristic (ROC) analysis was used in which percent change in rCBV greater than 0% or 0% or lower was used. This analysis showed an area under the ROC curve of 0.85 with 76.9% sensitivity and 85.7% specificity.

A 2012 retrospective study by Baek and colleagues[82] of 135 patients with newly diagnosed glioblastomas who were treated with chemoradiation found 79 patients with new or enlarging contrast-enhancing lesions concerning for TEP versus PsP. They found that changes in the shape (percent change of skewness and kurtosis) of normalized rCBV histograms between the first and second postchemoradiation MR imaging may be a potential technique to differentiate TEP from PsP. Four categories were created based on whether the histograms derived from a region of interest (ROI) of the contrast-enhancing lesion showed negative or positive skewness and leptokurtic or platykurtic kurtosis. The histographic pattern of normalized rCBV represented the largest area under the ROC curve of 0.934 and a sensitivity of 85.7% and a specificity of 89.2%. This method outperformed quantitative continuous variables using each percent change in skewness and kurtosis.

In 25 patients with glioblastoma undergoing surgical reresection for newly developed or enlarging lesions on follow-up MR imaging, Hu and colleagues[83] recently showed that a DSC perfusion thresholding metric called perfusion MR imaging–fractional tumor burden (pMRI-FTB) was strongly correlated with histologic tumor fraction and seemed to be correlated with OS. This type of approach could be significant because virtually all studies view contrast-enhancing MR imaging lesions as either tumor or posttreatment radiation effect (PsP and RN), even though most lesions are an admixture with variable amounts of tumor fraction. Using stereotactic coregistration, they showed that an rCBV threshold of 1.0 could differentiate posttreatment radiation effect from tumor with 100% accuracy. This threshold was higher than what the same group had reported earlier,[71] which could be because of technical differences in perfusion data postprocessing. The results of this study suggest that using pMRI-FTB to noninvasively quantify tumor burden relative to posttreatment radiation effect could prove useful to predict tumor progression and survival.

To account for the heterogeneity of DSC perfusion MR imaging values within tumors, parametric response mapping (PRM) was introduced by Galban and colleagues[84] as a voxel-wise method for analyzing perfusion maps. It differs from traditional whole-tumor ROI analysis methods in that it retains spatial alteration in perfusion metrics after the start of therapy. They measured the change in coregistered rCBV on a voxel-wise basis, designated as PRM_{rCBV}, before treatment and 1 and 3 weeks after treatment initiation. These values were then compared with standard whole-tumor ROI analysis for their accuracy in predicting OS. Percentage change of ROI-based mean rCBF and rCBF did not predict survival, probably because of varying changes in these parameters throughout the tumor that desensitizes the measurement. However, PRM_{rCBV} predicted OS, probably because of its ability to detect and quantify variations of increased, decreased, and unchanged voxels following treatment initiation. This finding held true even when accounting for baseline rCBV, which is also known to be prognostic. The investigators acknowledged a potential limitation that accurate image registration is required, which could introduce error if

large changes in tumor volume occur between examinations.

A follow-up study by the same group also evaluated PRM in PsP and seemed to show a significant difference in PRM_{rCBV} in patients with PsP compared with TEP at week 3 during chemoradiation. However, percent change in whole tumor rCBV or rCBF, extent of resection MR tumor volume changes, and Radiation Therapy Oncology Group recursive partitioning analysis classification could not make this distinction.[81] This study found significantly decreased rCBV based on PRM in those with TEP compared with PsP at 3 weeks, which is counterintuitive. Decreased perfusion could result in hypoxia and treatment resistance, although it is unclear to what extent underestimation of rCBV caused by T1 GBCA leakage effects could have influenced these results.[46,84,85] Nonetheless, this technique seems to be promising and more validation of this method is necessary.

A prospective study in 14 patients by Gahramanov and colleagues[86] compared the GBCA gadoteridol (without leakage correction) with the blood pool agent ferumoxytol, an ultrasmall superparamagnetic iron oxide nanoparticle, in determining rCBV in patients with HGG following chemoradiation. Because of its larger molecular size, the leakage rate of ferumoxytol is lower than that of GBCAs and their results suggest that a low rCBV derived from ferumoxytol may be a better discriminator of PsP than an rCBV derived with a GBCA. A high ferumoxytol rCBV may similarly be a better indicator of TEP. They also suggest that the use of a blood pool agent may be a simpler and more reliable method to minimize GBCA leakage effect compared with other proposed methods.[71,87]

In a retrospective study of 16 patients with recurrent glioblastoma treated with bevacizumab, Sawlani and colleagues[88] examined mean rCBV, mean leakage coefficient K_2, and hyperperfusion volume (HPV), defined as the fraction of tumor with an rCBV greater than a predefined threshold, as potential imaging biomarkers of therapeutic response. A statistically significant hazard ratio of 1.077 was found that correlated with time to progression when examining the percent change in HPV (rCBV threshold of 1.00). Given the small sample size and that hazard ratio was just greater than 1, further validation and modification of this technique may be needed.[37]

Although OS or duration of response or PFS may be a better indicator of true antitumoral effect of antiangiogenic agents, the amount of initial response may also correlate with survival.[11] Changes in microvascular permeability (volume transfer constant [K^{trans}]), rCBV, and circulating collagen IV were recently combined to produce a vascular normalization index in 31 patients with recurrent glioblastoma following a single dose of the antiangiogenic agent cediranib.[49] This index was closely associated with both PFS and OS in these patients.

In theory, the vascular normalization produced by antiangiogenic agents should result in improved perfusion and improved oxygenation and drug delivery. However, until now, clinical evidence for this has been lacking.[45,46] A recent study by Sorensen and colleagues[46] found a durable increase in perfusion for at least 1 month and longer survival in 7 out of 30 patients with recurrent glioblastoma treated with cediranib. These results suggest that decreases in permeability from vascular normalization could result in increased perfusion in some patients, with consequently improved antitumoral effect of cediranib caused by improved drug delivery.

In a longitudinal study of 13 patients with biopsy-proven LGG who were treated conservatively, Danchaivijitr and colleagues[65] noted that rCBV values at baseline were not significantly different between transformer and nontransformer groups. However, a significant increase in consecutive rCBV was found in patients who transformed to HGG. An increase in rCBV was noted up to 1 year before contrast enhancement was evident in those undergoing malignant degeneration. Law and colleagues[89] performed retrospective analysis in 189 patients with LGG and HGGs to determine whether baseline rCBV could predict clinical outcome. They concluded that both patients with HGG and LGG with increased rCBV (>1.75) had significantly more rapid time to progression compared with those with low rCBV, independent of pathologic findings. The development and validation of rCBV threshold values in the future may result in an earlier diagnosis of progression, or stage migration, the clinical significance of which is unclear.[62] Oligodendrogliomas, especially the 1p/19q loss of heterozygosity genotype, may be problematic with this approach given their propensity to show increased rCBV regardless of grade because of their chicken-wire vasculature.[69,90] Because of the low rCBV of nontransforming LGG, it is unlikely to be a sensitive biomarker of treatment response because of this floor effect.[62]

Permeability MR Imaging

Permeability dynamic contrast-enhanced (DCE) MR imaging is a technique that can measure the integrity and leakiness of tumoral microvasculature.[91] By assuming a 2-compartment model composed of intravascular and extravascular space, common variables reported using pharmacokinetic modeling, variables including the K^{trans}, blood plasma volume (V_p), and volume of extravascular-extracellular space (V_e) can be measured.[67,92,93] Semiquantitative model-free parameters include initial area under the curve (iAUC), time to peak (TTP), and slope of the initial phase or washout curve. Although iAUC is easier to calculate and correlated with the quantitative variables K^{trans}, V_e, and V_p, it is less physiologically specific and seems to represent a combination of the three parameters.[91]

Most DCE MR imaging studies have focused on K^{trans} and, although it seems that K^{trans} represents a potentially intractable combination of microvascular permeability, blood flow, and endothelial surface area, it seems to be reproducible.[94,95] There are comparatively few studies using DCE MR imaging to diagnose RN compared with DSC MR imaging. Early work by Hazle and colleagues[96] in 1997 seemed to indicate that RN had lower permeability than recurrent tumor. A recent study by Bisdas and colleagues[97] used DCE MR imaging in 18 patients with HGG who developed postradiation enhancement questionable for recurrent tumor or RN. Both K^{trans} and iAUC were significantly higher for the recurrent glioma group, with K^{trans} showing a superior sensitivity and specificity compared with iAUC. Another recent study by Narang and colleagues[98] found that iAUC at both 60 and 120 seconds, maximum slope of enhancement in the initial vascular phase (MSIVP), and normalized MSIVP (nMSIVP) were all significantly higher in the recurrent tumor group, whereas normalized slope of the delayed equilibrium phase (nSDEP) was significantly lower. nMSIVP seemed to be the single best predictor of recurrent tumor, with a sensitivity of 95% and specificity of 78%. They postulated that semiquantitative, non–model-based metrics derived from DCE MR imaging could serve as alternatives to more complex pharmacokinetic-based methods.

Diffusion MR Imaging

Diffusion MR imaging is commonly performed in both academic and community settings. Compared with DCE and DSC MR imaging, it has some advantages in that it does not require the use of an exogenous contrast agent and may be easier to implement and more reproducible.[99,100] It can allow insight into cellular architecture at the millimeter scale by being sensitive to thermally driven molecular water motion.[101] In vivo, water motion is thought to be impeded by cellular packing, membranes, intracellular elements, and macromolecules, although there is still an incomplete understanding and consensus regarding the biophysical basis of apparent diffusion coefficient (ADC) values.[102]

In general, increases in ADC following therapy can be seen as evidence of successful therapy in most malignancies, including brain tumors.[101,103–106] However, the cellular processes resulting from successful therapy, particularly antiangiogenic/cytostatic rather than cytotoxic/radiotherapies that kill tumor cells, can produce variable, occasionally opposing, effects on ADC.[107–110] Early cellular swelling in cell death mediated by necrosis can produce diffusion restriction, whereas later cell lysis can result in increased water diffusion.[104,111] Early cell shrinkage associated with apoptosis can also result in increased ADC.[112] Tumor progression may manifest as a decrease in ADC caused by an increase in tumor cell density, although an increase in ADC could also be seen in tumor progression secondary to vasogenic edema that accompanies tumor cell infiltration along intact white matter tracts.[113–115]

There is currently limited and conflicting evidence regarding the use of diffusion MR imaging to differentiate RN or PsP from recurrent tumor.[32,33] A recent preclinical diffusion tensor imaging (DTI) study by Wang and colleagues[30] used rat models of RN as well as 2 orthotopic glioma models. Compared with viable glioma, RN had significantly lower ADC in the central zone of necrosis and lower fractional anisotropy (FA) in the peripheral zone of necrosis. These changes were thought to be caused by coagulative necrosis in the central zone and random microstructures of necrosis in the peripheral zone. Parallel diffusivity ($\lambda_{\parallel}$) in the central and peripheral zone and perpendicular diffusivity ($\lambda_{\perp}$) in the central zone were also significantly lower in RN compared with glioma; in addition, their diagnostic powers seemed to be nearly equal to those of ADC and higher than those of FA, although further validation in clinical cases is needed. An earlier clinical study in 28 patients by Sundgren and colleagues[116] found lower ADC, $\lambda_{\parallel}$, and $\lambda_{\perp}$ in RN compared with tumor recurrence and no difference in FA. Other reports have suggested that ADC may be increased and that FA may be decreased in RN compared with recurrence.[117–119]

A recent study in 15 patients with recurrent glioblastoma showed that a change in any direction in mean ADC in the FLAIR signal abnormality region after bevacizumab and irinotecan therapy was associated with decreased survival.[120] This finding suggests the importance of disease stability to be a favorable prognostic factor and that an increase or decrease of ADC could correspond with tumor progression. Another study in 20 patients with recurrent/progressive glioblastoma treated with bevacizumab alone or with concurrent chemotherapy found that those with tumor progression showed a trend of decreasing ADC in both the contrast-enhancing and FLAIR hyperintense signal regions, whereas those without progression seemed to show a trend of stable to slightly progressive increase over time.[121]

Histogram analysis is an alternative to traditional ROI analysis that allows documentation of tumor heterogeneity, although no spatial specificity can be extracted. In 2 separate studies, Pope and colleagues[100] showed that ADC histogram analysis derived from contrast-enhancing tumor and fitted to a 2 normal distribution curve seemed to show that the mean ADC from the lower curve (ADC-L) and the mean lower curve proportion (LCP) were able to predict PFS and OS.[122] The Pope and colleagues[100] study from 2012 is notable because it was performed in a multicenter setting in 97 patients without standardization of imaging technique. The longest surviving patients (living more than 600 days) were all identified with their method.

Functional diffusion maps (fDMs) were proposed in 2005 in which multiple ADC maps are generated at multiple time points and coregistered with a first-scan baseline.[106,108] Then, voxel-wise changes are isolated and computed according to the magnitude of their change. As opposed to conventional ROI analysis, in which the ADC values are averaged over the ROI, fDM does not assume homogeneity within the lesion, a factor that is critical because many tumors show quite a bit of spatial heterogeneity.

This technique has been shown to be a sensitive early biomarker for brain tumor responses to therapy and specific to progression of HGG.[123,124] Different degrees of cell density change may be reflected by using graded thresholds in fDM.[125] This modification of fDM allows quantification and tracking of the volume of tissue showing changes between different ADC thresholds and this may be more predictive of OS than traditional fDMs in patients with recurrent glioblastoma treated with bevacizumab.[110]

Like the potential difficulties seen with PRM-based perfusion MR imaging, fDM is limited by the proper registration of diffusion MR images from subsequent scans. Slight misregistration between the datasets caused by image distortion or edema may confound quantification and interpretation of the fDM-classified tumor regions.[126]

At present, only linear image registration techniques have been used to match the DWI sets. Ellingson and colleagues[126] hypothesized that an additional nonlinear (elastic) registration step after linear registration could improve the clinical sensitivity and reduce misregistration and misclassification of fDMs (Fig. 4). In patients undergoing antiangiogenic therapy, nonlinear fDMs provide improved clinical predictability, sensitivity, and specificity for PFS and OS compared with the linear fDMs.[126]

The significance of new diffusion restriction lesions in patients with glioblastoma during therapy is unclear. Gupta and colleagues[127] reported that some patients with glioblastoma who develop a new focus of nonenhancing diffusion restriction during therapy (chemoradiation with TMZ or bevacizumab with or without chemotherapy) may evolve into a region of enhancing tumor, although histopathologic correlation was lacking. Gerstner and colleagues[128] described a case report of pathologically confirmed diffusion-restricting, nonenhancing tumor in a patient with recurrent glioblastoma treated with bevacizumab, possibly reflecting vascular cooption by tumor. Rieger and colleagues[129] showed the presence of persistent diffusion-restricting lesions in 13 out of 18 patients with recurrent glioblastoma treated with bevacizumab. In the 1 patient for whom pathologic confirmation was available, only atypical necrosis and upregulation of hypoxia-inducible factor 1 alpha without recurrent tumor was found. A recent retrospective study by Mong and colleagues[130] found that 20 patients with malignant glioma treated with bevacizumab had significantly greater time to progression, time

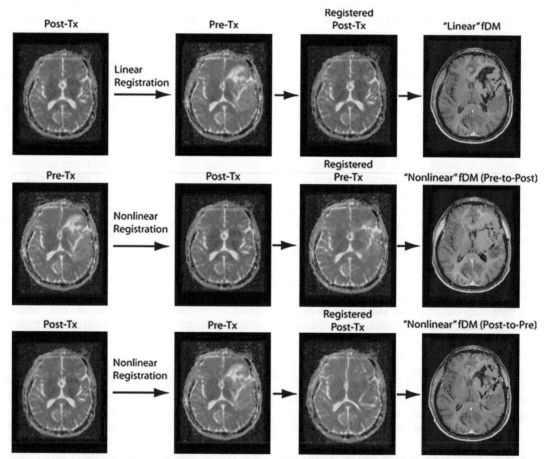

Fig. 4. Linear and nonlinear fDM calculations. Top row: linear (traditional) fDMs consisting of a linear registration algorithm to align posttreatment ADC maps to pretreatment ADC maps. Middle row: before to after nonlinear fDMs consisting of nonlinear registration of pretreatment ADC maps to posttreatment ADC maps. Bottom row: after to before nonlinear fDMs consisting of nonlinear registration of posttreatment ADC maps to pretreatment ADC maps. For fDMs, blue voxels represent a significant decrease in ADC (beyond 0.4 mm^2/ms), red voxels represent a significant increase in ADC (beyond 0.4 mm^2/ms), and green voxels are those with no significant change in ADC. (*Reproduced from* Ellingson BM, et al. Nonlinear registration of diffusion-weighted images improves clinical sensitivity of functional diffusion maps in recurrent glioblastoma treated with bevacizumab. Magn Reson Med 2012;67(1):237–45; with permission.)

to survival from bevacizumab initiation, and OS compared with matched controls. Gelatinous necrotic tissue was found in the 1 diffusion-restricting patient in whom surgical resection was performed and, where available, perfusion MR imaging and 3,4-dihydroxy-6-[18F]fluoro-phenylal-anine (18F-FDOPA) PET scans also were not consistent with tumor. The investigators concluded that these persistent diffusion-restricting lesions may be related to atypical necrosis rather than active tumor.

Smith and colleagues[131] reported that diffusion restriction can occur in or around the resection cavity in patients with glioma immediately following surgery. The diffusion restriction typically resolves and is followed by contrast enhancement on follow-up imaging. Over time, this region of contrast enhancement evolves into encephalomalacia. Therefore, it seems that contrast enhancement that is preceded by diffusion restriction is be more consistent with postresection injury than with tumor recurrence. As stated earlier, routine inclusion of DWI has been recommended by the Surgery Working Group of RANO.[10]

PET

PET imaging can provide quantitative metabolic information about gliomas.[132] Various radiotracers can be used to characterize different molecular processes within glioma, most of which are concerned with increased metabolism and cell proliferation. Some disadvantages of PET imaging relate to its increased expense as well as its decreased availability compared with MR imaging.

The first oncologic application of PET was in the imaging of brain tumors with 18F-fluorodeoxyglucose (FDG).[133–136] To date, there is little known regarding use of 18F-FDG and PsP directly. However, literature does exist on attempts to use 18F-FDG to differentiate RN from tumor progression. These studies typically display low or disputed sensitivities and specificities, largely because of high background activity within the brain parenchyma.[24,28,137–140] A study by Ricci and colleagues[137] found that 18F-FDG had a sensitivity of 73% and specificity of 56% when the contralateral gray matter was used as reference standard. Using contralateral white matter as a reference, sensitivity was 86% and specificity was 22%, respectively. Based on their study, nearly one-third of patients would have been treated inappropriately if 18F-FDG were the sole determinant of treatment response.

A recent meta-analysis by Nihashi and colleagues[140] examined the diagnostic accuracy of various PET radiotracers to diagnose recurrent glioma. They conducted database searches of Scopus and PubMed from inception until June 30, 2011. Their analysis found wide-ranging sensitivities and specificities for the 2 radiotracers that satisfied their search criteria: 18F-FDG (16 studies) and the amino acid–based 11C-methionine (11C-MET) (7 studies). Results were based primarily on visual assessment of 18F-FDG and quantitative assessment of 11C-MET. Various thresholds and diagnostic criteria were used across studies. For 18F-FDG in HGG, sensitivities ranged between 18% and 100% and specificity ranged between 25% and 100%. For 11C-MET, sensitivity ranged between 44% and 93% and specificity ranged between 50% and 100%. When summary estimates of sensitivity and specificity with their 95% confidence intervals (CIs) were calculated by using bivariate random effects meta-analysis with the exact binomial likelihood, 18F-FDG had a summary sensitivity of 77% (95% CI, 66%–85%) and specificity of 78% (95% CI, 54%–91%) for any glioma histology, whereas 11C-MET had a summary sensitivity of 70% (95% CI, 50%–84%) and specificity of 93% (95% CI, 44%–100%) for HGG. The investigators concluded that both 18F-FDG and 11C-MET had moderately good accuracy for detecting recurrent glioma as add-on tests for diagnosing recurrent glioma. However, they cautioned that these estimates may not be replicable or relevant to other clinical settings given that most studies had limited internal and external validity. Other limitations were that the number of studies was small and few studies used current standard-of-care therapies. Their study also revealed limited data on other radiotracers such as 18F-FLT, 18F-fluoroethyl-L-tyrosine (18F-FET), and 18F-boronophenylalanine. They also found few direct comparison studies examining different PET radiotracers and of PET versus other non-PET imaging modalities.

Numerous novel radiotracers have been developed because of the limitations of 18F-FDG-PET in the brain. Amino acid–based PET, such as 11C-MET or 18F-FET, seem to be more useful in brain imaging because of lower baseline uptake.[132] Both of these modalities have been promising in determining tumor progression from RN, and may be potentially useful to diagnose PsP.[141–147] 11C-MET is the most widely used non–18F-FDG-PET radiotracer in use because of its localization precision and higher sensitivity than 18F-FDG.[139] However, its major limitation is the requirement of an on-site cyclotron because of its short half-life.[143] Terakawa and colleagues[142] examined the diagnostic accuracy of 11C-MET in 77 patients with metastatic brain tumors (n = 51) and glioma (n = 26) and determined that uptake of ^{11}C-MET tended to be increased for tumor recurrence compared with RN. Using a lesion to normal to mean ratio (L/N_{mean}) of mean standardized uptake values, ROC analysis found that, for metastatic tumor, an L/N_{mean} cutoff value greater than 1.41 had a sensitivity of 79% and specificity of 75%, whereas, for glioma, an L/N_{mean} greater than 1.58 had a sensitivity of 75% and specificity of 75%. A limitation of ^{11}C-MET that was raised by this study was that a reduction of specificity could result from accumulation of ^{11}C-MET in necrotic tissue because of disruption of the BBB. Potzi and colleagues[148] studied both ^{18}F-FDG and ^{11}C-MET in 28 patients with glioblastoma following surgery and/or conservative treatment and found that ^{11}C-MET was able to show increased uptake in tumor in 24 patients compared with only 2 for ^{18}F-FDG. However, neither radiotracer correlated with survival. Focusing on volumetric data, Gallidkis and colleagues[149] found that ^{11}C-MET may be able to show that the volume of recurrent glioblastoma may be underestimated by contrast-enhanced MR imaging. ^{11}C-MET may offer complementary information to MR imaging, which can be helpful for therapeutic planning.

As discussed previously, the major disadvantage of ^{11}C-MET relates to its short half-life of 20 minutes, making it unavailable in PET centers without a cyclotron. ^{18}F-amino acid analogs such as ^{18}F-FDOPA with longer half-lives may be attractive alternatives to ^{11}C-MET. Becherer and colleagues[150] compared ^{18}F-FDOPA with ^{11}C-MET and found that it could serve as an accurate surrogate for ^{11}C-MET in brain tumors. Chen and colleagues[151] examined 81 patients with brain tumors and found that ^{18}F-FDOPA was more sensitive and specific for evaluation of recurrent tumors than ^{18}F-FDG-PET. It may be particularly useful for detection of recurrent low-grade tumors and for differentiating RN from recurrent tumor.

In a retrospective study comparing conventional MR imaging and ^{18}F-FET during routine posttreatment follow-up, ^{18}F-FET had a sensitivity of 100% and specificity of 92.9% to distinguish treatment response versus recurrent glioma, compared with conventional MR imaging's specificity of 50%.[147] Another study using ^{11}C-MET on a patient population that, on average, was almost 7 months after treatment resulted in a sensitivity of 100% and accuracy of 82% to differentiate recurrent glioma and RN, although specificity was 60%.[143] Grosu and colleagues[146] found that ^{18}F-FET and ^{11}C-MET had equal efficacy when performed on the same day, with an equal sensitivity of 91% and specificity of 100%. The lack of congruence

among these studies could be caused by variations in the timing of posttreatment imaging and variations in technique, underscoring the need for a large multicenter trial focusing on PsP. A study of 24 patients with HGG who underwent intracavitary radioimmunotherapy found that nodular foci of uptake of ^{18}F-FET indicated recurrent glioma, as opposed to slightly increased, homogeneous uptake around the resection cavity that seemed to indicate benign, therapy-related changes.[152]

^{18}F-FLT is a newer PET alternative that also shows promise. It is thought to show cellular proliferation by tracking DNA synthesis; however, its analysis can be complicated by the status of the BBB.[153] It seems to be advantageous compared with ^{18}F-FDG in that there is minimal uptake and retention in normal brain tissue.[154] In a prospective study of 25 patients, Chen and colleagues[155] performed side-by-side comparison of ^{18}F-FLT with ^{18}F-FDG in newly diagnosed or treated patients with glioma and found that ^{18}F-FLT may have greater sensitivity than ^{18}F-FDG to detect recurrent glioma, likely secondary to the low background uptake of ^{18}F-FLT in normal brain tissue. ^{18}F-FLT was also better correlated with Ki-67 proliferation index values and was also a better predictor of tumor progression and survival. There were limited data on the specificity of ^{18}F-FLT PET in the differential diagnosis of RN versus tumor because they did not have a case of RN in their study group. A later prospective study by the same group in 19 patients with recurrent gliomas treated with irinotecan and bevacizumab found that ^{18}F-FLT PET responses seemed to be significant predictors of OS and outperformed conventional MR imaging.[156] In LGGs, there is preliminary evidence to suggest that ^{18}F-FET may be able to show metabolic responses earlier than changes seen on MR imaging in patients treated with TMZ. This finding may prove to be significant given the slow growth rate of LGG.[157]

A recent study by Laymon and colleagues[154] investigated treatment response by imaging patients with glioblastoma before, during, and after therapy with voxel-wise analysis of ^{18}F-FLT PET, (^{23}Na) sodium MR imaging, and 3-T MR imaging. Sodium MR imaging may be useful for brain tumor imaging because an increase in intracellular and total ^{23}Na concentration caused by depolarization of the cell membrane precedes increased cell division. However, analysis is complicated because the ^{23}Na signal is a result of a combination of both intracellular and extracellular regions. The investigators found that both ^{18}F-FLT and (^{23}Na) MR imaging were promising for evaluating tumor progression/response and may provide complementary information because, unlike ^{18}F-FLT, ([23]Na) MR imaging is not affected by changes in the BBB.

In tumors, structurally and functionally abnormal microvasculature, impaired ability of oxygen to diffuse through tissues, competition between different regions within a tumor, and decreased oxygen carrying capacity of blood caused by treatment-related or disease-related anemia results in hypoxia.[158] Hypoxia has been linked to tumor progression and treatment resistance, with much attention in the literature devoted to hypoxia within head and neck tumors.[139] ^{18}F-Fluoromisonidazole (MISO) is probably the most widely used PET radiotracer that has been used to quantify hypoxia in tumors.[158,159] Uptake of ^{18}F-MISO has been seen in HGG but not in LGG and a significant relationship was seen between ^{18}F-MISO or ^{18}F-FDG and expression of VEGF-R1 and Ki-67 expression and ^{18}F-MISO.[160] It also seemed to be prognostic of treatment outcomes in most of their patients. Bruehlmeier and colleagues[161] showed that, in 11 patients with various brain tumors, ^{18}F-MISO could depict hypoxic regions in tumors independently of BBB disruption or tumor perfusion. The investigators suggest that the development of hypoxia in glioblastomas may occur regardless of the magnitude of perfusion. There is also some evidence to show that ^{18}F-MISO may be beneficial before surgery and radiotherapy to quantify tumor volume and degree of hypoxia and following therapy to predict outcome.[139] Although the full potential of ^{18}F-MISO has yet to be realized, there is a search for other hypoxia imaging radiotracers because ^{18}F-MISO is not widely available and it also exhibits slow clearance from normoxic tissues. Other radiotracers that are in development include Cu-diacetyl-bis(N4-methylthiosemicarbazone) (^{64}Cu-ATSM), ^{99m}Tc-labeled and ^{68}Ga-labeled metronidazole (MN), ^{99m}Tc-labeled iminodiacetic acid (IDA) derivative of 2-methyl-5-nitroimidazole and 1-(2-[^{18}F] fluoro-1-[hydroxymethyl]ethoxy) methyl-2-nitroimidazole, an ^{18}F-labeled 2-nitroimidazole analog.[158]

MR Spectroscopy

Although different heteronuclei such as sodium ([11]Na) and phosphorus (^{31}P) MR spectroscopy have been used to evaluate brain tumor metabolism, the most common method involves use of proton (^{1}H) MR spectroscopy.[162] [1]H MR spectroscopy is capable of assessing membrane turnover and proliferation (choline), energy homeostasis (creatine), glioneural structures (N-acetyl-aspartate), and necrosis (lactate or lipids).[132] It has been used in both adult and pediatric brain tumor populations to distinguish recurrent tumor from RN. Multiple studies have shown that tumor recurrence can be suggested in the presence of increased Cho signal (ie, Cho levels relative to Cho signal in normal-appearing tissue, Cho/Cr or Cho/NAA ratios), whereas reduced Cho (and Cr) levels suggest RN.[163–171] However, there can be difficulty in determining whether increased choline is caused by membrane production or degradation, which can lead to temporary choline peaks after treatment.[172] False-positive results for recurrent tumor can occur from radiation-induced inflammation, demyelination, or gliosis, whereas false-negatives are typically secondary to partial-volume effects (such as small tumor cell clusters within nonneoplastic tissues).[164] A substantial limitation of MR spectroscopy is its inability to properly evaluate masses composed of mixed tumor and RN.[167,173] The addition of ADC measurements does not seem to improve the ability to distinguish between mixed-tissue versus pure tumor or RN, although it can improve the distinction between pure tumor versus RN.[168,173] The grade of glioma may also influence the accuracy of spectroscopy. A recent study reported that ^{1}H MR spectroscopy seems to be more accurate when predicting tumor recurrence versus RN for LGG, whereas FDG-PET seemed to be more accurate than MR spectroscopy in HGG recurrences.[174] Fink and colleagues[175] recently compared both single-voxel and multivoxel MR spectroscopy in a multiparametric evaluation of patients with suspicion for recurrent glioblastoma using 3-T MR imaging. They found that single-voxel MR spectroscopy parameters could not reliably differentiate tumor recurrence compared with posttreatment effects, whereas multivoxel MR spectroscopy Cho/Cr peak area and Cho/NAA PH ratios seemed to show good diagnostic performance (Fig. 5). The differentiation between PsP and TEP is likely to be challenging in most clinical settings given that both may present with increased choline, decreased NAA, and increased lipid/lactate.[32]

Changes in metabolite signatures may be able to predict changes in tumor volume. A decrease in Cho may suggest response to treatment, whereas stable or increased Cho may indicate progression.[12,170,171,176–180] Increases in Cho/NAA may also predict areas of new contrast enhancement on MR imaging following chemoradiation in patients with glioblastoma.[181] For patients undergoing Gamma knife radiosurgery for recurrent glioblastoma, MR spectroscopy may be able to predict survival.[182] There was significantly shorter survival in patients whose metabolic lesion was outside the Gamma knife

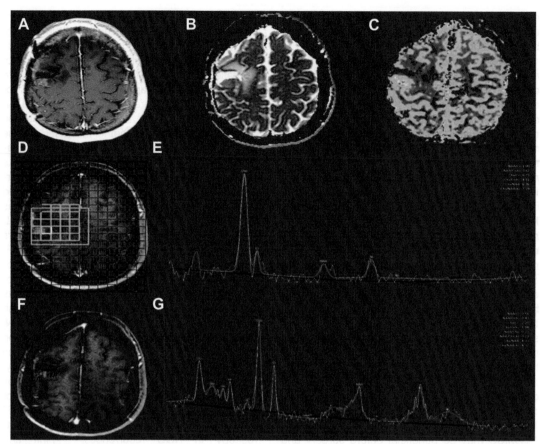

Fig. 5. A 45-year-old woman with right frontal anaplastic oligoastrocytoma status post subtotal resection, followed by external beam radiation therapy completed 7 years before surveillance 3-T MR imaging. Postcontrast axial T1-weighted image shows a new enhancing lesion at the resection site (*A*) with corresponding intermediate to low ADC (*B*). The 3-T DSC and multivoxel MR spectroscopy (TE = 144) acquired 1 week later show marked corresponding CBV increase (*C*) and Cho peak increase (*D, E*) relative to Cr and NAA. Single-voxel MR spectroscopy (TE = 36) acquired during the same session (*F, G*) shows improved metabolic peak resolution compared with multivoxel MR spectroscopy, but Cho/Cr and Cho/NAA ratios (which should be higher at short TE than at long TE) are lower because of greater volume averaging with adjacent tissue. Three weeks after physiologic 3-T MR imaging, surgical reoperation confirmed high-grade glioma recurrence. (*Reproduced from* Fink JR, et al. Comparison of 3 Tesla proton MR spectroscopy, MR perfusion and MR diffusion for distinguishing glioma recurrence from post-treatment effects. J Magn Reson Imaging 2012;35(1):56–63; with permission.)

target compared with those whose lesions were confined to the target. These results suggested that MR spectroscopy could be used to define the Gamma knife target and that alternative forms of therapy such as chemotherapy or surgical resection should be considered in Gamma knife candidates who possessed very large metabolic lesions.

Emerging MR imaging techniques

In addition to the more familiar advanced imaging methods mentioned previously, a few newer imaging methods such as molecular MR imaging and radiogenomics have gained recent attention. A brief overview is provided.

Molecular MR imaging Nuclear medicine techniques such as PET have traditionally been the dominant method of clinical molecular imaging. Although MR imaging has been thought of as a less-than-ideal molecular imaging technique because of its inherently low sensitivity to depict contrast agents (orders of magnitude lower than PET), advances in MR imaging contrast agents have made molecular MR imaging a viable technique.[183]

The functional MR imaging techniques mentioned earlier can generally be thought of as indirect approaches to measuring changes in molecular processes in tissues. However, more direct molecular imaging using MR imaging are in development and have been reviewed recently.[183,184] General approaches to detecting molecular MR imaging probes involve the use of direct detection of a nuclear species that is a component of an imaging probe or indirect detection through the effects of an agent on the large signal from the hydrogen protons in tissue water, either by introducing new pathways for magnetization transfer or altering the water relaxation rate.[184]

The direct approach is most analogous to radionuclear techniques. However, using MR imaging is less sensitive than detecting high-energy photons. The most promising nuclear species without hyperpolarization seems to be ^{19}F (found in perfluorocarbons) because it has the greatest gyromagnetic ratio following hydrogen and so produces stronger signals than any other species at a given field strength and concentration.[184] Also, under normal physiologic conditions, no background fluorine signal exists, and so detection only requires that the signal be greater than ambient noise.

The indirect approach can use either paramagnetic or superparamagnetic (ie, iron oxide nanoparticle) agents that alter T1, T2, or T2* (the basis of conventional MR imaging contrast agents) or manipulation of the water signal magnitude using radiofrequency irradiation to label one species of protons, which then transfers the label to water through magnetization exchange.[183,184] Examples include paramagnetic chemical exchange saturation transfer (PARACEST) and chemical exchange saturation transfer (CEST) agents. Amide proton transfer (APT) MR imaging is a new molecular MR imaging technique based on CEST.[185] APT MR imaging allows indirect detection of the amide proton signals in the backbone of endogenous proteins and peptides. In preclinical work by Zhou and colleagues,[186] APT MR imaging was able to distinguish between viable glioma and RN in rat models. Increased APT signal in tumors is thought to be caused by a highly cellular environment with increased cytosolic protein and peptide content, whereas the decreased APT signal in RN is probably the result of the absence of mobile cytosolic proteins and peptides caused by loss of the cytoplasm.

Radiogenomics The diagnosis of glioblastoma is still primarily based on histopathology and immunohistochemistry. Histologically grouped tumors often similarly display widely variant clinical behavior and methods to better characterize the molecular differences between tumors may improve diagnosis and individualize therapy.[186] High-throughput methods such as microarray analysis of gene expression are now able to provide a wealth of molecular information about cancer. Current conventional imaging techniques are histopathologically based and provide anatomic and morphologic information. Much of the information in MR imaging of a tumor remains unaccounted for and incompletely understood on a molecular level.[186] Radiogenomics is a developing field that seeks to associate specific imaging traits with specific gene expression patterns to gain a better understanding of cellular and molecular disorders.[187] Recent work by Zinn and colleagues,[186] Diehn and colleagues,[187] Pope and colleagues,[190] and Barajas and colleagues[191] has been published examining the relationship between gene expression and its influence on both conventional and physiologic imaging parameters such as edema, contrast enhancement, mass effect, perfusion, and diffusion metrics in glioblastoma.[188–191] In a radiogenomic approach, specific radiological tumor phenotypes referred to as radiophenotypes may serve as surrogates for gene expression to provide an accurate, but noninvasive, diagnosis of tumor subtype and molecular biology.[187]

SUMMARY

Although conventional contrast-enhanced MR imaging remains the standard-of-care imaging method in the posttreatment evaluation of gliomas, recent developments in therapeutic options such as chemoradiation and antiangiogenic agents have caused the neuro-oncology community to rethink traditional imaging criteria. This article highlights the latest RANO Working Group recommendations, with particular attention to PsP and PsR. These recommendations should be viewed as works in progress. As more is learned about the pathophysiology of glioma treatment response, quantitative imaging biomarkers will be validated within this context. There will likely be further refinements and modifications to glioma response criteria, although the lack of technical standardization in image acquisition, postprocessing, and interpretation also need to be addressed.

REFERENCES

1. Wen PY, Kesari S. Malignant gliomas in adults. N Engl J Med 2008;359(5):492–507.
2. Walker MD. Evaluation of BCNU and/or radiotherapy in the treatment of anaplastic gliomas. A cooperative clinical trial. J Neurosurg 1978;49(3): 333–43.
3. Heesters MA. Brain tumor delineation based on CT and MR imaging. Implications for radiotherapy

treatment planning. Strahlenther Onkol 1993; 169(12):729–33.

4. Nieder C. Radiotherapy for high-grade gliomas. Does altered fractionation improve the outcome? Strahlenther Onkol 2004;180(7):401–7.

5. Stupp R. Radiotherapy plus concomitant and adjuvant temozolomide for glioblastoma. N Engl J Med 2005;352(10):987–96.

6. Wong ET. Outcomes and prognostic factors in recurrent glioma patients enrolled onto phase II clinical trials. J Clin Oncol 1999;17(8):2572–8.

7. Lamborn KR. Progression-free survival: an important end point in evaluating therapy for recurrent high-grade gliomas. Neuro Oncol 2008;10(2): 162–70.

8. Macdonald DR. Response criteria for phase II studies of supratentorial malignant glioma. J Clin Oncol 1990;8(7):1277–80.

9. van den Bent MJ. End point assessment in gliomas: novel treatments limit usefulness of classical Macdonald's Criteria. J Clin Oncol 2009; 27(18):2905–8.

10. Vogelbaum MA. Application of novel response/ progression measures for surgically delivered therapies for gliomas: Response Assessment in Neuro-Oncology (RANO) Working Group. Neurosurgery 2012;70(1):234–43 [discussion: 243–4].

11. Wen PY. Updated response assessment criteria for high-grade gliomas: Response Assessment in Neuro-Oncology Working Group. J Clin Oncol 2010;28(11):1963–72.

12. Kumar AJ. Malignant gliomas: MR imaging spectrum of radiation therapy- and chemotherapy-induced necrosis of the brain after treatment. Radiology 2000;217(2):377–84.

13. Henegar MM, Moran CJ, Silbergeld DL. Early postoperative magnetic resonance imaging following nonneoplastic cortical resection. J Neurosurg 1996;84(2):174–9.

14. Finn MA. Transient postictal MRI changes in patients with brain tumors may mimic disease progression. Surg Neurol 2007;67(3):246–50 [discussion: 250].

15. Ulmer S. Clinical and radiographic features of peritumoral infarction following resection of glioblastoma. Neurology 2006;67(9):1668–70.

16. Valk PE, Dillon WP. Radiation injury of the brain. AJNR Am J Neuroradiol 1991;12(1):45–62.

17. Watling CJ. Corticosteroid-induced magnetic resonance imaging changes in patients with recurrent malignant glioma. J Clin Oncol 1994;12(9): 1886–9.

18. Cairncross JG. Steroid-induced CT changes in patients with recurrent malignant glioma. Neurology 1988;38(5):724–6.

19. Brandsma D, van den Bent MJ. Pseudoprogression and pseudoresponse in the treatment of gliomas. Curr Opin Neurol 2009;22(6):633–8.

20. Young RJ. Potential utility of conventional MRI signs in diagnosing pseudoprogression in glioblastoma. Neurology 2011;76(22):1918–24.

21. Lacerda S, Law M. Magnetic resonance perfusion and permeability imaging in brain tumors. Neuroimaging Clin N Am 2009;19(4):527–57.

22. Tofilon PJ, Fike JR. The radioresponse of the central nervous system: a dynamic process. Radiat Res 2000;153(4):357–70.

23. Wong CS, Van der Kogel AJ. Mechanisms of radiation injury to the central nervous system: implications for neuroprotection. Mol Interv 2004;4(5): 273–84.

24. Brandsma D. Clinical features, mechanisms, and management of pseudoprogression in malignant gliomas. Lancet Oncol 2008;9(5):453–61.

25. Lampert PW, Davis RL. Delayed effects of radiation on the human central nervous system; "early" and "late" delayed reactions. Neurology 1964;14: 912–7.

26. Burger PC, BO. The pathology of central nervous system radiation injury. In: LS, Gutin PH, Sheline GE, editors. Radiation injury to the nervous system. New York: Raven; 1991.

27. Clarke JL, Chang S. Pseudoprogression and pseudoresponse: challenges in brain tumor imaging. Curr Neurol Neurosci Rep 2009;9(3):241–6.

28. Hustinx R. PET imaging for differentiating recurrent brain tumor from radiation necrosis. Radiol Clin North Am 2005;43(1):35–47.

29. Siu A. Radiation necrosis following treatment of high grade glioma–a review of the literature and current understanding. Acta Neurochir (Wien) 2012;154(2):191–201 [discussion: 201].

30. Wang S. Evaluation of radiation necrosis and malignant glioma in rat models using diffusion tensor MR imaging. J Neurooncol 2012;107(1):51–60.

31. Brandes AA. Disease progression or pseudoprogression after concomitant radiochemotherapy treatment: pitfalls in neurooncology. Neuro Oncol 2008; 10(3):361–7.

32. Hygino da Cruz LC Jr. Pseudoprogression and pseudoresponse: imaging challenges in the assessment of posttreatment glioma. AJNR Am J Neuroradiol 2011;32(11):1978–85.

33. Fink J, Born D, Chamberlain MC. Pseudoprogression: relevance with respect to treatment of high-grade gliomas. Curr Treat Options Oncol 2011; 12(3):240–52.

34. Brandes AA. MGMT promoter methylation status can predict the incidence and outcome of pseudoprogression after concomitant radiochemotherapy in newly diagnosed glioblastoma patients. J Clin Oncol 2008;26(13):2192–7.

35. Chan DT. Pseudoprogression of malignant glioma in Chinese patients receiving concomitant chemoradiotherapy. Hong Kong Med J 2012;18(3):221–5.

36. Gunjur A. Early post-treatment pseudo-progression amongst glioblastoma multiforme patients treated with radiotherapy and temozolomide: a retrospective analysis. J Med Imaging Radiat Oncol 2011; 55(6):603–10.

37. Pope WB, Young JR, Ellingson BM. Advances in MRI assessment of gliomas and response to anti-VEGF therapy. Curr Neurol Neurosci Rep 2011; 11(3):336–44.

38. Chamberlain MC. Early necrosis following concurrent Temodar and radiotherapy in patients with glioblastoma. J Neurooncol 2007;82(1):81–3.

39. Taal W. Incidence of early pseudo-progression in a cohort of malignant glioma patients treated with chemoirradiation with temozolomide. Cancer 2008;113(2):405–10.

40. de Wit MC. Immediate post-radiotherapy changes in malignant glioma can mimic tumor progression. Neurology 2004;63(3):535–7.

41. Hegi ME. MGMT gene silencing and benefit from temozolomide in glioblastoma. N Engl J Med 2005;352(10):997–1003.

42. Esteller M. Inactivation of the DNA-repair gene MGMT and the clinical response of gliomas to alkylating agents. N Engl J Med 2000;343(19): 1350–4.

43. Hegi ME. Clinical trial substantiates the predictive value of O-6-methylguanine-DNA methyltransferase promoter methylation in glioblastoma patients treated with temozolomide. Clin Cancer Res 2004;10(6):1871–4.

44. Hegi ME. Correlation of O6-methylguanine methyltransferase (MGMT) promoter methylation with clinical outcomes in glioblastoma and clinical strategies to modulate MGMT activity. J Clin Oncol 2008;26(25):4189–99.

45. Goel S. Normalization of the vasculature for treatment of cancer and other diseases. Physiol Rev 2011;91(3):1071–121.

46. Sorensen AG. Increased survival of glioblastoma patients who respond to antiangiogenic therapy with elevated blood perfusion. Cancer Res 2012; 72(2):402–7.

47. Jain RK. Normalizing tumor vasculature with anti-angiogenic therapy: a new paradigm for combination therapy. Nat Med 2001;7(9):987–9.

48. Batchelor TT. AZD2171, a pan-VEGF receptor tyrosine kinase inhibitor, normalizes tumor vasculature and alleviates edema in glioblastoma patients. Cancer Cell 2007;11(1):83–95.

49. Sorensen AG. A "vascular normalization index" as potential mechanistic biomarker to predict survival after a single dose of cediranib in recurrent glioblastoma patients. Cancer Res 2009;69(13): 5296–300.

50. Winkler F. Kinetics of vascular normalization by VEGFR2 blockade governs brain tumor response to radiation: role of oxygenation, angiopoietin-1, and matrix metalloproteinases. Cancer Cell 2004; 6(6):553–63.

51. Jain RK. Normalization of tumor vasculature: an emerging concept in antiangiogenic therapy. Science 2005;307(5706):58–62.

52. Gerstner ER. VEGF inhibitors in the treatment of cerebral edema in patients with brain cancer. Nat Rev Clin Oncol 2009;6(4):229–36.

53. Norden AD. Bevacizumab for recurrent malignant gliomas: efficacy, toxicity, and patterns of recurrence. Neurology 2008;70(10):779–87.

54. Raymond E. Phase II study of imatinib in patients with recurrent gliomas of various histologies: a European Organisation for Research and Treatment of Cancer Brain Tumor Group study. J Clin Oncol 2008;26(28):4659–65.

55. Rubenstein JL. Anti-VEGF antibody treatment of glioblastoma prolongs survival but results in increased vascular cooption. Neoplasia 2000;2(4): 306–14.

56. Paez-Ribes M. Antiangiogenic therapy elicits malignant progression of tumors to increased local invasion and distant metastasis. Cancer Cell 2009; 15(3):220–31.

57. Bergers G, Hanahan D. Modes of resistance to anti-angiogenic therapy. Nat Rev Cancer 2008; 8(8):592–603.

58. Jain RK. Biomarkers of response and resistance to antiangiogenic therapy. Nat Rev Clin Oncol 2009; 6(6):327–38.

59. Pope WB, Hessel C. Response assessment in neuro-oncology criteria: implementation challenges in multicenter neuro-oncology trials. AJNR Am J Neuroradiol 2011;32(5):794–7.

60. Forsyth PA. Radiation necrosis or glioma recurrence: is computer-assisted stereotactic biopsy useful? J Neurosurg 1995;82(3):436–44.

61. Tihan T. Prognostic value of detecting recurrent glioblastoma multiforme in surgical specimens from patients after radiotherapy: should pathology evaluation alter treatment decisions? Hum Pathol 2006;37(3):272–82.

62. van den Bent MJ. Response assessment in neuro-oncology (a report of the RANO group): assessment of outcome in trials of diffuse low-grade gliomas. Lancet Oncol 2011;12(6):583–93.

63. Mason WP, Krol GS, DeAngelis LM. Low-grade oligodendroglioma responds to chemotherapy. Neurology 1996;46(1):203–7.

64. Pallud J. Prognostic significance of imaging contrast enhancement for WHO grade II gliomas. Neuro Oncol 2009;11(2):176–82.

65. Danchaivijitr N. Low-grade gliomas: do changes in rCBV measurements at longitudinal perfusion-weighted MR imaging predict malignant transformation? Radiology 2008;247(1):170–8.

66. Stege EM. Successful treatment of low-grade oligodendroglial tumors with a chemotherapy regimen of procarbazine, lomustine, and vincristine. Cancer 2005;103(4):802–9.

67. Essig M. Perfusion MRI: the five most frequently asked technical questions. AJR Am J Roentgenol 2013;200(1):24–34.

68. Cha S. Intracranial mass lesions: dynamic contrast-enhanced susceptibility-weighted echo-planar perfusion MR imaging. Radiology 2002;223(1):11–29.

69. Cha S. Update on brain tumor imaging: from anatomy to physiology. AJNR Am J Neuroradiol 2006;27(3):475–87.

70. Barajas RF Jr. Differentiation of recurrent glioblastoma multiforme from radiation necrosis after external beam radiation therapy with dynamic susceptibility-weighted contrast-enhanced perfusion MR imaging. Radiology 2009;253(2):486–96.

71. Hu LS. Relative cerebral blood volume values to differentiate high-grade glioma recurrence from posttreatment radiation effect: direct correlation between image-guided tissue histopathology and localized dynamic susceptibility-weighted contrast-enhanced perfusion MR imaging measurements. AJNR Am J Neuroradiol 2009;30(3):552–8.

72. Sugahara T. Posttherapeutic intraaxial brain tumor: the value of perfusion-sensitive contrast-enhanced MR imaging for differentiating tumor recurrence from nonneoplastic contrast-enhancing tissue. AJNR Am J Neuroradiol 2000;21(5):901–9.

73. Hopewell JW. Microvasculature and radiation damage. Recent Results Cancer Res 1993;130: 1–16.

74. Wesseling P, Ruiter DJ, Burger PC. Angiogenesis in brain tumors; pathobiological and clinical aspects. J Neurooncol 1997;32(3):253–65.

75. Oh BC. Stereotactic radiosurgery: adjacent tissue injury and response after high-dose single fraction radiation: part I–Histology, imaging, and molecular events. Neurosurgery 2007;60(1):31–44 [discussion: 44–5].

76. Hoefnagels FW. Radiological progression of cerebral metastases after radiosurgery: assessment of perfusion MRI for differentiating between necrosis and recurrence. J Neurol 2009;256(6):878–87.

77. Hu LS. Optimized preload leakage-correction methods to improve the diagnostic accuracy of dynamic susceptibility-weighted contrast-enhanced perfusion MR imaging in posttreatment gliomas. AJNR Am J Neuroradiol 2010;31(1):40–8.

78. Ozsunar Y. Glioma recurrence versus radiation necrosis? A pilot comparison of arterial spin-labeled, dynamic susceptibility contrast enhanced MRI, and FDG-PET imaging. Acad Radiol 2010; 17(3):282–90.

79. Mangla R. Changes in relative cerebral blood volume 1 month after radiation-temozolomide therapy can help predict overall survival in patients with glioblastoma. Radiology 2010;256(2):575–84.

80. Kong DS. Diagnostic dilemma of pseudoprogression in the treatment of newly diagnosed glioblastomas: the role of assessing relative cerebral blood flow volume and oxygen-6-methylguanine-DNA methyltransferase promoter methylation status. AJNR Am J Neuroradiol 2011;32(2):382–7.

81. Tsien C. Parametric response map as an imaging biomarker to distinguish progression from pseudo-progression in high-grade glioma. J Clin Oncol 2010;28(13):2293–9.

82. Baek HJ. Percent change of perfusion skewness and kurtosis: a potential imaging biomarker for early treatment response in patients with newly diagnosed glioblastomas. Radiology 2012;264(3): 834–43.

83. Hu LS. Reevaluating the imaging definition of tumor progression: perfusion MRI quantifies recurrent glioblastoma tumor fraction, pseudoprogression, and radiation necrosis to predict survival. Neuro Oncol 2012;14(7):919–30.

84. Galban CJ. The parametric response map is an imaging biomarker for early cancer treatment outcome. Nat Med 2009;15(5):572–6.

85. Radbruch A. Comment to: parametric response map as an imaging biomarker to distinguish progression from pseudoprogression in high-grade glioma: pitfalls in perfusion MRI in brain tumors: Tsien C, Galban CJ, Chenevert TL, Johnson TD, Hamstra DA, Sundgren PC, Junck L, Meyer CR, Rehemtulla A, Lawrence T, Ross BD. J Clin Oncol. 2010;28:2293-9. Clin Neuroradiol 2010;20(3):183–4.

86. Gahramanov S. Potential for differentiation of pseudoprogression from true tumor progression with dynamic susceptibility-weighted contrast-enhanced magnetic resonance imaging using feru-moxytol vs. gadoteridol: a pilot study. Int J Radiat Oncol Biol Phys 2011;79(2):514–23.

87. Paulson ES, Schmainda KM. Comparison of dynamic susceptibility-weighted contrast-enhanced MR methods: recommendations for measuring relative cerebral blood volume in brain tumors. Radiology 2008;249(2):601–13.

88. Sawlani RN. Glioblastoma: a method for predicting response to antiangiogenic chemotherapy by using MR perfusion imaging–pilot study. Radiology 2010;255(2):622–8.

89. Law M. Gliomas: predicting time to progression or survival with cerebral blood volume measurements at dynamic susceptibility-weighted contrast-enhanced perfusion MR imaging. Radiology 2008;247(2):490–8.

90. Cha S. Differentiation of low-grade oligodendrogliomas from low-grade astrocytomas by using quantitative blood-volume measurements derived

from dynamic susceptibility contrast-enhanced MR imaging. AJNR Am J Neuroradiol 2005;26(2): 266–73.

91. Yankeelov TE, Gore JC. Dynamic contrast enhanced magnetic resonance imaging in oncology: theory, data acquisition, analysis, and examples. Curr Med Imaging Rev 2009;3(2):91–107.

92. Tofts PS. Estimating kinetic parameters from dynamic contrast-enhanced T(1)-weighted MRI of a diffusable tracer: standardized quantities and symbols. J Magn Reson Imaging 1999;10(3): 223–32.

93. Paldino MJ, Barboriak DP. Fundamentals of quantitative dynamic contrast-enhanced MR imaging. Magn Reson Imaging Clin N Am 2009;17(2): 277–89.

94. Jackson A. Reproducibility of quantitative dynamic contrast-enhanced MRI in newly presenting glioma. Br J Radiol 2003;76(903):153–62.

95. Gribbestad IS, GK, Nilsen G. An introduction to dynamic contrast-enhanced MRI in oncology. In: BD, Jackson A, Parker GJ, editors. Dynamic contrast-enhanced MRI in oncology, vol. 1, 1st edition. Berlin, Heidelberg (NY): Springer; 2005.

96. Hazle JD. Dynamic imaging of intracranial lesions using fast spin-echo imaging: differentiation of brain tumors and treatment effects. J Magn Reson Imaging 1997;7(6):1084–93.

97. Bisdas S. Distinguishing recurrent high-grade gliomas from radiation injury: a pilot study using dynamic contrast-enhanced MR imaging. Acad Radiol 2011;18(5):575–83.

98. Narang J. Differentiating treatment-induced necrosis from recurrent/progressive brain tumor using nonmodel-based semiquantitative indices derived from dynamic contrast-enhanced T1-weighted MR perfusion. Neuro Oncol 2011;13(9): 1037–46.

99. Bedekar D, Jensen T, Schmainda KM. Standardization of relative cerebral blood volume (rCBV) image maps for ease of both inter- and intrapatient comparisons. Magn Reson Med 2010;64(3): 907–13.

100. Pope WB. Apparent diffusion coefficient histogram analysis stratifies progression-free and overall survival in patients with recurrent GBM treated with bevacizumab: a multi-center study. J Neurooncol 2012;108(3):491–8.

101. Padhani AR. Diffusion-weighted magnetic resonance imaging as a cancer biomarker: consensus and recommendations. Neoplasia 2009;11(2):102–25.

102. Lee JH, Springer CS Jr. Effects of equilibrium exchange on diffusion-weighted NMR signals: the diffusigraphic "shutter-speed". Magn Reson Med 2003;49(3):450–8.

103. Mardor Y. Early detection of response to radiation therapy in patients with brain malignancies using conventional and high b-value diffusion-weighted magnetic resonance imaging. J Clin Oncol 2003; 21(6):1094–100.

104. Chenevert TL. Diffusion magnetic resonance imaging: an early surrogate marker of therapeutic efficacy in brain tumors. J Natl Cancer Inst 2000; 92(24):2029–36.

105. Sijens PE. Diffusion tensor imaging and chemical shift imaging assessment of heterogeneity in low grade glioma under temozolomide chemotherapy. Cancer Invest 2007;25(8):706–10.

106. Hamstra DA. Evaluation of the functional diffusion map as an early biomarker of time-to-progression and overall survival in high-grade glioma. Proc Natl Acad Sci U S A 2005;102(46):16759–64.

107. Chenevert TL, McKeever PE, Ross BD. Monitoring early response of experimental brain tumors to therapy using diffusion magnetic resonance imaging. Clin Cancer Res 1997;3(9):1457–66.

108. Moffat BA. Functional diffusion map: a noninvasive MRI biomarker for early stratification of clinical brain tumor response. Proc Natl Acad Sci U S A 2005; 102(15):5524–9.

109. Lee KC. Dynamic imaging of emerging resistance during cancer therapy. Cancer Res 2006;66(9): 4687–92.

110. Ellingson BM. Graded functional diffusion map-defined characteristics of apparent diffusion coefficients predict overall survival in recurrent glioblastoma treated with bevacizumab. Neuro Oncol 2011;13(10):1151–61.

111. Le Bihan D. The 'wet mind': water and functional neuroimaging. Phys Med Biol 2007;52:R57–90.

112. Lee KC. Noninvasive molecular imaging sheds light on the synergy between 5-fluorouracil and TRAIL/Apo2L for cancer therapy. Clin Cancer Res 2007;13(6):1839–46.

113. Guo AC. Lymphomas and high-grade astrocytomas: comparison of water diffusibility and histologic characteristics. Radiology 2002;224(1):177–83.

114. Stadlbauer A. Gliomas: histopathologic evaluation of changes in directionality and magnitude of water diffusion at diffusion-tensor MR imaging. Radiology 2006;240(3):803–10.

115. Goebell E. Low-grade and anaplastic gliomas: differences in architecture evaluated with diffusion-tensor MR imaging. Radiology 2006;239(1):217–22.

116. Sundgren PC. Differentiation of recurrent brain tumor versus radiation injury using diffusion tensor imaging in patients with new contrast-enhancing lesions. Magn Reson Imaging 2006;24(9):1131–42.

117. Hein PA. Diffusion-weighted imaging in the follow-up of treated high-grade gliomas: tumor recurrence versus radiation injury. AJNR Am J Neuroradiol 2004;25(2):201–9.

118. Asao C. Diffusion-weighted imaging of radiation-induced brain injury for differentiation from tumor

recurrence. AJNR Am J Neuroradiol 2005;26(6): 1455–60.

119. Kashimura H. Diffusion tensor imaging for differentiation of recurrent brain tumor and radiation necrosis after radiotherapy–three case reports. Clin Neurol Neurosurg 2007;109(1):106–10.

120. Paldino MJ. A change in the apparent diffusion coefficient after treatment with bevacizumab is associated with decreased survival in patients with recurrent glioblastoma multiforme. Br J Radiol 2012;85(1012):382–9.

121. Jain R. Imaging response criteria for recurrent gliomas treated with bevacizumab: role of diffusion weighted imaging as an imaging biomarker. J Neurooncol 2010;96(3):423–31.

122. Pope WB. Recurrent glioblastoma multiforme: ADC histogram analysis predicts response to bevacizumab treatment. Radiology 2009;252(1):182–9.

123. Moffat BA. The functional diffusion map: an imaging biomarker for the early prediction of cancer treatment outcome. Neoplasia 2006;8(4):259–67.

124. Hamstra DA. Functional diffusion map as an early imaging biomarker for high-grade glioma: correlation with conventional radiologic response and overall survival. J Clin Oncol 2008;26(20):3387–94.

125. Ellingson BM. Validation of functional diffusion maps (fDMs) as a biomarker for human glioma cellularity. J Magn Reson Imaging 2010;31(3):538–48.

126. Ellingson BM. Nonlinear registration of diffusion-weighted images improves clinical sensitivity of functional diffusion maps in recurrent glioblastoma treated with bevacizumab. Magn Reson Med 2012; 67(1):237–45.

127. Gupta A. Isolated diffusion restriction precedes the development of enhancing tumor in a subset of patients with glioblastoma. AJNR Am J Neuroradiol 2011;32(7):1301–6.

128. Gerstner ER, Frosch MP, Batchelor TT. Diffusion magnetic resonance imaging detects pathologically confirmed, nonenhancing tumor progression in a patient with recurrent glioblastoma receiving bevacizumab. J Clin Oncol 2010;28(6):e91–3.

129. Rieger J. Bevacizumab-induced diffusion-restricted lesions in malignant glioma patients. J Neurooncol 2010;99(1):49–56.

130. Mong S. Persistent diffusion-restricted lesions in bevacizumab-treated malignant gliomas are associated with improved survival compared with matched controls. AJNR Am J Neuroradiol 2012; 33(9):1763–70.

131. Smith JS. Serial diffusion-weighted magnetic resonance imaging in cases of glioma: distinguishing tumor recurrence from postresection injury. J Neurosurg 2005;103(3):428–38.

132. Dhermain FG. Advanced MRI and PET imaging for assessment of treatment response in patients with gliomas. Lancet Neurol 2010;9(9):906–20.

133. Patronas NJ. Work in progress: [18F] fluorodeoxyglucose and positron emission tomography in the evaluation of radiation necrosis of the brain. Radiology 1982;144(4):885–9.

134. Di Chiro G. Cerebral necrosis after radiotherapy and/or intraarterial chemotherapy for brain tumors: PET and neuropathologic studies. AJR Am J Roentgenol 1988;150(1):189–97.

135. Doyle WK. Differentiation of cerebral radiation necrosis from tumor recurrence by [18F]FDG and 82Rb positron emission tomography. J Comput Assist Tomogr 1987;11(4):563–70.

136. Wong TZ, van der Westhuizen GJ, Coleman RE. Positron emission tomography imaging of brain tumors. Neuroimaging Clin N Am 2002;12(4): 615–26.

137. Ricci PE. Differentiating recurrent tumor from radiation necrosis: time for re-evaluation of positron emission tomography? AJNR Am J Neuroradiol 1998;19(3):407–13.

138. Chao ST. The sensitivity and specificity of FDG PET in distinguishing recurrent brain tumor from radionecrosis in patients treated with stereotactic radiosurgery. Int J Cancer 2001;96(3):191–7.

139. Gulyas B, Halldin C. New PET radiopharmaceuticals beyond FDG for brain tumor imaging. Q J Nucl Med Mol Imaging 2012;56(2):173–90.

140. Nihashi T, Dahabreh IJ, Terasawa T. Diagnostic accuracy of PET for recurrent glioma diagnosis: a meta-analysis. AJNR Am J Neuroradiol 2012. [Epub ahead of print].

141. Thiel A. Enhanced accuracy in differential diagnosis of radiation necrosis by positron emission tomography-magnetic resonance imaging coregistration: technical case report. Neurosurgery 2000; 46(1):232–4.

142. Terakawa Y. Diagnostic accuracy of 11C-methionine PET for differentiation of recurrent brain tumors from radiation necrosis after radiotherapy. J Nucl Med 2008;49(5):694–9.

143. Tsuyuguchi N. Methionine positron emission tomography for differentiation of recurrent brain tumor and radiation necrosis after stereotactic radiosurgery–in malignant glioma. Ann Nucl Med 2004;18(4):291–6.

144. Van Laere K. Direct comparison of 18F-FDG and 11C-methionine PET in suspected recurrence of glioma: sensitivity, inter-observer variability and prognostic value. Eur J Nucl Med Mol Imaging 2005;32(1):39–51.

145. Mehrkens JH. The positive predictive value of O-(2-[18F]fluoroethyl)-L-tyrosine (FET) PET in the diagnosis of a glioma recurrence after multimodal treatment. J Neurooncol 2008;88(1):27–35.

146. Grosu AL. An interindividual comparison of O-(2-[18F]fluoroethyl)-L-tyrosine (FET)- and L-[methyl-11C]methionine (MET)-PET in patients with brain

gliomas and metastases. Int J Radiat Oncol Biol Phys 2011;81(4):1049–58.

147. Rachinger W. Positron emission tomography with O-(2-[18F]fluoroethyl)-L-tyrosine versus magnetic resonance imaging in the diagnosis of recurrent gliomas. Neurosurgery 2005;57(3):505–11 [discussion: 505–11].

148. Potzi C. [11C] methionine and [18F] fluorodeoxyglucose PET in the follow-up of glioblastoma multiforme. J Neurooncol 2007;84(3):305–14.

149. Galldiks N. Volumetry of [(11)C]-methionine PET uptake and MRI contrast enhancement in patients with recurrent glioblastoma multiforme. Eur J Nucl Med Mol Imaging 2010;37(1):84–92.

150. Becherer A. Brain tumour imaging with PET: a comparison between [18F]fluorodopa and [11C]methionine. Eur J Nucl Med Mol Imaging 2003;30(11):1561–7.

151. Chen W. 18F-FDOPA PET imaging of brain tumors: comparison study with 18F-FDG PET and evaluation of diagnostic accuracy. J Nucl Med 2006; 47(6):904–11.

152. Popperl G. Serial O-(2-[(18)F]fluoroethyl)-L: -tyrosine PET for monitoring the effects of intracavitary radioimmunotherapy in patients with malignant glioma. Eur J Nucl Med Mol Imaging 2006;33(7): 792–800.

153. Muzi M. Kinetic analysis of 3'-deoxy-3'-18F-fluorothymidine in patients with gliomas. J Nucl Med 2006;47(10):1612–21.

154. Laymon CM. Combined imaging biomarkers for therapy evaluation in glioblastoma multiforme: correlating sodium MRI and F-18 FLT PET on a voxel-wise basis. Magn Reson Imaging 2012; 30(9):1268–78.

155. Chen W. Imaging proliferation in brain tumors with 18F-FLT PET: comparison with 18F-FDG. J Nucl Med 2005;46(6):945–52.

156. Chen W. Predicting treatment response of malignant gliomas to bevacizumab and irinotecan by imaging proliferation with [18F] fluorothymidine positron emission tomography: a pilot study. J Clin Oncol 2007;25(30):4714–21.

157. Wyss M. Early metabolic responses in temozolomide treated low-grade glioma patients. J Neurooncol 2009;95(1):87–93.

158. Mendichovszky I, Jackson A. Imaging hypoxia in gliomas. Br J Radiol 2011;84(2):S145–58.

159. Rasey JS. Quantifying regional hypoxia in human tumors with positron emission tomography of [18F] fluoromisonidazole: a pretherapy study of 37 patients. Int J Radiat Oncol Biol Phys 1996;36(2):417–28.

160. Cher LM. Correlation of hypoxic cell fraction and angiogenesis with glucose metabolic rate in gliomas using 18F-fluoromisonidazole, 18F-FDG PET, and immunohistochemical studies. J Nucl Med 2006;47(3):410–8.

161. Bruehlmeier M. Assessment of hypoxia and perfusion in human brain tumors using PET with 18F-fluoromisonidazole and 15O-H2O. J Nucl Med 2004; 45(11):1851–9.

162. Horska A, Barker PB. Imaging of brain tumors: MR spectroscopy and metabolic imaging. Neuroimaging Clin N Am 2010;20(3):293–310.

163. Schlemmer HP. Differentiation of radiation necrosis from tumor progression using proton magnetic resonance spectroscopy. Neuroradiology 2002; 44(3):216–22.

164. Schlemmer HP. Proton MR spectroscopic evaluation of suspicious brain lesions after stereotactic radiotherapy. AJNR Am J Neuroradiol 2001;22(7): 1316–24.

165. Weybright P. Differentiation between brain tumor recurrence and radiation injury using MR spectroscopy. AJR Am J Roentgenol 2005;185(6):1471–6.

166. Zeng QS. Multivoxel 3D proton MR spectroscopy in the distinction of recurrent glioma from radiation injury. J Neurooncol 2007;84(1):63–9.

167. Rock JP. Correlations between magnetic resonance spectroscopy and image-guided histopathology, with special attention to radiation necrosis. Neurosurgery 2002;51(4):912–9 [discussion: 919–20].

168. Zeng QS. Distinction between recurrent glioma and radiation injury using magnetic resonance spectroscopy in combination with diffusion-weighted imaging. Int J Radiat Oncol Biol Phys 2007;68(1): 151–8.

169. Preul MC. Magnetic resonance spectroscopy guided brain tumor resection: differentiation between recurrent glioma and radiation change in two diagnostically difficult cases. Can J Neurol Sci 1998;25(1):13–22.

170. Taylor JS. Clinical value of proton magnetic resonance spectroscopy for differentiating recurrent or residual brain tumor from delayed cerebral necrosis. Int J Radiat Oncol Biol Phys 1996;36(5):1251–61.

171. Wald LL. Serial proton magnetic resonance spectroscopy imaging of glioblastoma multiforme after brachytherapy. J Neurosurg 1997;87(4):525–34.

172. Nakajima T. Differential diagnosis between radiation necrosis and glioma progression using sequential proton magnetic resonance spectroscopy and methionine positron emission tomography. Neurol Med Chir (Tokyo) 2009;49(9):394–401.

173. Rock JP. Associations among magnetic resonance spectroscopy, apparent diffusion coefficients, and image-guided histopathology with special attention to radiation necrosis. Neurosurgery 2004;54(5): 1111–7 [discussion: 1117–9].

174. Imani F. Comparison of proton magnetic resonance spectroscopy with fluorine-18 2-fluorodeoxyglucose positron emission tomography for assessment of brain tumor progression. J Neuroimaging 2012;22(2):184–90.

175. Fink JR. Comparison of 3 Tesla proton MR spectroscopy, MR perfusion and MR diffusion for distinguishing glioma recurrence from posttreatment effects. J Magn Reson Imaging 2012;35(1):56–63.

176. Sijens PE. Hydrogen magnetic resonance spectroscopy follow-up after radiation therapy of human brain cancer. Unexpected inverse correlation between the changes in tumor choline level and post-gadolinium magnetic resonance imaging contrast. Invest Radiol 1995;30(12):738–44.

177. Heesters MA. Localized proton spectroscopy of inoperable brain gliomas. Response to radiation therapy. J Neurooncol 1993;17(1):27–35.

178. Lazareff JA, Gupta RK, Alger J. Variation of post-treatment H-MRSI choline intensity in pediatric gliomas. J Neurooncol 1999;41(3):291–8.

179. Graves EE. Serial proton MR spectroscopic imaging of recurrent malignant gliomas after gamma knife radiosurgery. AJNR Am J Neuroradiol 2001;22(4):613–24.

180. Lichy MP. Follow-up gliomas after radiotherapy: 1H MR spectroscopic imaging for increasing diagnostic accuracy. Neuroradiology 2005;47(11):826–34.

181. Laprie A. Proton magnetic resonance spectroscopic imaging in newly diagnosed glioblastoma: predictive value for the site of postradiotherapy relapse in a prospective longitudinal study. Int J Radiat Oncol Biol Phys 2008;70(3):773–81.

182. Nelson SJ, Vigneron DB, Dillon WP. Serial evaluation of patients with brain tumors using volume MRI and 3D 1H MRSI. NMR Biomed 1999;12(3):123–38.

183. Kircher MF, Willmann JK. Molecular body imaging: MR imaging, CT, and US. Part I. Principles. Radiology 2012;263(3):633–43.

184. Gore JC. Magnetic resonance in the era of molecular imaging of cancer. Magn Reson Imaging 2011;29(5):587–600.

185. Ward KM, Aletras AH, Balaban RS. A new class of contrast agents for MRI based on proton chemical exchange dependent saturation transfer (CEST). J Magn Reson 2000;143(1):79–87.

186. Zhou J. Differentiation between glioma and radiation necrosis using molecular magnetic resonance imaging of endogenous proteins and peptides. Nat Med 2011;17(1):130–4.

187. Diehn M. Identification of noninvasive imaging surrogates for brain tumor gene-expression modules. Proc Natl Acad Sci U S A 2008;105(13):5213–8.

188. Rutman AM, Kuo MD. Radiogenomics: creating a link between molecular diagnostics and diagnostic imaging. Eur J Radiol 2009;70(2):232–41.

189. Zinn PO. Radiogenomic mapping of edema/cellular invasion MRI-phenotypes in glioblastoma multiforme. PLoS One 2011;6(10):e25451.

190. Pope WB. Relationship between gene expression and enhancement in glioblastoma multiforme: exploratory DNA microarray analysis. Radiology 2008;249(1):268–77.

191. Barajas RF Jr. Glioblastoma multiforme regional genetic and cellular expression patterns: influence on anatomic and physiologic MR imaging. Radiology 2010;254(2):564–76.

Clinical Applications of Functional MR Imaging

Artem S. Belyaev, BA[a], Kyung K. Peck, PhD[a,b],
Nicole M. Petrovich Brennan, BA[a], Andrei I. Holodny, MD[c],*

KEYWORDS

- Functional MRI • Neuroanatomy • Motor and language function
- Paradigm delivery and modification

KEY POINTS

- The use of functional magnetic resonance (fMR) imaging in the preoperative setting allows neurosurgeons to identify the location of patient-specific eloquent cortices adjacent to brain tumors with a high degree of certainty.
- fMR imaging helps neurosurgeons plan the operation and maximize the resection of the lesion while at the same time avoiding the adjacent eloquent cortex, thus, diminishing neurologic complications, including motor or speech function.
- Good patient performance is very important to achieve optimal fMR imaging results. Patients with neurologic deficits may need to have the paradigms modified.
- The blood oxygenation level–dependent fMR imaging method has several limitations that can make it difficult to acquire consistent and accurate data or to correctly interpret images. Knowledge of these pitfalls and artifacts will allow the radiologist to optimize the performance and interpretation of the fMR imaging scans.

IMPORTANCE OF FUNCTIONAL MAGNETIC RESONANCE IMAGING

The main clinical application of functional magnetic resonance (fMR) imaging has been in preoperative brain tumor surgery planning. In brain surgery, it is essential to maximize the resection of the lesion (tumor or arteriovenous malformation) while at the same time avoiding the adjacent eloquent cortex. An eloquent cortex is defined as an area of gray matter essential for performing specific functions, such as sensation; movement; speech; vision; and higher cortical function, including memory.

Traditionally, before the advent of fMR imaging, the eloquent cortices were identified intraoperatively by physiologic methods, such as electrocorticography or somatosensory-evoked potentials. However, direct cortical stimulation has several drawbacks. First, this procedure requires a craniotomy and carries associated risks. Cortical mapping is restricted to the exposed surface of the brain; as a result, the cortex in the deep sulci cannot be adequately mapped. Also, cortical mapping occurs following a craniotomy, with the brain exposed, when patients are brought out of anesthesia. This mapping is known as *awake mapping*. In this setting, patients may have difficulty cooperating with task performance during cortical stimulation, especially when mapping higher function, such as language.

The authors have nothing to disclose.
[a] Functional MRI Laboratory, Department of Radiology, Memorial Sloan-Kettering Cancer Center, 1275 York Avenue, New York, NY 10065, USA; [b] Functional MRI Laboratory, Department of Medical Physics and Radiology, Memorial Sloan-Kettering Cancer Center, 1275 York Avenue, New York, NY 10065, USA; [c] Department of Radiology, Memorial Sloan-Kettering Cancer Center, Weill Medical College of Cornell University, 1275 York Avenue, New York, NY 10065, USA
* Corresponding author.
E-mail address: holodnya@mskcc.org

mri.theclinics.com

Performing preoperative fMR imaging, however, has several distinct advantages. First, preoperative fMR imaging does not require the use radioisotopes like positron emission tomography, which means that patients can be scanned multiple times without risk before the surgery. Second, using specific functional tasks decided by the location of the tumor, fMR imaging could generate cortical activity maps showing activated voxels adjacent to the tumor. With the meaningful functional maps, neurosurgeons can decide whether to perform a resection, biopsy, or not to operate at all. Thus, fMR imaging can help avoid an unnecessary craniotomy. Third, fMR imaging can elucidate whether the lesion is ipsilateral or contralateral to patients' dominant language areas. If one can establish with a high degree of certainty that the lesion is contralateral to the dominant language areas, then the neurosurgeon can avoid awake mapping. Fourth, preoperative fMR imaging may influence the trajectory that a surgeon will take for resecting the tumor to bypass an important functional area and maximize tumor resection[1-3] while minimizing damage to surrounding areas. However, it should be stressed that fMR imaging does not eliminate the need for intraoperative cortical mapping. If the tumor involves or is adjacent to the motor cortex or the language areas, the surgeon will most likely have to resort to cortical mapping to optimize the resection and avoid iatrogenic injury.

BASIC FMR IMAGING PRINCIPLES

Blood oxygenation level–dependent (BOLD) fMR imaging, discovered by Seiji Ogawa,[4] is a brain-mapping technique using oxyhemoglobin and deoxyhemoglobin in the blood vessels as an endogenous contrast agent to generate functional activation maps. BOLD fMR imaging is based on the following principle: an increase in neuronal activity causes an increase in the local oxygen extraction from the blood because of an increase of the cerebral metabolic rate of oxygen. This increase leads to an increase in paramagnetic deoxyhemoglobin, which drops the signal intensity. However, after several seconds, neuronal activity also causes an increase in cerebral blood flow (CBF) and cerebral blood volume, which leads to an increase in the flow of oxygenated blood and a consequential increase in oxyhemoglobin. For yet unknown reasons, the amount of oxygenated blood that arrives to support the active neurons far exceeds the metabolic need. This overcompensation of oxyhemoglobin leads to a reduction in the ratio of deoxyhemoglobin to oxyhemoglobin, which is measureable and is the basis for the BOLD fMR imaging signal.[5-8]

NEUROANATOMY (FUNCTIONAL AREAS)
Motor

The primary motor cortex (M1) is involved in performing movement and is located in the posterior portion of the frontal lobe in the precentral gyrus. The motor and sensory systems both have a topographic organization, which means that each portion of the body has a specific location on the cortex. The foot and leg are represented along the interhemispheric fissure, the hand lateral to that of the foot and leg, and the tongue and face at the most lateral level (**Fig. 1**). The motor hand region of the precentral gyrus can be identified in

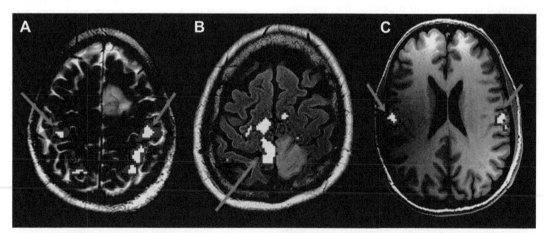

Fig. 1. BOLD fMR imaging of motor homunculus. Identification of the (*A*) hand, (*B*) foot, and (*C*) tongue motor homunculi in the motor cortex in patients with brain tumors (*arrows*). The patients performed a bilateral finger tapping, foot movement, and tongue movement tasks, respectively. The red and yellow areas depict the localization of where changes in the BOLD fMR imaging signal correlated to each functional task to a statistically significant degree ($P<.0001$).

the axial plane as a knoblike structure that is shaped like an upside down (or inverse) omega (Ω) (**Fig. 2**).[9]

The supplementary motor area (SMA) is involved in motor planning and organization.[10,11] Its location is on the midline surface of each hemisphere anterior to the primary motor cortex leg representation. The SMA consists of 2 parts: the rostral (pre-SMA) and the caudal (SMA proper). The SMA proper, anatomically closer to primary motor and sensory areas, is involved in sensory, motor planning, and word articulation. The main functions of pre-SMA are cognitive tasks and language.[10–16] Recently, Peck and colleagues[11] showed that a central SMA between the rostral and caudal SMA can be resolved using simultaneous motor and language functional tasks.

The primary somatosensory cortex, the main sensory receptive area for the sense of touch, is located in the postcentral gyrus, a prominent structure in anterior aspect of the parietal lobe of the human brain. The organization of the sensory homunculus parallels the organization of the motor homunculus.

Language

In most right-handed individuals, language function is predominantly located in the left hemisphere. However, left-handed people are more likely to be codominant (language function seen in both hemispheres) or, in rare cases, right-hemisphere dominant.[17–19]

Language can be subdivided into productive and receptive areas or frontal and temporoparietal areas (**Fig. 3**).

The frontal (productive or Broca) language area is responsible for the expressive component of language and is located in the inferolateral portion of the left frontal lobe. The Broca area contains 2 main parts: pars opercularis and pars triangularis of the inferior frontal gyrus (**Fig. 4**). However, these subdivisions are not particularly relevant in clinical practice because the inferior frontal operculum as a whole is traditionally considered eloquent. The pars triangularis is located in the anterior portion of Broca area. The pars opercularis is located in the posterior region of the Broca area. Damage to the Broca area can result in telegraphic, dysarthric, nonfluent speech; semantic and phonemic paraphasia; or even mutism.

The dominant receptive speech area (Wernicke area) resides mostly in the posterior superior temporal gyrus of the left hemisphere just posterior to the primary auditory gyrus. The Wernicke area is associated with the comprehension of language. Damage to this region may result in fluent aphasia; semantic, phonemic paraphasia; circumlocutions; and word-finding difficulty.

Secondary language areas include the middle frontal gyrus, the supplementary motor area, the insula, and the supramarginal and angular gyri. The middle frontal gyrus–premotor area, is a large area located just superior to the Broca area. Its function includes verbal working memory. Damage produces varied deficits ranging from nothing to dysarthria and anomia. The SMA is located in the superior frontal gyrus and is delimited posteriorly by the foot motor area. Damage to the anterior, language portion of the SMA causes a syndrome characterized by paucity of speech and occasionally mutism. However, patients often recover

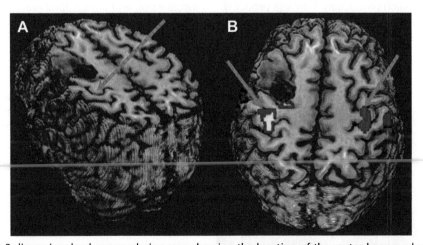

Fig. 2. (*A*) A 3-dimensional volume rendering map showing the location of the motor homunculus in the precentral gyrus (the reverse omega Ω [*arrow*]). (*B*) fMR imaging activation map showing the hand motor activity (*arrow*) overlaid onto the high-resolution anatomic image. It is clear that the functional activity is overlaid onto the precentral gyrus.

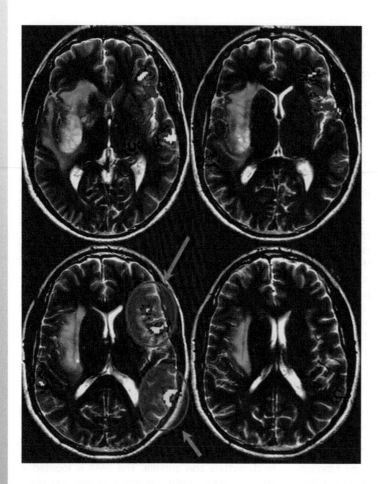

Fig. 3. An example showing a language activation map in a patient with a tumor in right hemisphere, contralateral to the tumor. fMR imaging visualizes a well-lateralized left-dominant language activity map. It clearly shows the frontal (Broca area: *top arrow*) and the temporal (Wernicke area: *bottom arrow*) language areas.

completely from damage to the language part of the SMA within weeks to months. The insula is located deep to the frontal operculum. It is likely involved in ventilatory needs during speech and end-stage speech production. Damage produces variable language deficits also ranging from nothing to word-finding difficulty and speech apraxia. The supramarginal and angular gyri are wrapped around the posterior portion of the sylvian fissure. The main functions of these areas include language perception, processing of auditory and visual input, and the comprehension of language. Damage to these areas usually results in alexia (inability to read) and agraphia (inability to write).

Pars triangularis

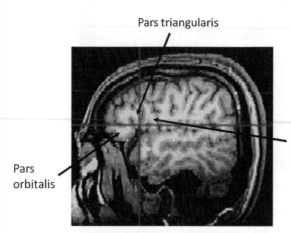

Pars opercularis

Pars orbitalis

Fig. 4. A sagittal MR image showing the anatomic localization of the pars opercularis and the pars triangularis of the Broca area (*arrows*). The crosshairs show the border between the pars triangularis and opercularis. Pars orbitalis is not technically part of the Broca area.

However, one must stress the great variability in language organization from one person to another. This point was recently emphasized in a careful study, conducted by Sanai and colleagues,[20] using direct cortical stimulation. This variability of language organization further stresses the need for preoperative fMR imaging and intraoperative cortical stimulation.

TASK AND PARADIGM SELECTION

Functional tasks are tasks specially designed for use with fMR imaging and are designed to increase neuronal activity in specific cortical areas. The functional tasks can be performed with one of 2 types of paradigms: block and event related. Each type of paradigm requires a resting and active state. The most common type in clinical fMR imaging is block-design paradigms. When performing a block paradigm, patients alternate between ON (active state) and OFF (resting state) periods of equal or unequal duration. Varying the duration of ON and OFF periods can be effective in decreasing noise from the scanner, heartbeat, and respiration.[2,21] For example, to identify the hand motor area, a block paradigm might consist of alternating finger tapping and resting periods, each lasting 20 seconds.[2,22] Usually, the paradigms repeat 5 to 6 times to increase power during statistical analysis.

In event-related paradigms, patients perform a single short event (usually, less than 4 seconds), such as swallowing or clenching a fist, followed by the rest period similar in duration to the block paradigms. This type of paradigm is used to investigate the neuronal or hemodynamic response to a specific single event.[23] Event-related paradigms are particularly useful when an estimation of the hemodynamic response is desirable; but their limitations include long acquisition times, low statistical power, and corresponding complicated statistical analyses. Hence, this type of paradigm is not commonly used with clinical fMR imaging. Block designs are more effective at detecting an averaged fMR imaging signal because patients perform the same task over a period, for example, a 10- or 20-second period, and the design will increase the power to detect activated regions associated with a specific task. So, this type of detection can be advantageous in patients who may have impaired function or cognitive capacity.

General Motor Paradigms

Motor fMR imaging paradigms should be performed if there is a close anatomic relationship between the lesion and the motor homunculus, even if there are no motor symptoms. Commonly used paradigms to localize the motor strip include finger tapping, tongue motion, wiggling toes, or sensory foot or hand stimulation. In the finger-tapping task, patients are asked to sequentially tap their fingers avoiding arm or shoulder motion. Also, finger tapping can be changed to fist clenching or to sequential motion of the fingers from thumb to pinky finger, which can better capture premotor areas as well as the primary motor gyrus.[15] However, in the authors' experience in the brain tumor patient population, there is little practical difference in the exact type of hand-motor paradigm that is performed. The hand homunculus takes up a large portion of the motor cortex and gives a good motor signal, so hand paradigms should always be performed when localization of the motor strip is in question.

When performing tongue movement, patients are asked to keep their mouth closed and make a small sweeping tongue motion against the back of their teeth. Even small motion can elicit a strong fMR imaging signal; so large mouth movements should be avoided because they make it difficult to keep the patients' head still during the fMR imaging scan.

The preservation of foot and leg mobility is essential in brain tumor surgery because loss of function will leave patients wheel-chair or bed bound. To complicate matters, the location of the foot motor homunculus is much more difficult from routine anatomic images. In addition, the foot motor homunculus is located deep in the interhemispheric sulcus making it inaccessible to direct cortical stimulation. As with other fMR imaging paradigms, it is very essential to keep the patients' head still. Therefore, the foot-motion paradigms must be performed carefully with no ankle motion. Extensive ankle movement (performed concurrently with the paradigm) can lead to movement of the entire body, including the head, which will cause artifacts in the fMR imaging data that are very difficult to eliminate, even with sophisticated software.

Passive sensory paradigms, such as foot or hand stimulation by the examiner, can be helpful with patients who are paretic or elderly patients. Sensory paradigms will preferentially activate the postcentral (sensory) gyrus, from which the location of the corresponding motor homunculus can be extrapolated. However, these results should be interpreted with caution because fMR imaging activity usually activates both the sensory and motor gyri.

Language

The main goal of language fMR imaging is to lateralize and localize the brain area processing language function relative to the tumor. Tasks should be designed to target productive or frontal areas as well as receptive or temporoparietal areas.

Productive speech tasks are generally tasks that require patients to generate words in response to specific cues. These tasks are considered fluency tasks. During a phonemic fluency task, patients are given a letter and asked to generate words that begin with that letter. In the semantic fluency task, patients are asked to generate words that fit a given category, for example, fruits or vegetables. Another productive paradigm is verb generation whereby patients are given nouns and are asked to generate verbs. An example can be the word *baby*, to which patients will generate words such as *cries*, *crawls*, *smiles*, and so forth. Verb-generation tasks show more specificity than fluency tasks but have less variability in measuring hemispheric dominance.[15]

Receptive speech tasks generally involve reading or listening to aurally presented words or reading a visually presented sentence and filling in the most appropriate answer. One more important receptive speech task requires patients to answer simple questions asked aurally, such as the following: What do you shave with? What color is grass? This type is generally known as *auditory responsive naming*.

It should be mentioned that despite tailoring the language paradigm to the lesion location, most language tasks will activate both frontal and posterior language areas to some degree because these areas are highly cooperative. However, it is more difficult to measure posterior language areas than frontal language areas.[2]

An important question when performing language paradigms is whether they should be performed silent (covert) or vocalized (overt). Certain investigators recommend overt paradigms.[24] The advantage of vocalized (overt) paradigms is that the investigator is able to confirm that patients are actually performing the required paradigm. Obviously, if patients are not performing the paradigm, the results of the fMR imaging will be useless. Additionally, the patients' responses can be quantified, for example, how many of the questions did the patient answer correctly. However, for patients with a clinical brain tumor, the authors recommend silent (covert) paradigms. The authors have found that the main problem in patients with brain tumors is head motion, which often results from articulation of responses. In the authors' practice, they use the real-time fMR imaging analysis to monitor patient responses and to ensure as much as possible that patients are performing the task correctly (see later discussion).[25]

PATIENT PREPARATION AND PARADIGM MODIFICATION

Good patient performance is very important to achieve optimal fMR imaging results. The most important parts are interviewing the patients, detailed pre-fMRI instructions, and paradigm practice. Usually the interview starts with checking the patients' handedness, including the question about having switched handedness as a child. Assessing the function that is to be tested during fMR imaging is essential during this phase. For example, testing for hand weakness is crucial because compromise in motor ability can adversely affect the fMR imaging results. The authors use the Boston Naming Test to evaluate language and also ask the patient to repeat a sentence, such as "no ifs ands or buts."

The examiner must explain the procedure, reviewing the timing of the paradigm, before placing patients in the scanner. Practicing the paradigm with patients to maximize compliance with the paradigm while patients are in the scanner is essential. Patients are not healthy graduate students. Patients often have neurologic deficits, which are sometimes severe. In addition, patients may have hearing problems, difficulties with following commands, or even language barriers. They may be claustrophobic, forgetful, or scared, and they may need premedication. These factors have to be accounted for when interviewing patients before the fMR imaging examination and when considering possible modifications of fMR imaging paradigms. One must keep these potential problems in mind when monitoring patients during the performance of the fMR imaging paradigms in the scanner. Therefore, paradigms may need to be modified to better suit patients' neurologic limitations.[2,3,15] For example, if patients are paralyzed, a sensory paradigm can be used to determine the location of the motor cortex. A sensory paradigm may include brushing, squeezing, or touching the patients' foot or hand.[3,15] A language paradigm may need to be simplified or the timing may need to be slowed to increase compliance with the task.

Properly positioning patients in the scanner to ensure comfort will also increase the compliance with the fMR imaging paradigm. No matter what paradigm is used, it is important that it is designed to minimize any type of unwanted head or body motion to achieve ideal results. For example, a toe paradigm should be performed with no ankle motion (we can also use a pillow under patients' knees). A tongue paradigm should be performed with a closed mouth.[15,26,27]

A useful way to monitor patient compliance and the successful completion of the fMR imaging test is *real-time fMR imaging*. This is available in most MR scanner manufacturers and involves rapid analysis of the fMR imaging data. The analysis is performed and displayed on the MR imaging console while the patient is being scanned, which allows the examiner to assess if the fMR imaging test has been successful. For example, if the examiner can identify the Broca area using real-time fMR imaging, then he or she can be reasonably confident that the fMR imaging test has been successfully acquired. On the other hand, if the Broca area is not visualized, this raises the possibility that the fMR imaging test has not been successfully acquired and should be repeated. Often, in the authors' clinical practice, questioning patients after an unsuccessful fMR imaging test, identified by real-time fMR imaging, allows us to pinpoint the problem, correct it, and acquire adequate fMR imaging data. For example, the authors have had cases whereby patients did not hear the instructions or did not follow them correctly. Seeing that the fMR imaging data were suboptimal, the authors addressed the issue with the patients and it allowed them to acquire adequate fMR imaging data. Without real-time fMR imaging, the authors would have been stuck with useless fMR imaging data when they tried to analyze it in the laboratory.

DATA ACQUISITION, ANALYSIS, AND INTERPRETATION

The goal of fMR imaging data analysis is to accurately identify the small-amplitude BOLD signal. Typically, the BOLD fMR imaging signal change is approximately 2% to 5% in the sensorimotor system and is even smaller for higher cognitive tasks. The problem is compounded by the fact that the BOLD signal is easily obscured by undesirable noise.[28]

One of the issues with fMR imaging is the signal-to-noise ratio. So, after acquiring fMR imaging data, one must optimize the signal associated with the specific functional tasks and minimize the noise. The quality of the preprocessed data more often than not determines the quality of the final result.

Data Processing and Analysis

Preprocessing must be performed to reduce the artifactual signal that is not associated with the patients' functional task and to improve the detectability of induced changes. The typical preprocessing steps applied in clinical fMR imaging include raw data quality check, motion correction, and spatial smoothing. Most software packages include ways to correct for motion. Head motion during the fMR imaging scan is the biggest practical problem in clinical fMR imaging. Even small head motion can lead to moving voxels of high signal intensity to locations of low signal intensity. Most software manufacturers allow one to monitor the degree of motion in the 3 orthogonal planes as well as pitch, yaw, and role. During data quality assessment, one should be able to find images affected by excessive head motion.

Notwithstanding the sophisticated programs available to counteract motion artifact, it is essential to understand that that motion is easier to prevent than to correct after the scan and during data processing.[3] Random noise must be reduced to improve the ability of a statistical technique to detect true activations. Spatial smoothing improves the signal-to-noise ratio; but it has several limitations, including reduction in the image resolution.

Once the data have been through a variety of preprocessing steps, a statistical method to identify the activated regions associated with the patients' functional task can be performed. When the statistics are calculated for each voxel and the resulting statistics are presented in an image in which intensity is used to represent the statistical value, the resulting image is called a *statistical parametric map* of brain activation. In such methods, either correlation or linear modeling algorithms can be used. From a statistical point of view, the analysis of fMR imaging data can be divided broadly into 2 types: (1) hypothesis driven (or model based for the BOLD response) and (2) data driven (model free). Hypothesis-driven analysis is the most popular method in clinical fMR imaging and includes parametric tests (require assumptions about the hemodynamic response timing and shape and about the noise characteristics), such as *t*-test,[29] cross-correlation,[30] and the general linear model.[31]

Coregistration and Neuronavigation Systems

After the statistical analysis, low-resolution fMR imaging activation images can be superimposed on high-resolution anatomic MR images. The coregistered images can be downloaded to the neurosurgical navigational system. The neurosurgeon can then visualize 3-dimensional reconstructions that help define the relationship between the lesion and the eloquent cortices during the resection.[32]

COMMON ARTIFACTS AND PITFALLS
Susceptibility Artifacts

The sequence for BOLD imaging is optimized to maximize the differences in susceptibility between oxyhemoglobin and deoxyhemoglobin concentration. However, this also means that BOLD fMR imaging is sensitive to susceptibility artifacts.

Magnetic susceptibility is a measure that indicates the amount of magnetization of a material in response to an applied external magnetic field. Different tissues have different magnetic susceptibilities. Tissues with large differences in magnetic susceptibility placed in close proximity can cause distortions in the local magnetic field and, therefore, produce artifacts. In patients without prior surgery, susceptibility artifacts are often located at air tissue interfaces, near cavities, or near moving tissues, such as the eyes, because of the rapid transition among different magnetic susceptibilities. In patients with prior surgery, this can be even more problematic. Titanium plates, metallic staples, hemorrhage and blood products, or any residual surgical metal can cause strong susceptibility artifacts increasing the risk of acquiring bad fMR imaging data. Notwithstanding such artifacts in patients who had undergone prior surgery, Peck and colleagues[33] determined that BOLD fMR imaging was able to correctly identify the location and lateralization of language areas correctly in most cases. However, some findings, especially potentially false negative results, should be interpreted with caution in the presence of postsurgical artifacts (**Fig. 5**).

Cortical Plasticity

Cortical reorganization is thought to occur when a disease process destroys part of the brain and this area of the brain is no longer able to perform its function, which causes another area of the brain to attempt to compensate in an effort to maintain function.[3,34] For example, when a primary motor area is damaged, other areas, such as the SMA, may start to play a larger role in normal motor function and movement execution.[10] The authors' group,[35,36] as well as others,[37–39] has demonstrated definite evidence for cortical reorganization of brain function in adults in response to a growing tumor. The interpreter of the fMR imaging results has to be cognizant of this possibility.

Loss of Autoregulation in Glioblastoma Multiforme

Studies have also shown that the presence of abnormal tumor neovasculature in high-grade lesions, such as glioblastoma multiforme, can lead to a decrease in the fMR imaging activation volume. Usually, an increase in neuronal activation leads to changes in blood flow, which lead to the BOLD effect. But in malignant brain tumors, the tumor neovasculature loses the ability to autoregulate, so an increase in neuronal activity does not lead to an increase in blood flow, which mutes the increase in BOLD signal.

The tumor neovasculature may cause decoupling of neuronal activity and the subsequent CBF response related specifically to that activity.[40] Increased blood flow to an area causes an increase in signal because of the increase in oxyhemoglobin (and decrease in deoxyhemoglobin) concentration; hence, a tumor neovasculature does not behave like a healthy neovasculature and may alter the reliability of the BOLD response. In addition, especially in areas of hypoxia in glioblastomas, the vasculature may already be maximally dilated and as a result will not be able to further increase the blood flow in response to an increased neuronal activity.[40] The interpreter must be aware

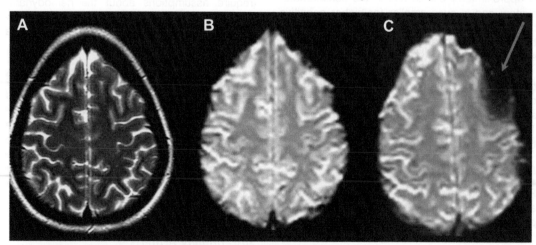

Fig. 5. Surgery-induced susceptibility artifact. (*A*) T2-weighted image, (*B*) T2* map before surgery, (*C*) T2* map after surgery. It is clear that there is a signal dropout (*arrow*) in areas of the prior surgery. T2* represents an image contrast that can be obtained from echo-planar imaging sequence.

of such potential limitations of fMR imaging, especially in the vicinity of high-grade gliomas.

OTHER MEDICAL APPLICATIONS

BOLD fMR imaging is not limited to brain tumors; there are many potential future applications, including stroke; brain injury; or degenerative diseases, such as Alzheimer disease.[41]

MR imaging provides a valuable tool in studying patients with early stage Alzheimer disease because MR imaging does not require ionizing radiation or exogenous contrast agents, making it a safe tool for performing longitudinal studies whereby patients can be tracked over time to understand the neurologic mechanisms of disease onset and progression.[42]

fMR imaging can measure the neural correlates of a seizure; study how the brain recovers from a stroke; test how well a drug or behavioral therapy works; and characterize disorders, like depression.[43] Recovered depressed patients have shown altered fMR imaging activity, which may indicate a tendency to relapse.[43] Lateralization of language and memory areas helps surgeons avoid resecting eloquent cortices in patients with intractable temporal lobe epilepsy.[44] Using fMR imaging in studies of pain can advance therapeutic approaches to acute and chronic pain.[45] Pharmacologic fMR imaging, measuring brain activity after drugs are administered, can be used to quantify dose versus effect information of the medication.[43]

SUMMARY

fMR imaging is a noninvasive, repeatable, and flexible technique for studying brain function in the clinical setting. Specifically, fMR imaging for neurosurgical planning has become the standard of care in centers where it is available. Although paradigms to measure eloquent cortices are not yet standardized, simple tasks elicit reliable maps for planning neurosurgical procedures. In addition, patient-specific paradigm design will further refine the usability of fMR imaging for prognostication and recovery of function. Certain pathologic conditions and technical issues limit the interpretation of fMR imaging maps in clinical use and should be considered carefully. However, given its ease of use and adaptability to the clinical environment, fMR imaging for neurosurgical planning continues to provide insights into how the brain works and how it responds to pathologic insults.

REFERENCES

1. Holodny A, Hou B. Physical principles of BOLD fMRI–what is important for the clinician. In: Holodny AI, editor. Functional neuroimaging: a clinical approach. New York: Informa Healthcare Inc; 2008. p. 1–12.

2. Bogomolny DL, Petrovich NM, Hou BL, et al. Functional MRI in the brain tumor patient. Top Magn Reson Imaging 2004;15(5):325–35.

3. Peck KK, Holodny AI. fMRI clinical applications. In: Reiser MF, Semmler W, Hricak H, editors. Magnetic resonance tomography. Berlin: Springer Verlag; 2007. p. 1308–31.

4. Ogawa S, Lee TM, Kay AR, et al. Biophysics brain magnetic resonance imaging with contrast dependent on blood oxygenation. Proc Natl Acad Sci U S A 1990;87:9868–72.

5. Ogawa S, Lee TM. Magnetic resonance imaging of blood vessels at high fields: in vivo and in vitro measurements and image simulation. Magn Reson Med 1990;16(1):9–18.

6. Ogawa S, Lee TM, Nayak AS, et al. Oxygenation-sensitive contrast in magnetic resonance image of rodent brain at high magnetic fields. Magn Reson Med 1990;14(1):68–78.

7. Buxton RB, Uludag K, Dubowitz DJ, et al. Modeling the hemodynamic response to brain activation. Neuroimage 2004;23(1):220–33.

8. Logothetis NK, Wandell BA. Interpreting the BOLD signal. Annu Rev Physiol 2004;66:735–69.

9. Yousry TA, Schmid UD, Alkadhi H, et al. Localization of the motor hand area to a knob on the precentral gyrus. A new landmark. Brain 1997;120: 141–57.

10. Peck KK, Bradbury MS, Hou BL, et al. The role of the supplementary motor area (SMA) in the execution of primary motor activities in brain tumor patients: functional MRI detection of time-resolved differences in the hemodynamic response. Med Sci Monit 2009; 15(4):MT55–62.

11. Peck KK, Bradbury M, Psaty EL, et al. Joint activation of the supplementary motor area and presupplementary motor area during simultaneous motor and language functional MRI. Neuroreport 2009; 20(5):487–91.

12. Picard N, Strick PL. Motor areas of the medial wall: a review of their location and functional activation. Cereb Cortex 1996;6(3):342–53.

13. Roland PE, Zilles K. Functions and structures of the motor cortices in humans. Curr Opin Neurobiol 1996;6(6):773–81.

14. Vorobiev V, Govoni P, Rizzolatti G, et al. Parcellation of human mesial area 6: cytoarchitectonic evidence for three separate areas. Eur J Neurosci 1998;10(6): 2199–203.

15. Brennan NP. Preparing the patient for the fMRI study and optimization of paradigm selection and delivery. In: Holodny AI, editor. Functional neuroimaging: a clinical approach. New York: Informa Healthcare Inc; 2008. p. 13–21.

16. Alario FX, Chainay H, Lehericy S, et al. The role of the supplementary motor area (SMA) in word production. Brain Res 2006;1076(1):129–43.

17. Knecht S, Drager B, Deppe M, et al. Handedness and hemispheric language dominance in healthy humans. Brain 2000;123(Pt 12):2512–8.

18. Issacs KL, Barr WB, Nelson PK, et al. Degree of handedness and cerebral dominance. Neurology 2006;66(12):1855–8.

19. Knecht S, Deppe M, Drager B, et al. Language lateralization in healthy right-handers. Brain 2000; 123(Pt 1):74–81.

20. Sanai N, Mirzadeh Z, Berger MS. Functional outcome after language mapping for glioma resection. N Engl J Med 2008;358:18–27.

21. Veltman DJ, Mechelli A, Friston KJ, et al. The importance of distributed sampling in blocked functional magnetic resonance imaging designs. Neuroimage 2002;17(3):1203–6.

22. Kesavadas C, Thomas B. Clinical applications of functional MRI in epilepsy. Indian J Radiol Imaging 2008;18(3):210–7.

23. Peck K, Galgano J, Branski R, et al. Event related functional MRI investigation of vocal pitch variation. Neuroimage 2009;14(1):175–81.

24. Gartus A, Foki T, Geissler A, et al. Improvement of clinical language localization with an overt semantic and syntactic language functional MR imaging paradigm. AJNR Am J Neuroradiol 2009;30(10): 1977–85.

25. Partovi S, Konrad F. Effects of covert and overt paradigms in clinical language fMRI. Acad Radiol 2012; 19(5):518–25.

26. Krings T, Reinges MH, Erberich S, et al. Functional MRI for presurgical planning: problems, artifacts, and solution strategies. J Neurol Neurosurg Psychiatry 2001;70(6):749–60.

27. Hoeller M, Krings T, Reinges MH, et al. Movement artifacts and MR BOLD signal increase during different paradigms for mapping the sensorimotor cortex. Acta Neurochir (Wien) 2002;144(3):279–84.

28. Parrish T, Gitelman D, LaBar K, et al. Impact of signal to noise on functional MRI. Magn Reson Med 2000;44:925–32.

29. Henriksen O, Larsson H, Ring P, et al. Functional MR imaging at 1.5T. Acta Radiol 1993;34:101–3.

30. Bendettini P, Jesmanowicz E, Wong E, et al. Processing strategies for time-course data sets in functional MRI of the human brain. Magn Reson Med 1993;30:161–73.

31. Friston K, Holmes A, Worseley K, et al. Statistical parametric maps in functional imaging: a general linear approach. Hum Brain Mapp 1995;3:165–89.

32. Brennan CW, Petrovich Brennan NM. Functional image-guided neurosurgery. In: Holodny AI, editor. Functional neuroimaging: a clinical approach. New York: Informa Healthcare Inc; 2008. p. 91–106.

33. Peck KK, Bradbury M, Petrovich N, et al. Presurgical evaluation of language using functional magnetic resonance imaging in brain tumor patients with previous surgery. Neurosurgery 2009;64(4):644–52 [discussion: 652–3].

34. Matthews PM, Honey GD, Bullmore ET. Applications of fMRI in translational medicine and clinical practice. Nat Rev Neurosci 2006;7(9):732–44.

35. Holodny AI, Schulder M, Ybasco A, et al. Translocation of Broca's area to the contralateral hemisphere as the result of the growth of a left inferior frontal glioma. J Comput Assist Tomogr 2002;26(6):941–3.

36. Petrovich NM, Holodny AI, Brennan CW, et al. Isolated translocation of Wernicke's area to the right hemisphere in a 62-year-man with a temporoparietal glioma. AJNR Am J Neuroradiol 2004; 25(1):130–3.

37. Robles SG, Gatignol P, Lehéricy S, et al. Long-term brain plasticity allowing a multistage surgical approach to World Health Organization grade II gliomas in eloquent areas. J Neurosurg 2008; 109(4):615–24.

38. Ius T, Angelini E, Thiebaut de Schotten M, et al. Evidence for potentials and limitations of brain plasticity using an atlas of functional resectability of WHO grade II gliomas: towards a "minimal common brain". Neuroimage 2011;56(3):992–1000.

39. Forster MT, Senft C, Hattingen E, et al. Motor cortex evaluation by nTMS after surgery of central region tumors: a feasibility study. Acta Neurochir (Wien) 2012;154(8):1351–9.

40. Hou BL, Bradbury M, Peck KK, et al. Effect of brain tumor neovasculature defined by rCBV on BOLD fMRI activation volume in the primary motor cortex. Neuroimage 2006;32(2):489–97.

41. Functional MR imaging (fMRI) - Brain, American College of Radiology, Radiological Society of North America, May 24, 2011, retrieved December 30, 2011. Available at: http://www.radiologyinfo.org/en/info.cfm?pg=fmribrain.

42. Jack CR Jr. Alzheimer disease: new concepts on its neurobiology and the clinical role imaging will play. Radiology 2012;263(2):344–61.

43. Rombouts SA, Barkhof F, Sheltens P. Clinical applications of functional brain MRI. Oxford UK: Oxford University Press; 2007. ISBN 978-0-19-856629-8.

44. Wang A, Peters TM, de Ribaupierre S, et al. Functional magnetic resonance imaging for language mapping in temporal lobe epilepsy. Hindawi Publishing Corporation. Epilepsy Res Treat 2012; 2012. http://dx.doi.org/10.1155/2012/198183. Article ID 198183, 8 pages.

45. Borsook D, Becerra LR. Breaking down the barriers: fMRI applications in pain, analgesia and analgesics. Mol Pain 2006;2:30.

Clinical Applications of Diffusion Tensor Imaging

Jason M. Huston, DO, Aaron S. Field, MD, PhD*

KEYWORDS

- Diffusion tensor imaging • Tractography • Tissue characterization • Lesion localization
- Tract mapping • Preoperative planning • Image guided therapy

KEY POINTS

- Clinical applications of diffusion tensor (DT) imaging and tractography include tissue characterization, lesion localization, and mapping of white matter tracts.
- DT imaging metrics are sensitive to microstructural changes associated with central nervous system disease; however, further research is needed to enhance specificity so as to facilitate more widespread clinical application.
- Preoperative tract mapping, with either directionally encoded color maps or tractography, provides useful information to the neurosurgeon and has been shown to improve clinical outcomes.

INTRODUCTION

Physical Principles

Since its introduction in the mid-1980s, the applications of diffusion in magnetic resonance (MR) imaging have rapidly evolved. Diffusion-weighted (DW) and diffusion tensor (DT) imaging are based on the inherently random, thermally driven motion of molecules, known as Brownian motion, initially described by the Scottish botanist Robert Brown[1] and mathematically characterized by Albert Einstein[2] and others. DW and DT imaging exploit this motion of water molecules in tissues to probe the underlying microstructure, which influences molecular motion in measurable ways. By acquiring DW imaging in at least 6 noncollinear directions, a mathematical "tensor" model of diffusion can be determined that approximates the 3-dimensional (3D) diffusion profile at a given voxel with a simple ellipsoid. Because the size and shape of a 3D ellipsoid are fully specified by its diameters (so-called eigenvalues) along its 3 principal axes (major, medium, and minor), and because the orientation of the ellipsoid in 3D space is determined by those axes (eigenvectors), the complete 3D diffusion profile can be described by just a few

measurable parameters. Isotropic diffusion occurs when the diffusion of water molecules occurs with equal probability in all directions (ie, the tensor ellipsoid is spherical), in contrast to anisotropic diffusion, which occurs when the structure of an underlying tissue creates a preferential axis (or axes) for molecular motion (nonspherical ellipsoid). The detailed physics of DT imaging is beyond the scope of this article, but several excellent review articles are available.[3–6]

DT Imaging Quantification and Display

Whereas DT imaging of course is used to generate images that may be qualitatively interpreted, the tensor model yields several quantitative parameters reflective of tissue microstructure. The most common are the scalar metrics, mean diffusivity (MD) and fractional anisotropy (FA), which are rotationally invariant parameters reflecting the degree of (directionally averaged) diffusivity and anisotropy, respectively.[7,8] MD is the tensor equivalent of the directionally averaged apparent diffusion coefficient (ADC) in common clinical use. The largest (major) eigenvalue is often called axial, longitudinal, or parallel diffusivity, as it is presumed

Department of Radiology, School of Medicine and Public Health, University of Wisconsin, 600 Highland Avenue M/C 3252, Madison, WI 53792, USA
* Corresponding author.
E-mail address: AField@uwhealth.org

Magn Reson Imaging Clin N Am 21 (2013) 279–298
http://dx.doi.org/10.1016/j.mric.2012.12.003
1064-9689/13/$ – see front matter © 2013 Elsevier Inc. All rights reserved.

mri.theclinics.com

to reflect the magnitude of diffusion parallel to axons. The average of the 2 lesser (medium and minor) eigenvalues is often called radial, transverse, or perpendicular diffusivity, as it is presumed to reflect the magnitude of diffusion perpendicular to axons (although this makes sense only under the assumption of a single population of unidirectional axons within an imaging voxel). Song and colleagues[9] have suggested that radial diffusivity is linked to the myelin content of fiber tracts, whereas axial diffusivity is reflective of axonal integrity. However, as pointed out by Wheeler-Kingshott and Cercignani,[10] multiple factors can affect the determination of axial and radial diffusivity such that these relationships may be less straightforward than often assumed.

Directionally encoded color (DEC) maps are commonly used to display the directionality of the major eigenvector (presumably paralleling local fiber bundles) using a red, green, and blue (RGB) color scheme to represent left-right, anterior-posterior, and superior-inferior directions, respectively.[11] Color intensity is often weighted by an index of diffusion anisotropy (most commonly FA), yielding a convenient summary map from which the degree of anisotropy and the local fiber direction can be determined. DEC maps are particularly appealing in clinical practice because anyone familiar with normal fiber-tract anatomy can readily survey the organization of the major tracts by paging through 2-dimensional sections just as standard clinical MR images are typically viewed. Moreover, the relationship of a lesion to specific tracts in the region is often readily assessed from these maps without the need for fiber tracking, or tractography, which requires additional processing as described in the next section.

Tractography

Tractography is another approach to depicting white matter (WM) connection patterns in which mathematical algorithms are used to map the trajectories of specific fiber tracts in 3D space. These trajectories are estimated from the tensor data by starting at specified locations (known as "seed" points) and iteratively taking incremental steps in the direction of maximum diffusivity. This process is repeated until some predetermined criterion for terminating the tract has been met. The resulting tractograms may be displayed in a variety of ways using 3D computer-graphic techniques.

Most tractography algorithms estimate a single discrete trajectory for each seed-point location and many use the major eigenvector to estimate the tangent of the trajectory for a WM fiber

bundle.[12–14] However, additional tracking methods based on the full DT field have also been developed.[15–17] Seed locations are usually defined either globally over the entire brain or in a user-specified region. Tracts are typically propagated in both forward and reverse directions until some termination criterion is met; commonly used criteria include intersecting a voxel where the anisotropy is below a specified threshold, or encountering an excessively sharp "bend" between steps along the putative tract. Tracts may be defined by constraining them to pass through 1 or more specified regions of interest.[18,19]

Tractography algorithms are capable of generating anatomically plausible estimates of WM trajectories in the brain, and they have been used to depict major projection pathways (eg, pyramidal tract, internal capsule, corona radiata), commissural pathways (eg, corpus callosum, anterior commissure), and association pathways (eg, arcuate, fronto-occipital, and uncinate fasciculi).[18–22] Additional quantitative tractography parameters have been proposed that take into account the rotational variance of DT imaging. These metrics include connectivity (the strength and/or likelihood of any functional connection between multiple cortical/subcortical areas)[23] and fiber density (the number of fiber trajectories identified per voxel in a region of interest).[24]

It must be noted that a given DT imaging–based trajectory is an imperfect model-based construct and does not (indeed cannot) directly correspond to a physical axonal fiber, given the marked discrepancy of scale between the microstructural anatomy and the spatial resolution of clinical imaging. This point is easily forgotten when admiring the aesthetic depictions of WM anatomy that tractography offers. Because of this and other limitations, tractography is most often applied qualitatively and with extreme caution in clinical practice, avoiding specific, quantitative conclusions regarding tissue integrity or character. Functional MR (fMR) imaging is considered a complementary adjunct to DT imaging, and fMR imaging activation centers can be used as seed points for tractography (**Fig. 1**).

Terminology

As clinical tractography is still in its infancy, published reports frequently use inconsistent terminology in describing pathologically altered tracts. Such descriptive terms as "disruption," "displacement," "deviation," "deformation," "destruction," "degeneration," "infiltration," "interruption," and "splaying" are frequently used in the context of DT imaging–tractography without precise definitions.

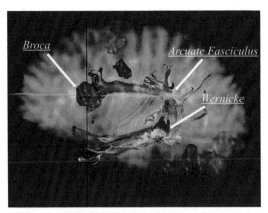

Fig. 1. Functional MR imaging–guided fiber tracking. The language activation centers (eg, Broca, Wernicke) in a normal healthy volunteer were used as seed points to perform tract mapping of the arcuate fasciculus.

In the spirit of encouraging consistency by DT imaging–tractography investigators, as well as radiologists reporting clinical DT imaging studies, the following terminology is suggested: Deviation,

Infiltration, Interruption, Degeneration, and Splaying (Box 1). Although these definitions are not perfect (eg, a severely deviated or infiltrated tract might be mistaken for an interrupted one), they represent a reasonable approach given the limitations inherent to DT imaging and tractography. Note also that these definitions are not mutually exclusive (eg, a tract may be both deviated and infiltrated, deviated and interrupted, and so forth) (Fig. 2).

CLINICAL APPLICATIONS

As already noted, DT imaging can exploit the magnitude and directionality of diffusion to provide exquisite noninvasive characterization of tissue architecture that is not feasible with standard MR imaging. Broadly categorized, clinical applications of DT imaging include: tissue characterization (eg, estimating the histology, grade, or margins of a neoplasm); lesion localization (eg, determining the specific anatomic fiber tract involved by an underlying pathologic condition); and tract mapping

---

Box 1
Recommended terminology For DT imaging–tractography

Deviation

Any portion of tract course is altered by bulk mass effect while maintaining tract coherence, with "coherence" implying that multiple adjacent fiber trajectories follow parallel pathways or they diverge/converge in an ordered fashion. "Deviation" is preferred over "displacement" because it is more specific and informative (eg, road repairs may "displace" traffic without providing an alternative route; "deviated" implies that the flow of traffic is maintained, routed around the repairs).

Infiltration

Any portion of a tract shows significantly reduced anisotropy while retaining sufficiently ordered structure to allow its identification on directional color maps and to allow fiber tracking to proceed. Note that infiltration by tumor is not discriminated from infiltration by edema, as this cannot yet be reliably done.

Interruption

Any portion of a tract is visibly discontinuous on anisotropy-weighted DEC maps, and/or fiber tracking is discontinuous despite reasonable relaxation of termination criteria. "Reasonable" termination criteria are those that impede the generation of recognizably spurious tracts but do not necessarily penalize fiber tracking for low anisotropy, provided excessively sharp turns are adequately avoided. "Interruption" is preferred over the more pathologically definitive "destruction" or the more ambiguous "disruption" (to disrupt can mean "to break apart" or to "throw into disorder," and these meanings would have very different implications for fiber tracts). Note also that a tract may be interrupted either partially or completely.

Degeneration

A tract characterized by significantly reduced size and/or anisotropy at a substantial distance from a lesion affecting the same neural pathway (either cortical or subcortical), such that secondary Wallerian degeneration rather than infiltration can reasonably be presumed (eg, a chronically atrophic-appearing pyramidal tract in the brainstem distal to a noninfiltrating lesion of the corona radiata).

Splaying

A tract separated by a lesion into distinct bundles deviated in different directions.

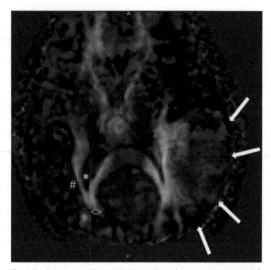

Fig. 2. Preoperative DT imaging in a patient with a presumed infiltrating glioma. Semitransparent DT imaging directionally encoded color (DEC) map overlaid onto T2 fluid-attenuated inversion recovery (FLAIR) image demonstrates an infiltrative hyperintense mass in the left parieto-occipital region. On the right there is a normal appearance of the arcuate fasciculus (*hash*), sagittal stratum (*lozenge*), and tapetum (*asterisk*). On the left, these tracts are both infiltrated and medially deviated by the mass (*arrows*). Of note, the hyperintensity of the tracts is a combination of anisotropy and T2-hyperintense signal.

(eg, preoperative mapping of a tract deviated by a space-occupying mass).

Tissue characterization is most often addressed using scalar metrics (most commonly MD, ADC, and FA) on a voxel-wise basis. Multiple studies have shown these parameters to be more sensitive to abnormalities than conventional MR imaging, based on changes found in the so-called normal-appearing white matter (NAWM). Unfortunately, this high sensitivity is accompanied by low specificity, particularly in the case of FA. Thus, although the common DT imaging metrics might have some appeal as imaging end points in clinical trials (based on their sensitivity to subclinical pathologic changes), their routine clinical utility currently is quite limited by their low specificity. Recent efforts to derive greater pathologic specificity from DT imaging parameters have focused on directionally specific (eg, axial and radial) diffusivities and other features of the diffusion tensor, but the clinical role of these emerging techniques is not yet defined. Lesion localization and tract mapping are more straightforward applications of DT imaging and tractography, a few anatomic controversies notwithstanding.[25,26] The ability to localize lesions and describe their relationship to specific tracts

on imaging has obvious importance to patient management.

Neoplasm

The interrogation of neoplasms has become one of the most frequent clinical applications of DT imaging and tractography. Many studies have evaluated the utility of scalar diffusion metrics (eg, MD, FA) in neoplastic tissue characterization, such as for estimating tumor type and grade[27–30] or discriminating tumor infiltration from peritumoral edema.[31–33] The inconsistent results of these studies overall make it difficult to apply quantitative DT imaging indices to these questions in routine clinical practice. Of all the potential relationships between DT imaging metrics and tissue properties that have been considered, the one supported by the most evidence is an inverse correlation between tumor cellularity and MD (or ADC). This relationship may have clinical utility in identifying tumors known for high cell density, such as lymphoma and medulloblastoma. However, other factors contribute to MD/ADC values such that reliable tumor identification before biopsy is usually not possible.

A more practical and frequently used application of DT imaging is to lesion localization and tract mapping (**Fig. 3**). Preoperative tractography can provide confirmation that a tumor-deviated tract remains intact and can potentially facilitate preservation of the tract during resection (**Fig. 4**).[34–36] This application is probably the best known to date, although studies clearly attributing improved clinical outcomes to DT imaging are still relatively few. In one of the largest published series to date, patients with high-grade gliomas survived an average of 7 months longer and were more functional postoperatively when DT imaging was added to standard neurosurgical navigation procedures.[34] Intraoperative DT imaging with tractography has also shown promise in monitoring the shift of WM tracts during resection.[37] The advantages of DT imaging as a technique that is complementary to preoperative fMR imaging were demonstrated by Ulmer and colleagues,[38] who identified twice as many functional systems near tumor margins when DT imaging and fMR imaging were combined in preoperative tumor planning, relative to fMR imaging alone.

Ischemic Stroke

Conventional DW imaging has become an invaluable tool in the evaluation of ischemic stroke, owing to its excellent sensitivity and ability to depict the infarct volume.[39] DT imaging is capable of providing additional tissue characterization of

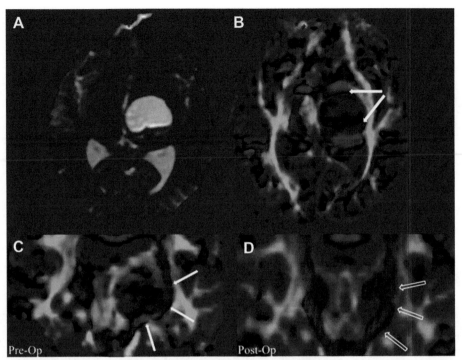

Fig. 3. (A–D) Preoperative DT imaging–tractography in a patient with a ganglioglioma. Conventional T2-weighted image (A) reveals a cystic mass centered in the left thalamus. Axial DEC map (B) demonstrates splaying and deviation of the left corticospinal tract (*solid arrows*). Preoperative coronal DEC map (C) also demonstrates infero-lateral displacement of the corticospinal tract just above the cerebral peduncle. Note the color change from blue to red as the superior-inferior oriented fibers are deviated into a more left-right orientation. Preoperative DT imaging, especially in the coronal plane shown here, helped the surgeon preserve the tract during resection. Note that the corticospinal tract is returned to anatomic position in a postoperative coronal DEC map (D) (*open arrows*). Preoperative motor deficit was 3-4/5 right upper/lower extremities, and there was no deficit postoperatively.

stroke (eg, improved temporal evaluation of ischemia).[40] In the acute phase of stroke, the MD is noted to initially decrease and the FA to increase. In the subacute phase, the MD will normalize while the FA begins to decrease. Subsequently, in the chronic phase of stroke there is an increase in MD and the FA continues to decline. Some investigators have also suggested that DT imaging may be more sensitive than conventional DW imaging in differentiating ischemia between gray matter and WM[41,42]; however, others have demonstrated conflicting results.[43,44] Following stroke, secondary (Wallerian) degeneration of WM tracts has been shown to correlate with the degree of motor dysfunction[45,46]; tractography allows lesion localization (eg, distance between ischemic tissue and WM tracts) as well as tract mapping that can depict Wallerian degeneration,[47–49] at times substantially better than conventional MR imaging. This technique has also been used to monitor reorganization of the WM architecture following stroke management.[50]

Epilepsy

Epilepsy is a chronic neurologic disorder, classified as generalized or partial (localized), in which abnormal or excessive neuronal activity results in an increased risk of recurrent seizures.[51] There are many potential causes of epilepsy including trauma, stroke, tumors, and congenital malformations. In temporal lobe epilepsy, a form of localized seizures, patients are frequently treated with anterior temporal lobectomy; a potential complication of this procedure is visual field deficits resulting from injury to the Meyer loop, the fibers of which have variable anterior extent.[52] Tractography has been demonstrated to be feasible in depicting the optic tracts (including the Meyer loop), which may improve surgical outcome (**Fig. 5**).[52–54] Scalar DT imaging metrics have also been used to lateralize seizure foci. In patients with mesial temporal sclerosis, MD is noted to be increased in the affected hippocampal formation.[55] The ability to lateralize the seizure focus has also been demonstrated in patients with unremarkable conventional

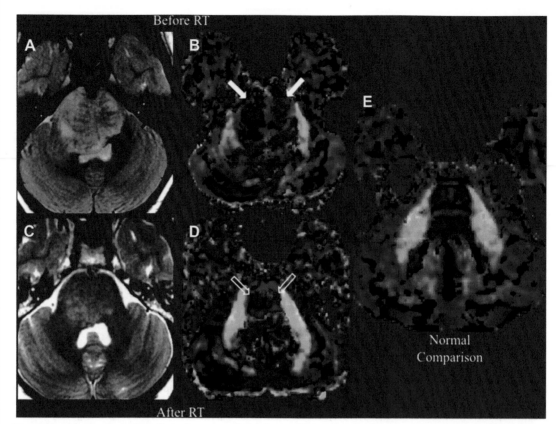

Fig. 4. (*A–E*) Evaluation of treatment response following radiation therapy for a brainstem glioma. Pretreatment T2-weighted image (*A*) reveals an expansile, infiltrative mass within the pons. Pretreatment DEC map (*B*) demonstrates infiltration of the bilateral pyramidal tracts (*solid arrows*). Posttreatment T2-weighted image (*C*) and DEC map (*D*) demonstrate decreased prominence of the brainstem glioma and improved visualization of the pyramidal tracts (*open arrows*). A normal volunteer (*E*) is provided for comparison. (*Courtesy of* Dr Lara A. Brandão, Clinical Radiology, Luiz Felippe Mattoso, Barra Da Tijuca, Rio de Janeiro, Brazil.)

MR imaging.[56,57] Additional studies have revealed alterations of anisotropy (eg, decreased FA) in normal-appearing WM beyond an identified seizure focus.[58,59]

Demyelinating Disease

Demyelinating diseases are a group of disorders in which there is loss of myelin as the sequela of inflammatory, autoimmune, infectious, nutritional, iatrogenic, toxic, or vascular causes.[60–62] Multiple sclerosis (MS) is the most common demyelinating disease of the central nervous system, and a major cause of chronic neurologic disability in the young and middle-aged.[62] Unfortunately the correlation between conventional MR imaging findings and clinical disability in MS is notoriously poor; this is due, at least in part, to the lack of functional specificity in standard estimates of disease burden (eg, the total number or volume of lesions on T1-/T2-weighted images). DT imaging has the potential to improve the characterization of demyelinating plaques. Studies using scalar metrics have revealed demyelinating lesions to have increased MD and decreased FA,[63] and FA changes extending significantly beyond lesion margins visible on conventional MR imaging.[64–66] In a widely cited study in a mouse retinal nerve ischemia model, Song and colleagues[67] suggested that axial and radial diffusivities are relatively specific for axonal and myelin degeneration, respectively; however, this relationship is unlikely to be as straightforward as is commonly assumed. Several studies have demonstrated that DT imaging reveals alterations in the diffusivity and anisotropy of NAWM.[63,66,68] For example, Werring and colleagues[69] demonstrated that acute demyelinating lesions are preceded by subtle diffusion changes in NAWM. These studies suggest that DT imaging may provide more meaningful imaging markers of demyelinating disease than conventional imaging, and thus enable more accurate and timely

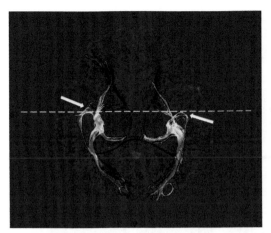

Fig. 5. Fiber tracking of the optic radiations. Seed points were placed in the regions of the lateral geniculate nuclei to depict the white matter (WM) fiber tracts of the bilateral optic radiations in a patient with left-sided mesial temporal sclerosis. The inferior/ventral component of the optic radiation corresponds to the Meyer loop as it courses anterior to the temporal horn (solid arrows). There is known variability in the anterior extent of the Meyer loop (demonstrated by the dashed white line), and preoperative tract mapping can provide useful information for the neurosurgeon planning temporal lobectomy.[52–54] A potential complication of surgical disruption of the Meyer loop is a superior homonymous quadrantanopia.

monitoring of disease progression and therapeutic effects. Lesion localization with tractography has also been shown to enable more functionally specific estimates of disease burden ("importance sampling"[70]), which better correlates with clinical disability (Fig. 6).

Dementia

Dementia is a group of disorders in which there is cognitive decline that significantly affects activities of daily living through alterations of memory, language, visuospatial function, or executive function.[71] There are many potential causes, including neurodegenerative, vascular, toxic, nutritional, and infectious etiology. A frequent application of DT imaging is for tissue characterization of patients with Alzheimer disease (AD), the most common of the dementias, and in mild cognitive impairment (MCI), considered a cognitive state intermediate between normal cognition and dementia. Studies have shown the effects of AD to be most pronounced in the medial temporal lobes, measurable as decreased FA and increased MD in hippocampus and adjacent gray matter. Higher MD is also observable in widespread portions of frontal, lateral and medial parietal, and lateral temporal cortices.[72–74] DT imaging indices have also allowed greater understanding of the effects of AD in the commissural (eg, corpus callosum) and association (eg, cingulum and inferior fronto-occipital/uncinate/superior longitudinal fasciculi) WM tracts that connect these regions (Fig. 7).[72,75] In addition, tractography has been shown to be feasible in characterizing association fibers (eg, cingulum) that may play a role in the progressive impairment in AD patients.[76–78] A meta-analysis performed by

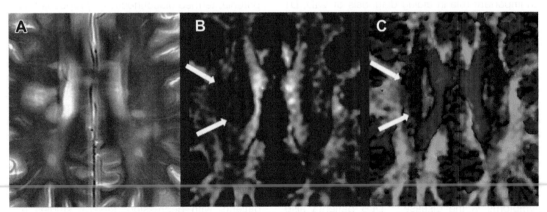

Fig. 6. (A–C) Improved lesion localization using DT imaging in demyelinating disease. A conventional T2-weighted image (A) reveals multiple demyelinating plaques in the bilateral periventricular WM. The correlation between conventional MR imaging findings and clinical disability in multiple sclerosis is notoriously poor, at least in part because of the lack of functional specificity in standard estimates of disease burden. Diffusion tensor fractional anisotropy (FA) (B) and DEC (C) maps more accurately depict that the 2 largest plaques are located within the right corona radiata (solid arrows). This improved lesion localization has also been shown to enable more functionally specific estimates of disease burden ("importance sampling"), which better correlates with clinical disability.[70]

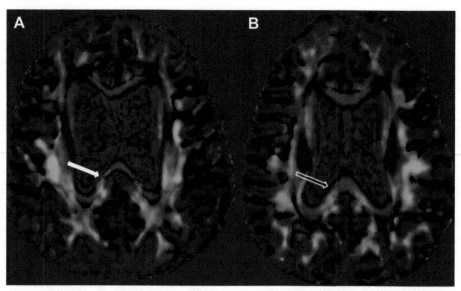

Fig. 7. (A, B) DT imaging in Alzheimer disease (AD). DEC map in an 83-year-old with AD (A) demonstrates prominent thinning of the corpus callosum (*solid arrow*), compared with an 86-year-old normal volunteer (B) (*open arrow*). DT imaging has allowed greater understanding of the effects of AD in the commissural and association WM tracts. (*Courtesy of* Dr Barbara B. Bendlin, University of Wisconsin, Madison, WI.)

Sexton and colleagues[79] revealed similar degeneration in patients with MCI, albeit with a reduced extent of differences.

DT imaging has also furthered our understanding of non-AD dementias. Vascular dementia (VaD) is the second most common dementia, and patients often show severe WM abnormality characterized by ischemic lesions that are highly visible on T2-weighted scans. Although conventional MR imaging has played an important role in aiding diagnosis of VaD, DT imaging shows high sensitivity for detecting vascular damage even in NAWM. Furthermore, DT imaging indices have been shown to have better correspondence with cognitive deficits in ischemic vascular disease when compared with conventional MR imaging.[80] Dementia with Lewy body (DLB) makes up about 10% to 15% of dementia, with patients showing fluctuating cognitive impairment, visual hallucinations, and features of Parkinsonism.[81] In contrast to AD, whereby occipital cortices are relatively spared, DLB patients show alterations in occipital gray and WM[82] that is potentially linked with visual symptoms in the disease.[83] DLB patients also show alterations in extended frontal temporal, insular, and posterior cingular WM, and in the inferior longitudinal fasciculus.[83,84] Similar to DLB, patients with Parkinson dementia show alterations in orbitofrontal regions, in addition to cingulum, and dorsolateral prefrontal, left anterior temporal, and left parietal WM. However, these changes are somewhat less extensive than those found in DLB.[85]

Psychiatric Disorders

Studies have demonstrated alterations within WM (eg, abnormal regulation of genes involved with myelination) in several major psychiatric diseases, including schizophrenia and chronic depression.[86] A prominent theory in schizophrenia, termed disconnectivity, proposes that an alteration in fiber-bundle connectivity of the brain is a potential cause of the disease.[87] Many researchers have applied DT imaging in schizophrenia to determine whether improved tissue characterization can aid in diagnosis or treatment. Several of these investigations have demonstrated alteration in scalar DT imaging metrics (eg, decreased FA) in multiple regions of the brain, including the frontal lobes, temporal lobes, cingulum, and corpus callosum.[88–90] However, a literature review by White and colleagues[88] revealed marked heterogeneity of these findings, even in such frequently identified locations. In patients with depression, several studies have revealed decreased FA in the superior longitudinal fasciculus.[91–93] However, contrary to these findings, a recent meta-analysis by Liao and colleagues[94] demonstrated the inferior longitudinal and inferior fronto-occipital fasciculi to be more commonly affected. Additional research is ongoing in several other psychiatric disorders (eg, obsessive-compulsive disorder, anxiety disorder, posttraumatic stress disorder).

Brain Development

MR imaging is commonly used to evaluate brain development and maturation, with T1-weighted and T2-weighted imaging demonstrating signal change that correlates with progressive myelination in the first few years of life.[95,96] However, there is often limited additional information that can be obtained after the age of 2 years. The application of DT imaging has created a new method for observing brain development and maturation beyond infancy (**Fig. 8**). Multiple studies have demonstrated a pattern of increasing FA and decreasing MD from infancy to adulthood.[97–101] Excellent review articles by Huppi[97,102] have described how this improved tissue characterization can aid in the evaluation of brain injury during development (eg, hypoperfusion, hypoxemia). In addition, the alteration of WM architecture observed by DT imaging has been noted to correlate with cognitive development in childhood.[98,103,104]

In adolescence, Asato and colleagues[105] demonstrated that increased FA is primarily noted in the intrahemispheric connections (eg, superior longitudinal and inferior fronto-occipital fasciculi)

and projection fibers (eg, corticospinal tracts and corona radiata). A recent meta-analysis by Peters and colleagues[106] demonstrated similar findings, with the most consistent location of increased FA being the superior longitudinal fasciculus. In adulthood there is a gradual decrease in the FA that corresponds to age-related volume loss, with several studies revealing frontal lobe predominance.[107,108] However, other studies have demonstrated conflicting results with a more widespread distribution.[100,109] Despite mixed results, DT imaging has considerable potential in allowing researchers to discover vulnerabilities of the aging brain.

An additional use of DT imaging is in the evaluation of autism, which is a form of pervasive developmental disorder thought to be related to abnormal connectivity.[110–113] Studies have revealed a decrease in FA within the prefrontal and temporal regions,[114,115] as well as within frontostriatal pathways that connect these regions.[115,116] Other investigators, however, have proposed that the abnormal connectivity is a more global process rather than being limited to particular regions of the brain.[117] In a study by Alexander and colleagues,[118] autism was noted to affect the macrostructure (eg, decreased volume) and microstructure (eg, decreased FA, increased MD)

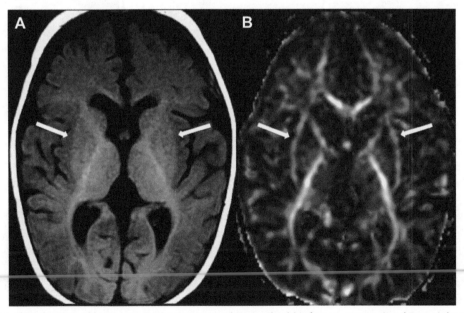

Fig. 8. (A, B) Evaluation of brain maturation in a normal 9-month-old infant. A conventional T1-weighted image (A) reveals age-appropriate myelination manifested by T1-hyperintense signal in the WM. Note that the external capsules (*solid arrows*) and anterior limbs of the internal capsules appear relatively isointense. A gray-scale FA map (B) demonstrates that anisotropy in WM tracts precedes the development of T1 hyperintensity related to myelination. Studies have shown a pattern of increasing FA and decreasing mean diffusivity in WM from infancy to adulthood. (*Courtesy of* Dr Lara A. Brandão, Clinical Radiology, Luiz Felippe Mattoso, Barra Da Tijuca, Rio de Janeiro, Brazil.)

of the corpus callosum. The alterations of the FA and MD were noted to be a result of significantly increased radial diffusivity that corresponded with slower processing speeds (ie, nonverbal cognitive performance).

Congenital Anomalies

Congenital brain anomalies constitute a broad group of malformations that can affect normal development. These anomalies can result in aberrant connections that can be imaged with DT and tractography. One of the more common applications of DT imaging is tract mapping of patients with agenesis of the corpus callosum. While conventional MR imaging can often easily depict complete or partial agenesis, DT imaging allows further characterization of aberrant intrahemispheric (eg, Probst bundles) and dysplastic interhemispheric connections (**Fig. 9**).[119–121] Similarly,

tractography has been shown to be feasible in the depiction of aberrant connections in holoprosencephaly.[122] DT imaging has also been used for tissue characterization of abnormalities in cortical development (eg, heterotopias and cortical dysplasia). In band heterotopia, studies have demonstrated increased FA in the heterotopic gray matter relative to cortex.[119,123] However, in contrast to these findings, alterations of anisotropy in subependymal heterotopia yielded no statistical significance.[119,124] Abnormalities of focal cortical dysplasia are often apparent on conventional MR imaging, but the application of DT imaging has demonstrated that there is additional reduction of FA in NAWM beyond the visible lesion (**Fig. 10**).[125–127] The potential benefit of DT imaging is still being explored; further research may allow greater understanding of how the brain adapts to congenital malformations.

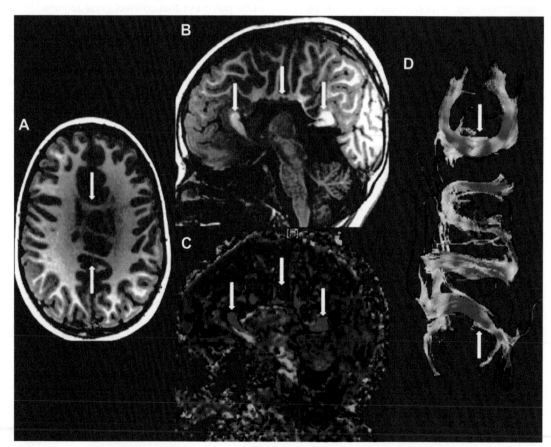

Fig. 9. (*A–D*) DT imaging–tractography in the evaluation of callosal dysgenesis. Axial (*A*) and sagittal (*B*) T1-weighted images demonstrate the presence of the genu and splenium of the corpus callosum; the body is absent, characterizing callosal dysgenesis (*solid arrows*). Although conventional MR imaging can often easily depict complete or partial agenesis, a sagittal DEC map (*C*) and tractography (*D*) allow further characterization of the callosal abnormality, with WM tracts from both hemispheres crossing the midline in the region of the absent body of the corpus callosum. (*Courtesy of Dr Lara A. Brandão, Clinical Radiology, Luiz Felippe Mattoso, Barra Da Tijuca, Rio de Janeiro, Brazil.*)

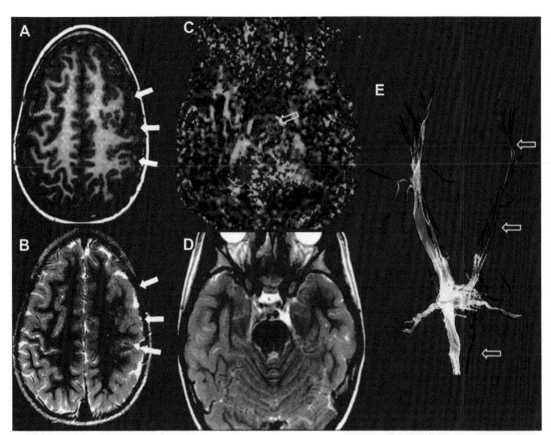

Fig. 10. (*A–E*) A 6-year-old child with right-sided motor delay and hemiparesis. Conventional T1-weighted (*A*) and T2-weighted (*B*) images demonstrate profound left frontoparietal polymicrogyria (*solid arrows*). However, conventional MR imaging does not clearly explain the patient's motor delay and hemiparesis. A DEC map (*C*) and tractography (*E*) demonstrate that there is loss of anisotropy and thinning of the left pyramidal tracts related to Wallerian degeneration (*open arrows*). Note that the pyramidal tracts at the level of the pons appear normal on conventional MR imaging (*D*). (*Courtesy of* Dr Lara A. Brandão, Clinical Radiology, Luiz Felippe Mattoso, Barra Da Tijuca, Rio de Janeiro, Brazil.)

Trauma

Traumatic brain injury (TBI) is a significant cause of mortality and disability worldwide, with approximately 80% categorized as mild, 10% as moderate, and 10% as severe.[128,129] Mechanisms of traumatic and posttraumatic tissue injury are myriad and complex, often encompassing both primary (eg, contusion, diffuse axonal injury) and secondary (eg, hypoxia-ischemia, Wallerian degeneration) phenomena. One of the most important pathologic features of TBI is diffuse axonal injury (DAI), which is a dynamic shearing/strain injury resulting from acceleration and deceleration of the brain.[130] These pathologic changes occur hours to several days after the initial injury, and findings may be occult on conventional MR imaging.

Several studies have found DW imaging to detect DAI more sensitively and predict clinical outcomes more accurately than T2*-weighted imaging.[131,132] In similar fashion, DT imaging has been shown to demonstrate alterations in anisotropy (eg, decreased FA) when conventional MR imaging is unremarkable.[133,134] Specifically, numerous studies have identified the corpus callosum as a frequent site of injury in TBI.[133–138] However, these alterations vary between the genu, body, and splenium of the corpus callosum, and other researchers have demonstrated conflicting results with no statistical group differences.[139] Several studies have also suggested that FA can predict the severity of TBI,[140,141] as well as aid in predicting patient outcome.[135,142] DT imaging has also been (anecdotally) useful in detecting complex secondary phenomena of traumatic brain injury (**Fig. 11**).[143]

It is important to remember that alterations of the microarchitecture identified by DT imaging are not specific to TBI, and there are numerous

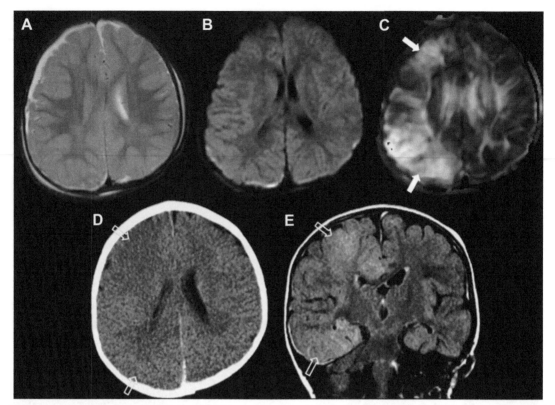

Fig. 11. (*A–E*) A 14-month-old infant with history of traumatic brain injury. Conventional T2-weighted (*A*) and diffusion-weighted (*B*) images, performed within 24 hours of the initial trauma, demonstrate no obvious parenchymal abnormality. However, a DT imaging gray-scale FA map (*C*) performed with the initial MR imaging reveals profound parenchymal abnormality that is manifested by increased anisotropy in the right cerebral hemisphere (*solid arrows*). Presumably reflecting complex secondary injury phenomena. Follow-up computed tomography (*D*) and T2 FLAIR (*E*) imaging, performed 4 days from the initial trauma, shows cerebral edema that correlates with the earlier detected abnormality on DT imaging (*open arrows*).

different variations in categorizing the severity of injury. Wortzel and colleagues[144] discuss these limitations and the difficulty of applying prior group differences to individual patients. Because of these and other pitfalls, caution is needed when applying DT imaging or tractography in routine clinical practice.

Brainstem and Spinal Cord

Conventional MR imaging has significantly improved the ability to evaluate the brainstem and spinal cord relative to computed tomography and traditional myelography. Using DT imaging and tractography in spinal cord imaging seems a logical extension given the multiple applications in the brain that have been previously discussed. However, there are several technical factors that have limited potential usefulness in clinical practice, including: (1) significant image distortion caused by prominent susceptibility artifact from the surrounding osseous structures

and/or chemical-shift artifact from the adjacent marrow; (2) ghosting artifact resulting from motion of the thoracic or abdominal organs as well as motion of the cord itself; and (3) partial volume averaging with surrounding cerebrospinal fluid.[145]

Continued technologic advances in MR imaging (eg, higher field strength leading to improved signal-to-noise ratio) have facilitated DT imaging research in spinal cord pathology. For example, DT imaging and fiber tractography have been shown to be feasible in the evaluation of spinal cord neoplasms.[146,147] In patients with MS, several studies have demonstrated altered anisotropy (eg, decreased FA) in both demyelinating lesions and the surrounding normal-appearing spinal cord.[148–150] In animal studies, Kim and colleagues[151,152] propose that DT imaging can aid in the evaluation of spinal cord injury as well as predict the degree of severity (**Fig. 12**). However, limited application in humans has yielded inconclusive results.[153,154] Further

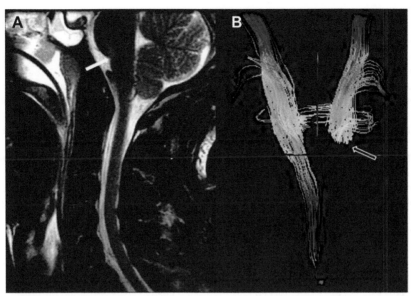

Fig. 12. (*A*, *B*) A 43-year-old person with history of a high-speed motor vehicle accident. Initial computed tomography of the head (not shown) demonstrated multifocal traumatic injury with a skull-base fracture, small epidural hematoma, subarachnoid hemorrhage, and frontotemporal contusions. Follow-up MR imaging of the cervical spine (*A*) revealed subtle T2-hyperintense signal abnormality at the pontomedullary junction (*solid arrow*). However, tractography (*B*) reveals interruption of the pyramidal tracts suggestive of a pontomedullary rent (*open arrow*). DT imaging–tractography can aid in the evaluation of spinal cord injury, as well as help predict the degree of severity.

research is needed to determine if DT imaging can be of any significant benefit in routine clinical practice.

LIMITATIONS AND PITFALLS

There are several limitations of DT imaging that should be considered. Estimates of the major eigenvector, and hence the local tract directions, are sensitive to image noise and assorted artifacts (eg, ghosting, misregistration, motion) that can reduce the accuracy of the DT imaging data and ultimately the tracts derived from these data. Even relatively straightforward ADC calculations in conventional DW imaging applications can be erroneous when "black-box" software is used carelessly, such as in a lesion having very low T2-weighted signal.[155] Crossing pathways are particularly problematic for DT imaging tractography, as most algorithms (particularly those based on the major eigenvector) are unable to resolve them. For example, the many intersecting pathways in the centrum semiovale (eg, corpus callosum, superior longitudinal fasciculus, and corona radiata) create problems for the mapping of trajectories through this region. As a result, most reconstructions of the corpus callosum and corticospinal tract show connections only to medial cortical areas, whereas lateral

connections are known to exist. New diffusion imaging methods, such as HARDI (High Angular Diffusion Imaging),[156,157] QBI (Q-Ball Imaging),[158] CHARMED (Composite Hindered and Restricted Model of Diffusion),[159] and DSI (Diffusion Spectrum Imaging),[158,160] promise more accurate depictions of intersecting tracts. Investigators have just begun to perform tractography using these advanced methods, with promising results.[161] Note, however, that these methods require much higher diffusion weighting (typically 3000–15000 s/mm^2) and take much more time to acquire.

Other technical problems remain to be solved before tractography can be considered a reliable technique in the setting of clinical pathology. Consider, for example, one of the best known and most promising clinical applications of DT imaging–tractography: the preoperative assessment of brain tumors. A fiber tract that is deviated by a noninfiltrating tumor with no associated edema presents the most straightforward case for DT imaging tract mapping. High anisotropy is generally preserved in such a tract, allowing it to be readily identified on DEC maps and traced around the tumor with fiber-tracking techniques. Such examples are now commonplace in the literature and at scientific meetings. However, intraoperative correlations and outcomes analyses are not so common, and the published experience of some investigators raises some serious concerns (eg, intraoperative tract mapping by evoked potentials analysis has revealed errors in preoperative DT imaging assessments of tract size and proximity to tumors[162]). There are also several potential sources of such error, including misregistration of multimodality images and shifting of the brain during craniotomy and tumor resection.[163]

Cases involving infiltrative tumors with associated edema can be even more problematic. Either edema or tumor infiltration may reduce the anisotropy of involved tracts without destroying them, posing a problem for tractography algorithms designed to terminate when the anisotropy falls below a designated threshold. It is difficult to know, in this setting, how to interpret an apparent loss of fiber trajectories. Relaxing the termination criteria may allow an algorithm to proceed through low-anisotropy regions, but this increases the risk of generating spurious tracts because estimates of major eigenvector become less reliable.[164] Moreover, tumor infiltration may cause tensor directional alterations that are more complex and less predictable than the bulk mass displacements of noninfiltrating tumors.[165,166] Finally, additional factors such as hemorrhage, calcification, surgical hardware, and postoperative pneumocephalus may cause susceptibility artifacts that are especially problematic for echoplanar imaging (EPI), the acquisition method used most commonly for DT imaging. Such cases would likely benefit from non-EPI acquisition schemes, such as DW fast spin-echo.[167]

SUMMARY

The potential utility of DT imaging in clinical practice is broad, and new applications continue to evolve as technology advances. DT imaging and tractography already have allowed unparalleled depiction of the WM architecture that is not feasible with conventional imaging. Nevertheless, it is important to remember that although these techniques are extremely sensitive, the alterations observed in a tissue's microarchitecture are not specific to any particular pathologic status. In addition, although many research studies have advocated the ability of DT imaging to provide quantifying metrics of diffusivity and anisotropy, it is difficult to apply findings derived from group data to an individual patient. As a result, in current clinical practice DT imaging and tractography are primarily used qualitatively. Despite these limitations, with further research these exciting techniques will likely lead to improved methods for diagnosis and monitoring of disease progression and treatment response.

REFERENCES

1. Brown R. A brief account of microscopical observations on the particles contained in the pollen of plants; and of the general existence of active molecules in organic and inorganic bodies. Edinburgh N Phil J 1828;4:358–71.
2. Einstein A. Investigations on the theory of Brownian movement. New York: Dover Publications; 1956. p. 17.
3. Mukherjee P, Berman JI, Chung SW, et al. Diffusion tensor MR imaging and fiber tractography: theoretic underpinnings. AJNR Am J Neuroradiol 2008;29:632–41.
4. Mukherjee P, Chung SW, Berman JI, et al. Diffusion tensor MR imaging and fiber tractography: technical considerations. AJNR Am J Neuroradiol 2008;29:843–52.
5. Le Bihan D, Mangin JF, Poupon C, et al. Diffusion tensor imaging: concepts and applications. J Magn Reson 2001;13:534–46.
6. Beaulieu C. The basis of anisotropic water diffusion in the nervous system: a technical review. NMR Biomed 2002;15:435–55.
7. Basser PJ. Inferring microstructural features and the physiological state of tissues from diffusion weighted images. NMR Biomed 1995;8:333–4.
8. Basser PJ, Pierpaoli C. Microstructural and physiological features of tissues elucidated by quantitative diffusion tensor MRI. J Magn Reson 1996; 111:209–19.
9. Song SK, Sun SW, Ramsbottom MJ, et al. Dysmyelination revealed through MRI as increased radial (but unchanged axial) diffusion of water. Neuroimage 2002;17:1429–36.
10. Wheeler-Kingshott CA, Cercignani M. About "axial" and "radial" diffusivities. Magn Reson Med 2009; 61:1255–60.
11. Pajevic S, Pierpaoli C. Color schemes to represent the orientation of anisotropic tissues from diffusion tensor data: application to white matter fiber tract mapping of the human brain. Magn Reson Med 1999;42:526–40.
12. Conturo TE, Lori NF, Cull TS, et al. Tracking neuronal fiber pathways in the living human brain. Proc Natl Acad Sci U S A 1999;96:10422–7.
13. Mori S, Crain BJ, Chacko VP, et al. Three-dimensional tracking of axonal projections in the brain by magnetic resonance imaging. Ann Neurol 1999; 45:265–9.
14. Basser PJ, Pajevic S, Pierpaoli C, et al. In vivo tractography using DT-MRI data. Magn Reson Med 2000;44:625–32.
15. Weinstein DM, Kindlmann GL, Lundberg EC. Tensorlines: advection-diffusion based propagation

through diffusion tensor fields. In: Proceedings of IEEE Visualization '99. San Francisco (CA): October 24-29, 1999. p. 249–53.

16. Westin CF, Maier SE, Mamata H, et al. Processing and visualization for diffusion tensor MRI. Med Image Anal 2002;6:93–108.

17. Lazar M, Weinstein DM, Tsuruda JS, et al. White matter tractography using tensor deflection. Hum Brain Mapp 2003;18:306–21.

18. Mori S, Kaufmann WE, Davatzikos C, et al. Imaging cortical association tracts in the human brain using diffusion-tensor-based axonal tracking. Magn Reson Med 2002;47:215–23.

19. Catani M, Howard RJ, Pajevic S, et al. Virtual in vivo interactive dissection of white matter fasciculi in the human brain. Neuroimage 2002;17:77–94.

20. Stieltjes B, Kaufmann WE, van Zijl PCM, et al. Diffusion tensor imaging and axonal tracking in the human brain. Neuroimage 2001;14:723–35.

21. Wakana S, Jiang H, Nagae-Poetscher LM, et al. Fiber tract-based atlas of human white matter anatomy. Radiology 2004;230:77–87.

22. Jellison BJ, Field AS, Medow J, et al. Diffusion tensor imaging of cerebral white matter: A pictorial review of physics, fiber tract anatomy, and tumor imaging patterns. AJNR Am J Neuroradiol 2004; 25:356–69.

23. Poupon C, Mangin J, Clark CA, et al. Towards inference of human brain connectivity from MR diffusion tensor data. Med Image Anal 2001;5:1–15.

24. Roberts TP, Liu F, Kassner A, et al. Fiber density index correlates with reduced fractional anisotropy in white matter of patients with glioblastoma. AJNR Am J Neuroradiol 2005;26:2183–6.

25. Ture U, Yasargil MG, Pait TG. Is there a superior occipitofrontal fasciculus? A microsurgical anatomic study. Neurosurgery 1997;40:1226–32.

26. Holodny AI, Gor DM, Watts R, et al. Diffusion-tensor MR tractography of somatotopic organization of corticospinal tracts in the internal capsule: initial anatomic results in contradistinction to prior reports. Radiology 2005;234:649–53.

27. Castillo M, Smith JK, Kwock L, et al. Apparent diffusion coefficients in the evaluation of high-grade cerebral gliomas. AJNR Am J Neuroradiol 2001; 22:60–4.

28. Lu S, Ahn D, Johnson G, et al. Peritumoral diffusion tensor imaging of high-grade gliomas and metastatic brain tumors. AJNR Am J Neuroradiol 2003; 24:937–41.

29. Lu S, Ahn D, Johnson G, et al. Diffusion-tensor MR imaging of intracranial neoplasia and associated peritumoral edema: introduction of the tumor infiltration index. Radiology 2004;232:221–8.

30. Stadnik TW, Chaskis C, Michotte A, et al. Diffusion-weighted MR imaging of intracerebral masses: comparison with conventional MR imaging and histologic findings. AJNR Am J Neuroradiol 2001; 22:969–76.

31. Bastin ME, Sinha S, Whittle IR, et al. Measurements of water diffusion and T1 values in peritumoral oedematous brain. Neuroreport 2002;13:1335–40.

32. Sinha S, Bastin ME, Whittle IR, et al. Diffusion tensor MR imaging of high-grade cerebral gliomas. AJNR Am J Neuroradiol 2002;23:520–7.

33. Provenzale JM, McGraw P, Mhatre P, et al. Peritumoral brain regions in gliomas and meningiomas: investigation with isotropic diffusion-weighted MR imaging and diffusion-tensor MR imaging. Radiology 2004;232:451–60.

34. Wu JS, Zhou LF, Tang WJ, et al. Clinical evaluation and follow-up outcome of diffusion tensor imaging-based functional neuronavigation: a prospective, controlled study in patients with gliomas involving pyramidal tracts. Neurosurgery 2007;61:935–48.

35. Romano A, D'Andrea G, Minniti G, et al. Pre-surgical planning and MR-tractography utility in brain tumour resection. Eur Radiol 2009;19:2798–808.

36. Yu CS, Li KC, Xuan Y, et al. Diffusion tensor tractography in patients with cerebral tumors: a helpful technique for neurosurgical planning and postoperative assessment. Eur J Radiol 2005;56:197–204.

37. Nimsky C, Ganslandt O, Hastreiter P, et al. Preoperative and intraoperative diffusion tensor imaging-based fiber tracking in glioma surgery. Neurosurgery 2005;56:130–8.

38. Ulmer JL, Salvan CV, Mueller WM, et al. The role of diffusion tensor imaging in establishing the proximity of tumor borders to functional brain systems: implications for preoperative risk assessments and postoperative outcomes. Technol Cancer Res Treat 2004;3:567–76.

39. Davis DP, Robertson T, Imbesi SG. Diffusion-weighted magnetic resonance imaging versus computed tomography in the diagnosis of acute ischemic stroke. J Emerg Med 2006;31:269–77.

40. Sotak CH. The role of diffusion tensor imaging in the evaluation of ischemic brain injury—a review. NMR Biomed 2002;15:561–9.

41. Mukherjee P, Bahn MM, McKinstry RC, et al. Differences between gray matter and white matter water diffusion in stroke: diffusion-tensor MR imaging in 12 patients. Radiology 2000;215:211–20.

42. Maniega SM, Bastin ME, Armitage PA, et al. Temporal evolution of water diffusion parameters is different in gray and white matter in human ischaemic stroke. J Neurol Neurosurg Psychiatry 2004;75:1714–8.

43. Sorensen AG, Wu O, Copen WA, et al. Human acute cerebral ischemia: detection of changes in water diffusion anisotropy by using MR imaging. Radiology 1999;212:785–92.

44. Bastin ME, Rana AK, Wardlaw JM, et al. A study of the apparent diffusion coefficient of grey and white

matter in human stroke. Neuroreport 2000;11: 2867–74.

45. Radlinska B, Ghinani S, Leppert IR, et al. Diffusion tensor imaging, permanent pyramidal tract damage, and outcome in subcortical stroke. Neurology 2010;75:1048–54.

46. Werring DJ, Toosy AT, Clark CA, et al. Diffusion tensor imaging can detect and quantify corticospinal tract degeneration after stroke. J Neurol Neurosurg Psychiatry 2000;69:269–72.

47. Yamada K, Ito H, Nakamura H, et al. Stroke patients' evolving symptoms assessed by tractography. J Magn Reson Imaging 2004;20:923–9.

48. Konishi J, Yamada K, Kizu O, et al. MR tractography for the evaluation of functional recovery from lenticulostriate infarcts. Neurology 2005;64:108–13.

49. Chen Z, Ni P, Zhang J, et al. Evaluating ischemic stroke with diffusion tensor imaging. Neurol Res 2008;30:720–6.

50. Jiang Q, Zhang ZG, Chopp M. MRI of stroke recovery. Stroke 2010;41:410–4.

51. Chang BS, Lowenstein DH. Epilepsy. N Engl J Med 2003;349:1257–66.

52. Nilsson D, Starck G, Ljungberg M, et al. Intersubject variability in the anterior extent of the optic radiation assessed by tractography. Epilepsy Res 2007;77:11–6.

53. Taoka T, Sakamoto M, Nakagawa H, et al. Diffusion tensor tractography of the Meyer loop in cases of temporal lobe resection for temporal lobe epilepsy: correlation between postsurgical visual field defect and anterior limit of Meyer loop on tractography. AJNR Am J Neuroradiol 2008;29: 1329–34.

54. Yogarajah M, Focke NK, Bonelli S, et al. Defining Meyer's loop-temporal lobe resections, visual field deficits and diffusion tensor tractography. Brain 2009;132:1656–68.

55. Assaf BA, Mohamed FB, Abou-Khaled KJ, et al. Diffusion tensor imaging of the hippocampal formation in temporal lobe epilepsy. AJNR Am J Neuroradiol 2003;24:1857–62.

56. Rugg-Gunn FJ, Eriksson SH, Symms MR, et al. Diffusion tensor imaging of cryptogenic and acquired partial epilepsies. Brain 2001;124:627–36.

57. Widjaja E, Geibprasert S, Otsubo H, et al. Diffusion tensor imaging assessment of the epileptogenic zone in children with localization-related epilepsy. AJNR Am J Neuroradiol 2011;32:1789–94.

58. Gross DW. Diffusion tensor imaging in temporal lobe epilepsy. Epilepsia 2011;52:32–4.

59. Arfanakis K, Hermann BP, Rogers BP, et al. Diffusion tensor MRI in temporal lobe epilepsy. Magn Reson Imaging 2002;20:511–9.

60. Popescu BF, Lucchinetti CF. Pathology of demyelinating diseases. Annu Rev Pathol Mech Dis 2012;7: 185–217.

61. Love S. Demyelinating diseases. J Clin Pathol 2006;59:1151–9.

62. Ratcliffe MR, Al-Islam S, Stockley HM, et al. Demyelinating disorders of the adult central nervous system: a pictorial review of MR imaging findings. Neurographics 2011;1:17–30.

63. Ge Y, Law M, Grossman RI. Applications of diffusion tensor MR imaging in multiple sclerosis. Ann N Y Acad Sci 2005;1064:202–19.

64. Filippi M, Cercignami M, Inglese M, et al. Diffusion tensor magnetic resonance imaging in multiple sclerosis. Neurology 2001;56:304–11.

65. Werring DJ, Clark CA, Barker GJ, et al. Diffusion tensor imaging of lesions and normal-appearing white matter in multiple sclerosis. Neurology 1999; 52:1626–32.

66. Bammer R, Augustin M, Strasser-Fuchs S, et al. Magnetic resonance diffusion tensor imaging for characterizing diffuse and focal white matter abnormalities in multiple sclerosis. Magn Reson Med 2000;44:583–91.

67. Song SK, Sun SW, Ju SW, et al. Diffusion tensor imaging detects and differentiates axonal and myelin degeneration in mouse optic nerve after retinal ischemia. Neuroimage 2003;20:1714–22.

68. Roosendaal SD, Geurts JJG, Vrenken H, et al. Regional DTI differences in multiple sclerosis patients. Neuroimage 2009;44:1397–403.

69. Werring DJ, Brassat D, Droogan AG, et al. The pathogenesis of lesions and normal-appearing white matter changes in multiple sclerosis: a serial diffusion MRI study. Brain 2000;123:1667–76.

70. Lin X, Tench CR, Morgan PS, et al. 'Importance sampling' in MS: use of diffusion tensor tractography to quantify pathology related to specific impairment. J Neurol Sci 2005;237:13–9.

71. Knopman DS, Boeve BF, Peterson RC. Essentials of the proper diagnoses of mild cognitive impairment, dementia, and major subtypes of dementia. Mayo Clin Proc 2003;78:1290–308.

72. Chua TC, Wen W, Slavin MJ, et al. Diffusion tensor imaging in mild cognitive impairment and Alzheimer's disease: a review. Curr Opin Neurol 2008; 21:83–92.

73. Huang J, Friedland RP, Auchus AP. Diffusion tensor imaging of normal-appearing white matter in mild cognitive impairment and early Alzheimer disease: preliminary evidence of axonal degeneration in the temporal lobe. AJNR Am J Neuroradiol 2007;28: 1943–8.

74. Bozzali M, Falini A, Franceschi M, et al. White matter damage in Alzheimer's disease assessed in vivo using diffusion tensor magnetic resonance imaging. J Neurol Neurosurg Psychiatry 2002;72: 742–6.

75. Bosch B, Arenaza-Urquijo EM, Rami L, et al. Multiple DTI index analysis in normal aging,

amnestic MCI and AD. Relationship with neuropsychological performance. Neurobiol Aging 2012;33:61–74.

76. Lo CY, Wang PN, Chou KH, et al. Diffusion tensor tractography reveals abnormal topological organization in structural cortical networks in Alzheimer's disease. J Neurosci 2010;30:16876–85.

77. Fischer FU, Scheurich A, Wegrzyn M, et al. Automated tractography of the cingulate bundle in Alzheimer's disease: a multicenter DTI study. J Magn Reson Imaging 2012;36:84–91.

78. Bozzali M, Giulietti G, Basile B, et al. Damage to the cingulum contributes to Alzheimer's disease pathophysiology by deafferentation mechanism. Hum Brain Mapp 2012;33:1295–308.

79. Sexton CE, Kalu UG, Filippini N, et al. A meta-analysis of diffusion tensor imaging in mild cognitive impairment and Alzheimer's disease. Neurobiol Aging 2011;32:2322.e5–18.

80. Xu Q, Zhou Y, Li YS, et al. Diffusion tensor imaging changes correlate with cognition better than conventional MRI findings in patients with subcortical ischemic vascular disease. Dement Geriatr Cogn Disord 2010;30:317–26.

81. McKeith I. Dementia with Lewy bodies. Dialogues Clin Neurosci 2004;6:333–41.

82. Bozzali M, Cherubini A. Diffusion tensor MRI to investigate dementias: a brief review. Magn Reson Imaging 2007;25:969–77.

83. Tartaglia MC, Johnson DY, Thai JN, et al. Clinical overlap between Jakob-Creutzfeldt disease and Lewy body disease. Can J Neurol Sci 2012;39:304–10.

84. Ota M, Sato N, Ogawa M, et al. Degeneration of dementia with Lewy bodies measured by diffusion tensor imaging. NMR Biomed 2009;22:280–4.

85. Lee JE, Park HJ, Park BS, et al. A comparative analysis of cognitive profiles and white-matter alterations using voxel-based diffusion tensor imaging between patients with Parkinson's disease dementia and dementia with Lewy bodies. J Neurol Neurosurg Psychiatry 2010;81:320–6.

86. Fields RD. White matter in learning, cognition, and psychiatric disorders. Trends Neurosci 2008;31:361–70.

87. Whitford TJ, Kubicki M, Shenton ME. Diffusion tensor imaging, structural connectivity, and schizophrenia. Schizophr Res Treatment 2011;2011:709523. http://dx.doi.org/10.1155/2011/709523.

88. White T, Nelson M, Lim KO. Diffusion tensor imaging in psychiatric disorders. Top Magn Reson Imaging 2008;19:97–109.

89. Ellison-Wright I, Bullmore E. Meta-analysis of diffusion tensor imaging studies in schizophrenia. Schizophr Res 2009;108:3–10.

90. Kubicki M, McCarley R, Westin CF, et al. A review of diffusion tensor imaging studies in schizophrenia. J Psychiatr Res 2007;41:15–30.

91. Murphy ML, Frodl T. Meta-analysis of diffusion tensor imaging studies shows altered fraction anisotropy occurring in distinct brain areas in association with depression. Biol Mood Anxiety Disord 2011;1:3.

92. Zuo N, Fang J, Lv X, et al. White matter abnormalities in major depression: a tract-based spatial statistics and rumination study. PLoS One 2012;7:e37561. http://dx.doi.org/10.1371/journal.pone.0037561.

93. Tham MW, Woon PS, Sum MY, et al. White matter abnormalities in major depression: evidence from post-mortem, neuroimaging and genetic studies. J Affect Disord 2010;132(1–2):26–36. http://dx.doi.org/10.1016/j.jad.2010.09.013.

94. Liao Y, Huan X, Wu Q, et al. Is depression a disconnection syndrome? Meta-analysis of diffusion tensor imaging studies in patients with MDD. J Psychiatry Neurosci 2012;38(1):49–56. http://dx.doi.org/10.1503/jpn.110180.

95. Barkovich AJ, Mukherjee P. Normal development of the neonatal and infant brain, skull, and spine. In: Barkovich AJ, Raybaud C, editors. Pediatric neuroimaging. 5th edition. Philadelphia: Wolters Kluwer Health/Lippincott Williams & Wilkins; 2011. p. 20–80.

96. Welker KM, Patton A. Assessment of normal myelination with magnetic resonance imaging. Semin Neurol 2012;32:15–28.

97. Huppi PS, Dubois J. Diffusion tensor imaging of brain development. Semin Fetal Neonatal Med 2006;11:489–97.

98. Cascio CJ, Gerig G, Piven J. Diffusion tensor imaging: application to the study of the developing brain. J Am Acad Child Adolesc Psychiatry 2007;46:213–23.

99. Qui D, Tan LH, Zhou K, et al. Diffusion tensor imaging of normal white matter maturation from late childhood to young adulthood: voxel-wise evaluation of mean diffusivity, fractional anisotropy, radial and axial diffusivities, and correlation with reading development. Neuroimage 2008;41:223–32.

100. Westlye LT, Walhovd KB, Dale AM, et al. Life-span changes of the human brain white matter: diffusion tensor imaging (DTI) and volumetry. Cereb Cortex 2010;20:2055–68.

101. Faria AV, Zhang J, Oishi K, et al. Atlas-based analysis of neurodevelopment from infancy to adulthood using diffusion tensor imaging and applications for automated abnormality detection. Neuroimage 2010;52:415–28.

102. Huppi PS. Advances in postnatal neuroimaging; relevance to pathogenesis and treatment of brain injury. Clin Perinatol 2002;29:827–56.

103. Nagy Z, Westerberg H, Klingberg T. Maturation of white matter is associated with the development of cognitive functions during childhood. J Cogn Neurosci 2004;17:1227–33.

104. Schmithorst VJ, Wilke M, Bardzinski BJ, et al. Cognitive functions correlate with white matter architecture in a normal pediatric population: a diffusion tensor MR imaging study. Hum Brain Mapp 2005;26:139–47.

105. Asato MR, Terwilliger R, Woo J, et al. White matter development in adolescence: a DTI study. Cereb Cortex 2010;20:2122–31.

106. Peters BD, Szeszko PR, Radua J, et al. White matter development in adolescence: diffusion tensor imaging and meta-analytic results. Schizophr Bull 2012;38(6):1308–17. http://dx.doi.org/10.1093/schbul/sbs054.

107. Sullivan EV, Adalsteinsson E, Hedehus M, et al. Equivalent disruption of regional white matter microstructure in ageing healthy men and women. Neuroreport 2001;12:99–104.

108. Salat DH, Tuch DS, Greve DN, et al. Age-related alterations in white matter microstructure measured by diffusion tensor imaging. Neurobiol Aging 2005;26:1215–27.

109. Madden DJ, Whiting WL, Huettel SA, et al. Diffusion tensor imaging of adult age differences in cerebral white matter: relation to response time. Neuroimage 2004;21:1174–81.

110. Belmonte MK, Cook EH Jr, Anderson GM, et al. Autism as a disorder of neural information processing: directions for research and targets for therapy. Mol Psychiatry 2004;9:646–63.

111. Rippon G, Brock J, Brown C, et al. Disordered connectivity in the autistic brain: challenges for the 'new psychophysiology'. Int J Psychophysiol 2007;63:164–72.

112. Hughes JR. Autism: the first firm finding = underconnectivity? Epilepsy Behav 2007;11:20–4.

113. Hughes JR. Update on autism: a review of 1200 reports published in 2008. Epilepsy Behav 2009;16:569–89.

114. Barnea-Gorlay N, Kwon H, Menon V, et al. White matter structure in autism: preliminary evidence from diffusion tensor imaging. Biol Psychiatry 2004;55:323–6.

115. Cheung C, Chua SE, Cheung V, et al. White matter fractional anisotrophy differences and correlates of diagnostic symptoms in autism. J Child Psychol Psychiatry 2009;50:1102–12.

116. Langen M, Leemans A, Johnston P, et al. Frontostriatal circuitry and inhibitory control in autism: findings from diffusion tensor imaging tractography. Cortex 2011;48(2):183–93. http://dx.doi.org/10.1016/j.cortex.2011.05.018.

117. Groen WB, Buitelaar JK, van der Gaag RJ, et al. Pervasive microstructural abnormalities in autism: a DTI study. J Psychiatry Neurosci 2011;36:32–40.

118. Alexander AL, Lee JE, Lazar M, et al. Diffusion tensor imaging of the corpus callosum in autism. Neuroimage 2007;34:61–73.

119. Lee SK, Kim DI, Kim J, et al. Diffusion-tensor MR imaging and fiber tractography: a new method of describing aberrant fiber connections in developmental CNS anomalies. Radiographics 2005;25:53–68.

120. Wahl M, Strominger Z, Jeremy RJ, et al. Variability of homotopic and heterotopic callosal connectivity in partial agenesis of the corpus callosum: a 3T diffusion tensor imaging and Q-ball tractography study. AJNR Am J Neuroradiol 2009;30:282–9.

121. Wahl M, Barkovich AJ, Mukherjee P. Diffusion imaging and tractography of congenital brain malformations. Pediatr Radiol 2010;40:59–67.

122. Rollins N. Semilobar holoprosencephaly seen with diffusion tensor imaging and fiber tracking. AJNR Am J Neuroradiol 2005;26:2148–52.

123. Lee SK, Kim J. Diffusion tensor imaging of heterotopia: changes of fractional anisotropy during radial migration of neurons. Yonsei Med J 2010;51:590–3.

124. Briganti C, Navarra R, Celentano C, et al. Diffusion tensor imaging of subependymal heterotopia. Epilepsy Res 2012;98:251–4.

125. Lee SK, Kim DI, Mori S, et al. Diffusion tensor MRI visualized decreased subcortical fiber connectivity in focal cortical dysplasia. Neuroimage 2004;22:1826–9.

126. Widjaja E, Mahmoodabadi SZ, Otsubo H, et al. Subcortical alterations in tissue microstructure adjacent to focal cortical dysplasia: detection at diffusion-tensor MR imaging by using magnetoencephalographic dipole cluster localization. Radiology 2009;251:206–15.

127. Fonseca VC, Yasuda CL, Tedeschi GG, et al. White matter abnormalities in patients with focal cortical dysplasia revealed by diffusion tensor imaging analysis in a voxelwise approach. Front Neurol 2012;3:121. http://dx.doi.org/10.3389/fneuro.2012.00121.

128. Bruns J, Hauser WA. The epidemiology of traumatic brain injury: a review. Epilepsia 2003;44:2–10.

129. Dombovy ML. Traumatic brain injury. Continuum (Minneap Minn) 2011;17:584–605.

130. Smith DH, Meaney DF, Shull WH. Diffuse axonal injury in head trauma. J Head Trauma Rehabil 2003;18:307–16.

131. Huisman T, Sorensen AG, Hergan K, et al. Diffusion-weighted imaging for the evaluation of diffuse axonal injury in closed head injury. J Comput Assist Tomogr 2003;27:5–11.

132. Schaefer PW, Huisman T, Sorensen AG, et al. Diffusion-weighted MR imaging in closed head injury: high correlation with initial Glasgow Coma Scale score and score on Modified Rankin Scale at discharge. Radiology 2004;233:58–66.

133. Nakayama N, Okumura A, Shinoda J, et al. Evidence for white matter disruption in traumatic

brain injury without macroscopic lesions. J Neurol Neurosurg Psychiatry 2006;77:850–5.

134. Akpinar E, Koroglu M, Ptak T. Diffusion tensor MR imaging in pediatric head trauma. J Comput Assist Tomogr 2007;31:657–61.

135. Huisman TAGM, Schwamm LH, Schaefer PW, et al. Diffusion tensor imaging as potential biomarker of white matter injury in diffuse axonal injury. AJNR Am J Neuroradiol 2004;25:370–6.

136. Wilde EA, Chu Z, Bigler ED, et al. Diffusion tensor imaging in the corpus callosum in children after moderate to severe traumatic brain injury. J Neurotrauma 2006;23:1412–26.

137. Rutgers DR, Fillard P, Paradot G, et al. Diffusion tensor imaging characteristics of the corpus callosum in mild, moderate, and severe traumatic brain injury. AJNR Am J Neuroradiol 2008;29: 1730–5.

138. Aoki Y, Inokuchi R, Gunshin M, et al. Diffusion tensor imaging studies of mild traumatic brain injury: a meta-analysis. J Neurol Neurosurg Psychiatry 2012;83:870–6.

139. Wozniak JR, Krach L, Ward E, et al. Neurocognitive and neuroimaging correlates of pediatric traumatic brain injury: a diffusion tensor imaging (DTI) study. Arch Clin Neuropsychol 2007;22:555–68.

140. Benson RB, Meda SA, Vasudevan S, et al. Global white matter analysis of diffusion tensor images is predictive of injury severity in traumatic brain injury. J Neurotrauma 2007;24:446–59.

141. Yasokawa YT, Shinoda J, Okumura A, et al. Correlation between diffusion-tensor magnetic resonance imaging and motor-evoked potential in chronic severe diffuse axonal injury. J Neurotrauma 2007; 24:163–73.

142. Ptak T, Sheridan RL, Rhea JT, et al. Cerebral fractional anisotropy score in trauma patients: a new indicator of white matter injury after trauma. Am J Roentgenol 2003;181:1401–7.

143. Field AS, Hasan K, Jellison BJ, et al. Diffusion tensor imaging in an infant with traumatic brain swelling. AJNR Am J Neuroradiol 2003;24:1461–4.

144. Wortzel HS, Kraus MF, Filley CM, et al. Diffusion tensor imaging in mild traumatic brain injury litigation. J Am Acad Psychiatry Law 2011;39:511–23.

145. Maier SE, Mamata H. Diffusion tensor imaging of the spinal cord. Ann N Y Acad Sci 2005;1064: 50–60.

146. Ducreux D, Lepeintre JF, Fillard P, et al. MR diffusion tensor imaging and fiber tracking in 5 spinal cord astrocytomas. AJNR Am J Neuroradiol 2006; 27:214–6.

147. Vargas MI, Delavelle J, Jlassi H, et al. Clinical applications of diffusion tensor tractography of the spinal cord. Neuroradiology 2008;50:25–9.

148. Hesseltine SM, Law M, Babb J, et al. Diffusion tensor imaging in multiple sclerosis: assessment

of regional differences in the axial plane with normal-appearing cervical spinal cord. AJNR Am J Neuroradiol 2006;27:1189–93.

149. Ohgiya Y, Oka M, Hiwatashi A, et al. Diffusion tensor MR imaging of the cervical spinal cord in patients with multiple sclerosis. Eur Radiol 2007; 17:2499–504.

150. Cruz LC Jr, Domingues RC, Gasparetto EL. Diffusion tensor imaging of the cervical spinal cord of patients with relapsing-remising multiple sclerosis. Arq Neuropsiquiatr 2009;67:291–395.

151. Kim JH, Loy DN, Liang HF, et al. Noninvasive diffusion tensor imaging of evolving white matter pathology in a mouse model of acute spinal cord injury. Magn Reson Med 2007;58:253–60.

152. Loy DN, Kim JH, Xie M, et al. Diffusion tensor imaging predicts hyperacute spinal cord injury severity. J Neurotrauma 2007;24:979–90.

153. Shanmuganathan K, Gullapalli RP, Zhuo J, et al. Diffusion tensor MR imaging in cervical spine trauma. AJNR Am J Neuroradiol 2008;29:655–9.

154. Wei CW, Tharmakulasingam J, Crawley A, et al. Use of diffusion-tensor imaging in traumatic spinal cord injury to identify concomitant traumatic brain injury. Arch Phys Med Rehabil 2008;89:S85–91.

155. Maldjian JA, Listerud J, Moonis G, et al. Computing diffusion rates in T2-dark hematomas and areas of low T2 signal. AJNR Am J Neuroradiol 2001;22: 112–8.

156. Frank LR. Characterization of anisotropy in high angular resolution diffusion-weighted MRI. Magn Reson Med 2002;47:1083–99.

157. Alexander DC, Barker GJ, Arridge SR. Detection and modeling of non-Gaussian apparent diffusion coefficient profiles in human brain data. Magn Reson Med 2002;48:331–40.

158. Tuch DS, Reese TG, Wiegell MR, et al. Diffusion MRI of complex neural architecture. Neuron 2003; 40:885–95.

159. Assaf Y, Freidlin RZ, Rohde GK, et al. New modeling and experimental framework to characterize hindered and restricted water diffusion in brain white matter. Magn Reson Med 2004;52: 965–78.

160. Wedeen VJ, Hagmann P, Tseng WY, et al. Mapping complex tissue architecture with diffusion spectrum magnetic resonance imaging. Magn Reson Med 2005;54:1377–86.

161. Hagmann P, Reese TG, Tseng WY, et al. Diffusion spectrum imaging tractography in complex cerebral white matter: an investigation of the centrum semiovale. In: Proceedings of the ISMRM 12th Scientific Meeting and Exhibition. Kyoto (Japan): May 15-21, 2004. p. 623.

162. Kinoshita M, Yamada K, Hashimoto N, et al. Fiber-tracking does not accurately estimate size of fiber bundle in pathological condition: initial

neurosurgical experience using neuronavigation and subcortical white matter stimulation. Neuroimage 2005;25:424–9.

163. Nimsky C, Ganslandt O, Hastreiter P, et al. Intraoperative diffusion-tensor MR imaging: shifting of white matter tracts during neurosurgical procedures—initial experience. Radiology 2005; 234:218–25.

164. Basser PJ, Pajevic S. Statistical artifacts in diffusion tensor MRI (DT-MRI) caused by background noise. Magn Reson Med 2000;44:41–50.

165. Field AS, Alexander AL, Wu YC, et al. Diffusion tensor eigenvector directional color imaging patterns in the evaluation of cerebral white matter tracts altered by tumor. J Magn Reson Imaging 2004;20:555–62.

166. Wu YC, Field AS, Chung MK, et al. Quantitative analysis of diffusion tensor orientation: theoretical framework. Magn Reson Med 2004;52:1146–55.

167. Pipe JG, Farthing VG, Forbes KP. Multishot diffusion-weighted FSE using PROPELLER MRI. Magn Reson Med 2002;47:42–52.

Clinical Applications of Diffusion Imaging in the Spine

Lawrence N. Tanenbaum, MD

KEYWORDS

- Diffusion magnetic resonance imaging • Spine • Bone marrow • Demyelination • Neoplasm
- Infection • Fracture

KEY POINTS

- Diffusion imaging is a powerful technique in widespread use in whole-body imaging that is a valuable adjunct to routine imaging protocols for the spine.
- Diffusion imaging adds sensitivity and specificity in evaluating the osseous and soft tissue structures of the spine for neoplastic involvement.
- Diffusion imaging adds sensitivity and specificity in evaluating the osseous and soft tissue structures of the spine in cases of suspected infection.
- Diffusion imaging can contribute valuable information to the evaluation of lesions of the spinal cord.
- Protocol optimization and pending technical advances can and will provide critical improvements in image quality, which should lead to routine use in the evaluation of diseases of the spine.

INTRODUCTION

The imaging assessment of the diffusion characteristics of water molecules on an intracellular and extracellular space level can herald powerful information about normal and abnormal tissues and processes. Diffusion-weighted imaging (DWI), a technique typically based on echo planar imaging (EPI), has been widely available for clinical purposes since the early 1990s. DWI rapidly achieved universal use for the evaluation of brain diseases, improving sensitivity and specificity of magnetic resonance (MR) imaging for a variety of disease states, including infarction, infection, inflammation, and hemorrhage. Of late, DWI has achieved greater importance in evaluation of the abdomen, pelvis, prostate, and breast[1–3] with increasingly routine use in day-to-day practice. Although DWI should be equally sensitive to diseases of the spine, it has been used far less frequently in this region. This is mainly because of the challenges placed by the spine's

heterogeneous magnetic environment, the small size of the spinal cord, and motion in and around the spine.

There is, however, a range of current and potential applications for DWI in the spine. As in the brain, the sensitivity of DWI to ischemic damage in the spinal cord may provide early identification of infarction. Diffusion anisotropy may enhance the detection and understanding of damage to the long fiber tracts with clinical implications for diseases such as multiple sclerosis and amyotrophic lateral sclerosis. Diffusion anisotropy may also yield insight into damage that occurs with spondylotic and traumatic myelopathy. DWI has also been exploited for its ability to detect and characterize lesions of the spinal marrow and potentially differentiate between benign and malignant vertebral compression fractures. Although technical limitations persist to a varying degree, the applications for DWI in the spine have been extensively investigated. Despite challenges and lingering controversy over clinical utility for some

Disclosures: None.
Department of Diagnostic Imaging, Mount Sinai School of Medicine, 50 Murray Street, Apartment 1001, New York, NY 10007, USA
E-mail address: nuromri@gmail.com

Magn Reson Imaging Clin N Am 21 (2013) 299–320
http://dx.doi.org/10.1016/j.mric.2012.12.002
1064-9689/13/$ – see front matter © 2013 Elsevier Inc. All rights reserved.

applications, DWI is increasingly becoming part of the routine clinical spine MR imaging regimen. This article reviews the basis for DWI for the evaluation of the spinal cord, osseous, and soft tissues of the spine and reviews the imaging appearance of a variety of disease states.

DIFFUSION-WEIGHTED MR IMAGING

DWI is a powerful tool for tissue investigation with MR imaging. By sensitizing the MR image to perturbations of the random motion of water molecules in tissues, DWI provides unique insight into pathologic physiology.[4–6]

DWI revolutionized the evaluation of patients with suspected stroke by providing exquisite sensitivity to the presence of brain infarction, almost immediately after onset. DWI also provides the critical ability to differentiate chronic ischemic brain changes from those caused by recent stroke in patients who present in the subacute stroke setting. Perhaps the most impactful role of cranial DWI is in characterization of brain lesions—the differentiation of stroke and abscess from tumor and the assessment and surveillance of demyelinating disease. Of late, DWI has become popular for imaging outside the brain and is now commonly used in the routine MR imaging study of the breast, prostate, abdomen and pelvis, providing a boost in lesion detection. DWI also offers valuable characterization information useful in the differentiation of malignant from benign lesions as well as tumor from reactive and treatment-related changes.

Technical Considerations

Typically based on clinically available single-shot EPI scanning techniques, DWI is rapidly acquired

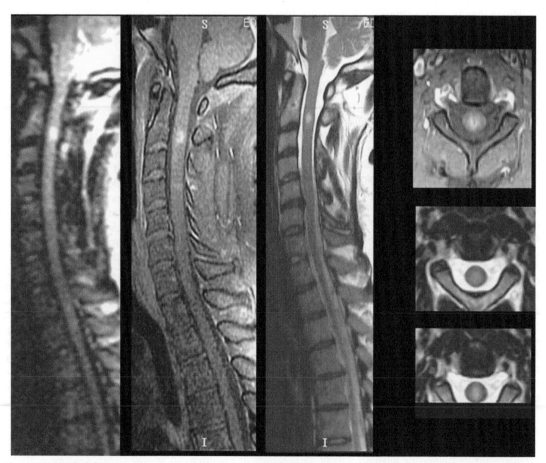

Fig. 1. Single shot fast spin echo (ssFSE) diffusion of an MS plaque. From left (sagittal): ssFSE DWI; fat-suppressed, contrast-enhanced spine echo (SE) T1; FSE T2. From top (axial): Fat-suppressed, contrast enhanced SE T1; FSE T2. Note the ovoid lesion at C2-3, which shows increased signal on DW and T2-weighted images as well as contrast enhancement.

and motion resistant. Although nearly ideal for imaging of the brain, EPI faces significant challenges in the spine. Bulk physiologic motion within the chest and abdomen or from swallowing and motion from the spinal cord itself are sources of artifact. Susceptibility variation associated with the osseous structures and field variations adjacent to the cervicothoracic junction and the lungs may cause severe distortion. The small size of the spinal cord and adjacent structures requires smaller voxel sizes and thus requires an inherently high signal-to-noise ratio (SNR) acquisition technique. As a result, application of DWI to the vertebral column and the spinal cord has been far less popular than elsewhere.

Alternative techniques based on single-shot and line scan fast spin echo (**Fig. 1**) have been investigated but have failed to achieve clinical availability despite potential advantages over EPI.[7,8] With minor modifications to current EPI-based protocol parameters, diagnostic quality studies of the spine can be obtained (**Fig. 2**). Reduced B values (400–500) and minimized frequency encoding each reduces echo times (TE) leading to improved SNR and reduced distortion (**Box 1**).

Recent and continuing technical innovations greatly affect EPI DWI of the spine. Applying the 3 diffusion gradients simultaneously instead of sequentially (3 in 1, GE, Waukesha, WI) allows

Box 1
Typical DW spine technique
Repetition time (TR), echo time (TE) minimum
Frequency (General Electric): minimum (64 if possible), Siemens 192
Phase 192–256
Field of view 26
3–4 mm, skip 1
4 nex, acquisitions
B value - 500

much shorter TE values, which boosts SNR, reduces distortion, and shortens scan times (**Fig. 3**). Parallel imaging–capable spine coils allow DWI at reduced TE values, preserving SNR and reducing susceptibility effects (**Fig. 4**). More powerful gradient systems also allow shorter TE values at a given B value, yielding either improved image quality or the use of higher B values. Recently available techniques such as multishot EPI (**Fig. 5**) and restricted field-of-view (FOV) DWI (**Fig. 6**) are practical and artifact resistant, promising better suitability to applications in body and spine.[9,10] As the quality of the clinical diffusion image improves, DWI will gain even wider use in the routine diagnostic workup of spinal disorders.

Scientific study of diffusion imaging has focused on assessment and often quantitative measures of the apparent diffusion coefficient (ADC). Individual direction and trace weighted or combined direction DW images routinely manifest T2 effects, which complicate assignment of diffusion imaging behavior. This finding has been cited as limiting the utility and scientific validity of early techniques that have been used in evaluating the spine.[11,12] In routine practice, it can be more useful to interrogate routine, combined, or trace diffusion images. These DW images additively combine T2 effects with diffusion alterations to significantly boost conspicuity (if not specificity) of lesions, which exhibit both diffusion restriction and T2 prolongation. As an example in the brain, although ADC values are lowest in the first few hours after stroke, it is only after T2 effects manifest that lesions are most conspicuous; when on (trace weighted) DWI the combined signal contributions manifest the characteristic light bulb high signal appearance. In contrast, chronic strokes have high diffusion values, which combine antagonistically with T2 prolongation to produce an isointense lesion. For clinical purposes, lower B values (eg, 500 s/mm^2) are typically used for spine

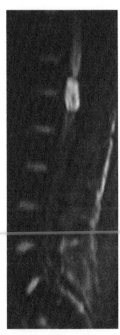

Fig. 2. Echoplanar (EPI) DW image of an ependymoma.

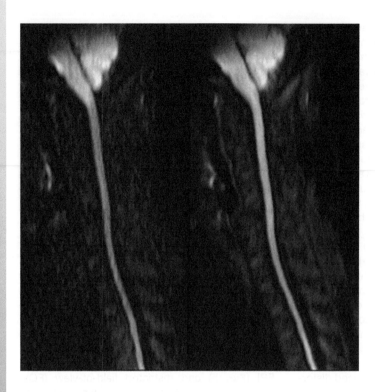

Fig. 3. Enhancements to spine DWI. Note the improvement in speed, SNR, and quality of depiction of the spinal cord when all 3 diffusion gradients are applied simultaneously (*right*, 3 in 1, scan time 0:38) when compared with the image obtained with traditional sequential (*left*, DTI 1:43) application. Both studies obtained at a parallel imaging factor of 2.

imaging, allowing for significant T2 contribution to the trace-weighted DWI. Although in the interest of diffusion image purity, use of higher B values can effectively minimize T2 contribution; with clinically available techniques, the proportional tradeoffs in increased distortion and reduced SNR are effectively limiting. On the other hand, the synergistic contribution of combined T2 prolongation and diffusion restriction is likely responsible for some of the contributions made by DWI to the clinical

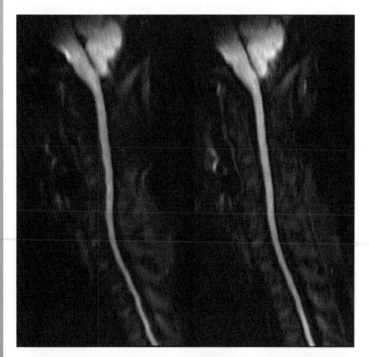

Fig. 4. Parallel imaging (PI) in spine DWI. Note the improvement in accuracy of anatomic depiction of the spinal cord with reduced distortion using a PI factor of 2 (*left*) when compared with the image obtained without PI. Both images obtained with a 3 in 1 DWI technique.

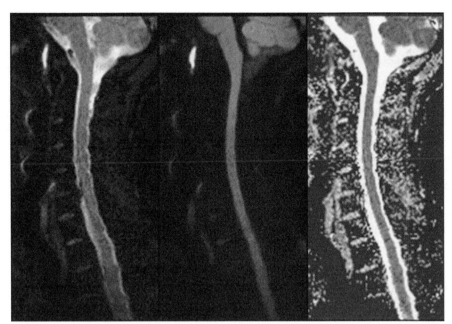

Fig. 5. Multishot EPI DW image (RESOLVE) at 3T. Note the striking lack of distortion and high spatial resolution.

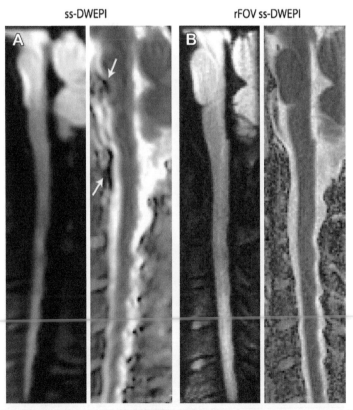

Fig. 6. Restricted FOV EPI DW image. Note the striking lack of distortion (*arrows*) and high spatial resolution. (*From* Saritas EU, Cunningham CH, Lee JH, et al. DWI of the spinal cord with reduced FOV single-shot EPI. Magn Reson Med 2008;60:468–73; with permission).

MR imaging of spine disease discussed in this article.

DIFFUSION TENSOR IMAGING

Using a matrix of diffusion measurements in 6 or more unique directions, a mathematical model of diffusion in 3-dimensional space can be created providing an assessment of diffusivity in any arbitrary direction as well as the direction of maximum diffusivity. In the brain and spinal cord, individual white matter fiber tracts impose directionality (anisotropy) on water motion—diffusion is relatively free along fibers and restricted across fibers. Anisotropy is the extent to which the ordered white matter water motion (ellipsoid in shape) deviates from that of unrestricted, random water motion (spherical in shape). The direction of maximum diffusivity is a result of the tract orientation. The directionality of diffusion is conveyed by relative or fractional anisotropy and ranges from values of 0, representing isotropic diffusion, and 1 representing complete directional preference along the major diffusion eigenvector or direction. The rate of diffusion is represented by mean diffusivity (analogous to the ADC). Quantitative and qualitative assessment of anisotropy may yield important information as to white matter integrity and tract count that can give insight into a variety of disease states.[13–15]

CLINICAL APPLICATIONS OF DWI OF THE SPINE

One of the most rewarding extracranial applications of DWI is for the evaluation of the spine. DWI provides diagnostic value similar to that provided in the brain when assessing diseases of the spinal cord. DWI also can contribute to the detection and characterization of intradural-extramedullary, and epidural lesions as well. Perhaps the most fruitful extracranial contribution of DWI is for the evaluation of marrow disease.

SPINAL CORD LESIONS

Using conventional MR imaging techniques, the myriad appearance of intramedullary lesions can be insufficiently specific for definitive diagnosis. DWI may assist in the differentiation of etiology between inflammatory, neoplastic, and ischemia-related changes.[16,17]

Neoplasm

Much as in the brain, DWI can be useful in the assessment of cord tumors.[18] Primary cord tumors tend to be close to isointense with the normal spinal cord (**Fig. 7**) as do metastatic lesions. When lesions are hemorrhagic (**Fig. 8**) or exhibit a dense cellularity because of a high

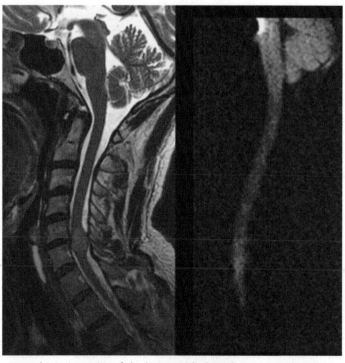

Fig. 7. Ependymoma. Note the isointensity of the lesion with the adjacent spinal cord.

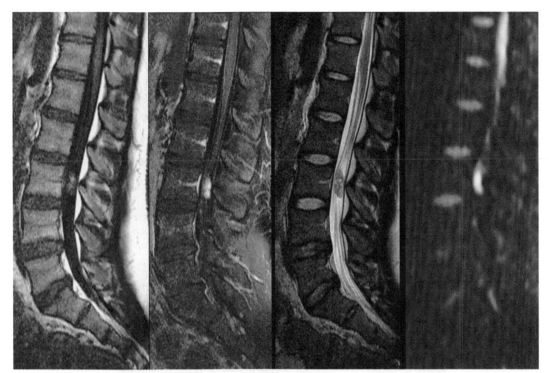

Fig. 8. Myxopapillary ependymoma. From left: Fat-suppressed, contrast enhanced T1 fluid attenuated inversion recovery (FLAIR), fast spin echo T2, and EPI DWI. Note the high signal on unenhanced T1-weighted image and the corresponding high signal on DWI.

nuclear-to-cytoplasmic ratio, some hyperintensity on DWI will result (**Fig. 9**). If dense cellularity or chronic blood products produce susceptibility effects on T2-weighted imaging, this can manifest as diminished signal on (particularly T2*-weighted EPI-based) DW images.

Infarction

As in the brain, acute infarctions of the cord will exhibit diffusion restriction (**Fig. 10**). Spinal infarctions are mainly central within the spinal cord and involve gray matter. As in the brain, diffusion abnormalities can be seen minutes after onset and begin to fade after about 1 week. Contrast enhancement is typically absent.[19,20] The characteristic hyperintensity on DWI correlated with an appropriate clinical presentation is useful in the differentiation of infarction from the somewhat overlapping appearance of neoplasm and demyelinating disease.

Demyelinating Disease

Multiple sclerosis (MS) is an inflammatory demyelinating disease of the central nervous system that is the most common cause of chronic disability in young adults in the United States. MS lesions are pathologically heterogeneous and show different imaging patterns on MR imaging, ranging from inflammatory changes to extensive tissue destruction. The highest diffusion values seem to be found in nonenhancing T1-hypointense lesions compared with enhancing lesions and nonenhancing T1-isointense lesions.[21–23] There is a variable degree of tissue damage during the period a lesion is active leading to a variable appearance on routine and DW MR imaging. Not uncommonly, active demyelinating lesions can be hyperintense on trace DWI (**Fig. 11**). Chronic demyelination, in which elevated diffusion coefficients tend to balance T2 contributions, is typically isointense with adjacent normal cord. DTI can improve sensitivity to a variety of disease states, including demyelinating disease, even detecting abnormalities in regions that are otherwise normal in imaging appearance.[24] Diffusion tensor anisotropy imaging can reveal abnormalities that are more severe and extensive than those apparent on routine imaging techniques based on T1- and T2-weighted imaging (**Fig. 12**).

Trauma, Spondylotic Myelopathy

DTI parameters are sensitive markers of cord injury compared with conventional MR imaging and may be more sensitive than routine MR

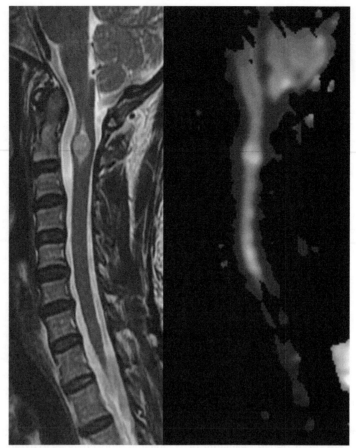

Fig. 9. Metastatic disease to the cord. FSE T2-weighted image (*left*) and EPI DWI show a well-circumscribed intramedullary lesion, which is slightly hyperintense on DWI, perhaps because of a high nucleus-to-cytoplasmic ratio.

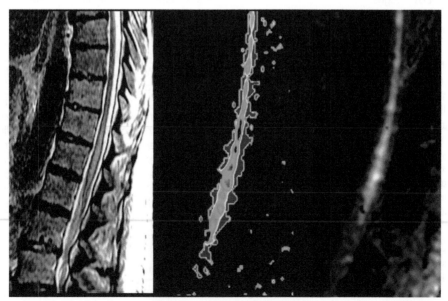

Fig. 10. Acute cord infarction after lumbar surgery. From left: T2-weighted image, ADC and isotropic DWI. Note the fusiform lesion at the conus, which reveals diffusion restriction.

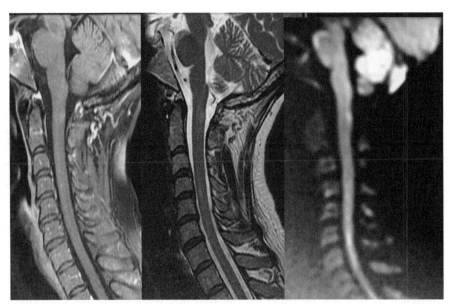

Fig. 11. Active demyelination. From left: fat-suppressed, contrast-enhanced T1 FLAIR, T2, and DWI. Note the subtle enhancement and DW hyperintensity associated with the ventral pontine and dorsal C2 cord lesions, which are presumed active. The absence of either enhancement or DWI increased signal suggests that the ventral cord lesion at C4-5 is chronic and inactive.

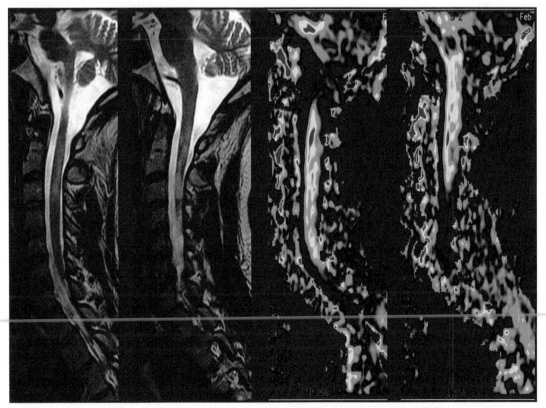

Fig. 12. Anisotropy imaging in MS. Sagittal T2 (*left*) and fractional anisotropy images of a diseased spinal cord in a patient with MS. Note the multifocal, patch cord involvement on the T2-weighted image that may be even more extensive on the anisotropy image.

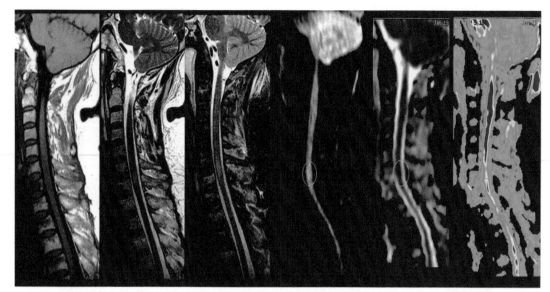

Fig. 13. Acute cord injury. From left: Sagittal T1, T2, STIR, DWI, ADC, and fractional anisotropy images. Note the C7 vertebral acute fracture associated with a cord contusion manifest as signal changes on routine imaging sequences as well as subtle diffusion restriction and a striking reduction in fractional anisotropy.

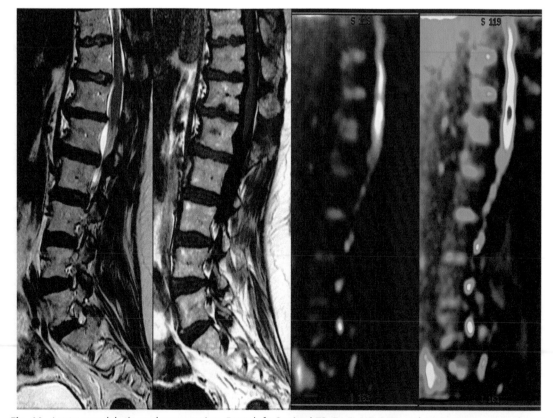

Fig. 14. Acute spondylotic cord compression. From left: Sagittal T2, T1 FLAIR, DW, and ADC images. Acute herniation (not well seen) compressing the cord with new onset of myelopathy. Note the clear diffusion restriction and subtle T2 signal changes.

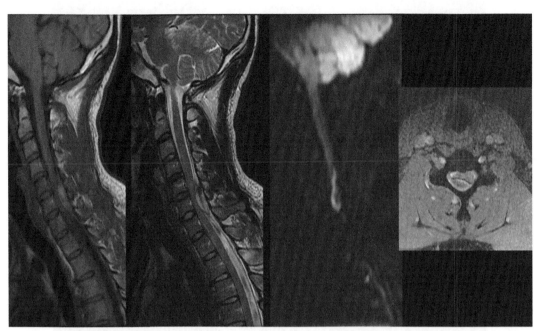

Fig. 15. Epidural hematoma. From left: Sagittal T1 FLAIR, T2, and DW, axial T2-weighted image. Note the fusiform, eccentrically left-sided epidural lesion with characteristic susceptibility and signal changes consistent with an epidural hematoma.

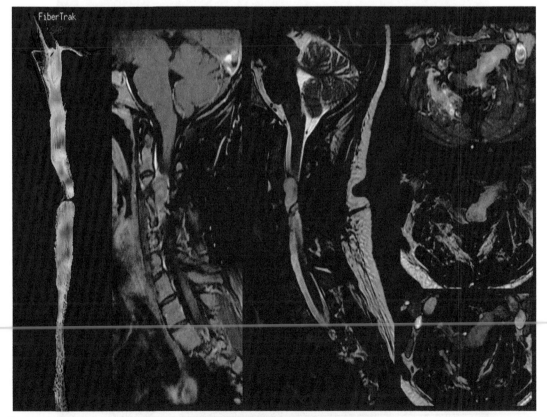

Fig. 16. Diffusion tensor myelogram neurofibroma. From left: diffusion tensor myelogram, contrast-enhanced, fat-suppressed T1 FLAIR, T2. From top: axial contrast-enhanced, fat-suppressed T1 fast spin echo; T2; gradient recalled (GRE). Note the extrinsic compression effects on the cord by the dumbbell-shaped extradural neurofibroma.

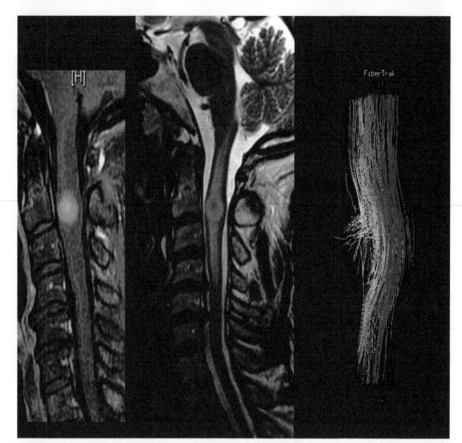

Fig. 17. DTM meningioma. From left: contrast-enhanced, fat-suppressed T1 FLAIR; T2; DTM. Although the lesion appearance with conventional techniques is suggestive of an intramedullary location, the clearly extrinsic appearance on DTM supports the final diagnosis of meningioma.

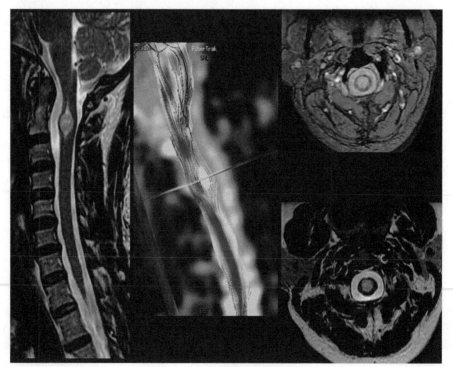

Fig. 18. Metastatic disease. Clockwise from upper left: sagittal T2, axial gradient recalled (GRE), and fast spin echo T2. Center: DTM. Note the intramedullary location of the lesion with apparent displacement of intact white matter fibers on the DTM.

imaging techniques. Studies have found that ADC and relative anisotropy values for patients with cervical spine contusions were significantly lower than comparative values in healthy individuals. Diffusion restriction (reduced ADC) is typically the most sensitive marker of cord injury. (**Fig. 13**) perhaps because of reduced diffusion coefficients and subtle hemorrhage.[25] Demonstration of abnormalities in the DTI parameters in areas of the spinal cord that seem normal on conventional MR imaging could be used to document the true extent of injury and help to correlate better the neurologic deficit with MR imaging. These results indicate that DTI parameters, in addition to the clinical examination, could be an independent predictor of the severity of spinal cord injury and may be used to monitor recovery after treatment.[26] Patients with electrophysiologic examination–confirmed spondylotic myelopathy can show increased ADC values and decreased anisotropy. Diffusion-weighted ADC maps can be more sensitive than T2-weighted images and have a higher negative predictive value.[27] Differentiation of edema from myelomalacia in the setting of spondylosis and cord compression is a common and perplexing diagnostic challenge. T2 signal changes within the compressed cord are nonspecific in etiology and can be caused by chronic myelomalacia or acute edema. Acute traumatic cord injuries tend to exhibit hyperintensity on DWI (**Fig. 14**), perhaps because of reduced diffusion coefficients and subtle hemorrhage. Myelomalacia, in which elevated diffusion coefficients tend to balance or slightly exceed T2 balancing T2 effects, appears isointense to hypointense with the adjacent normal cord. Definitive differentiation of acute compressive cord/injury edema from myelomalacia caused by chronic compression could drive clinical decision making. As they do intracranially, epidural hematomas reveal characteristic T1 and T2*-related signal changes (**Fig. 15**).

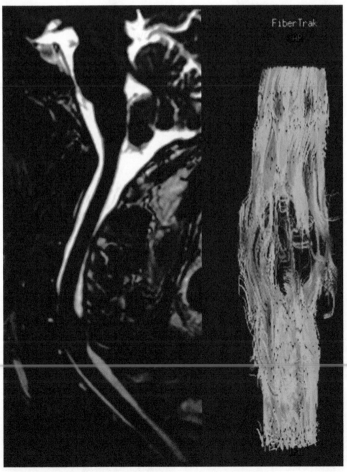

Fig. 19. Ependymoma. Sagittal T2 (*left*), DTM. Note the central, intramedullary location of the lesion with peripheral displacement of intact white matter fibers on the DTM.

312

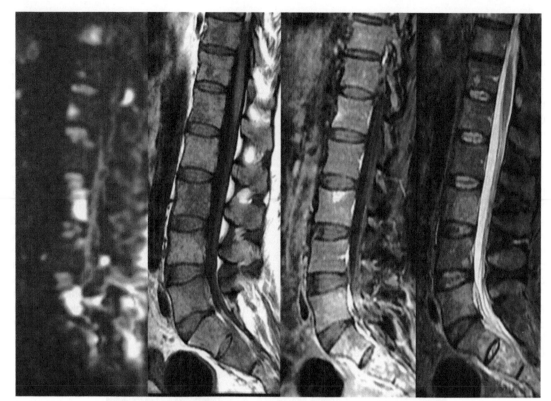

Fig. 20. Metastatic disease. From left: DWI; T1 FLAIR; fat-suppressed, contrast enhanced T1 FLAIR, STIR. Note the superior conspicuity of many of the metastatic lesions with DWI.

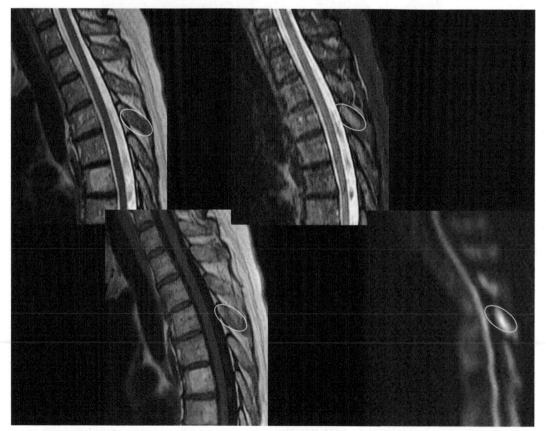

Fig. 21. Metastatic myeloma. Clockwise from upper left: T2, STIR, DWI, T1 FLAIR. Note the highest conspicuity of the spinous process lesion (*circle*) with DWI.

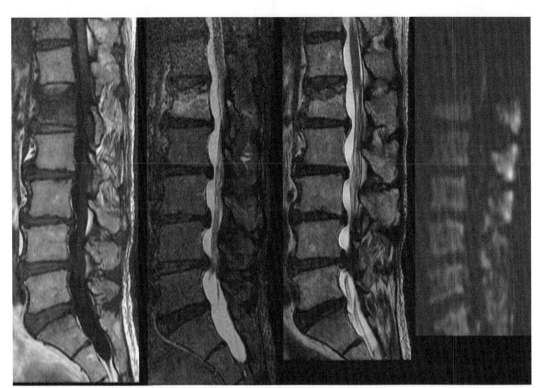

Fig. 22. Senescent compression fracture. From left: T1 FLAIR, STIR, T2, DWI. Note the diminished signal on DWI associated with the recent compression fracture involving the superior end plate of L1.

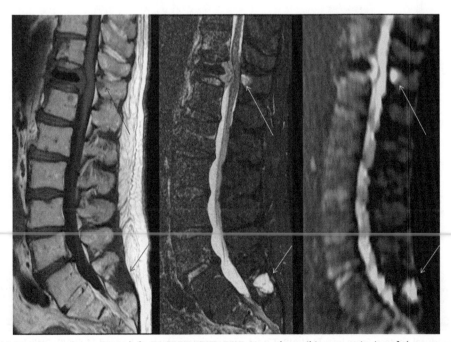

Fig. 23. Metastatic myeloma. From left: T1 FLAIR, STIR, DWI. Note the striking conspicuity of the tumor (*arrows*) within the compressed, T11 vertebral body, postvertebroplasty. Note also the posterior element tumor at L5.

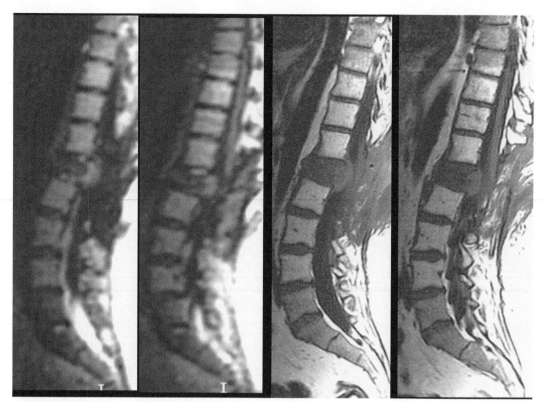

Fig. 24. Pathologic compression fracture, postdecompression. From left: single shot fast spin echo DWI and T1 SE. Note the residual tumor at L1 shows atypical isointensity and hypointensity rather than predicted diffusion restriction.

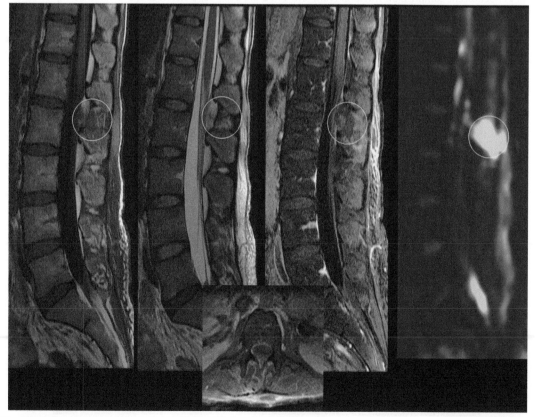

Fig. 25. Epidural abscess. From left: T1 FLAIR; T2; fat-suppressed, contrast-enhanced T1 FLAIR; DWI. Inset: Axial fat suppressed, contrast-enhanced T1. Note the characteristic striking diffusion hyperintensity involving the posterior epidural region at L1-2 (*circles*).

DIFFUSION TENSOR TRACT–BASED MYELOGRAPHY

Two and 3-dimensional representations with DTI have been used to visualize ordered white matter tracts in the brain and spine. Tract identification and display on a 2-dimensional and 3-dimensional basis can assist in revealing the relationship of lesions to adjacent eloquent structures in the brain and spine.

Diffusion tensor tract–based myelography (DTM) can be helpful with respect to localization of lesions intrinsic to or adjacent to the spinal cord (intramedullary or extramedullary) (**Figs. 16** and **17**). DTM may yield useful information in evaluation of intramedullary lesions[28] and assist in characterization (**Figs. 18** and **19**) as well as surgical planning.

EXTRADURAL LESIONS
Metastatic Disease and Myeloma

DWI is a powerful adjunct to the routine imaging regimen used to detect and characterize extradural lesions. Studies have found that diffusion is impaired within neoplastic tissue, and that a decrease in diffusion coefficient may indicate disease progression. Effective treatment may cause a transient decrease in diffusion, owing to cytotoxic edema, but eventually diffusion increases significantly.[29]

DWI adds sensitivity to the presence of osseous lesions of the spine. Added to the routine sequences used for the assessment of suspected metastatic disease and myeloma, DWI improves the detectability and conspicuity of many lesions.[30] In recently presented trials,[31,32] approximately 50% of lesions, identified as part of a neoplastic MR imaging spine survey, were most conspicuous on trace-weighted DWI compared with a combination of routine sequences including short inversion time inversion recovery (STIR) and T1 pre- and postcontrast techniques. Although approximately 20% of lesions were better seen on routine sequences, up to 10% of lesions were seen only on DWI or were solely evident in retrospect with routine scanning techniques (**Fig. 20**) DWI has gained wide use in whole-body screening

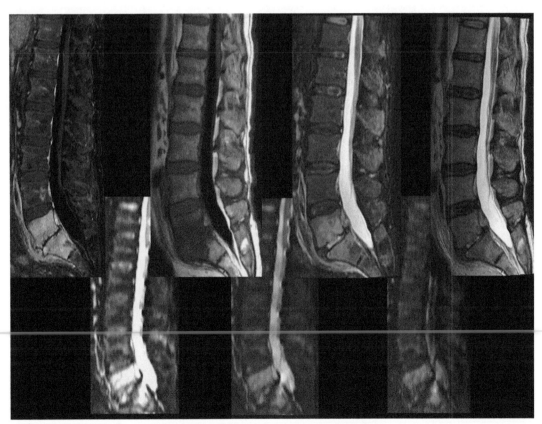

Fig. 26. Osteomyelitis and discitis. Clockwise from upper left: fat-suppressed, contrast-enhanced T1 FLAIR, T1 FLAIR, STIR, T2, DWI B = 500,150,0. Note the diffuse increase in signal within the L5 and S1 vertebral bodies on DWI. The signal changes and enhancement on routine imaging sequence are characteristic of infection.

MR imaging in part because of the boost in sensitivity to bone lesions it provides. Rib and posterior spinal element lesions can be difficult to detect with routine screening techniques because of morphologic and orientation issues on survey studies. The high lesion-to-background ratios provided by DWI can be particularly helpful in these circumstances (**Fig. 21**).

Compression Fractures

Acute vertebral fractures are a common clinical finding in elderly patients. Osteoporosis and tumor (primary and metastatic) are the most common causes, with the majority caused by osteoporosis. In the United States, approximately 35% of women older than 65 years have osteoporosis. More than 700,000 new vertebral compression fractures occur every year in the United States alone. Ten percent of vertebral fractures detected in patients with osteoporosis, however, are of malignant rather than senescent origin. On the other hand, 25% of the fractures in patients with a known malignancy are osteoporotic in origin.

Although MR is the most useful imaging technique for the evaluation and characterization of vertebral fractures in clinical practice, the differentiation of an osteoporotic or malignant fracture origin is challenging based on signal intensity criteria.[33,34] Morphologic criteria have been proposed for differentiation; however, these may not be sufficient to permit a definite diagnosis.[35,36] Because DWI is sensitive to presence of neoplastic lesions of bone, there have been numerous investigations of its potential in the characterization of the etiology of acute compression fractures. Using a variety of prototype and clinically available techniques, the efficacy remains controversial. Theory suggests that benign compression fractures would reveal manifestations of a rapid diffusion environment with water (edema) freely diffusing between the interstices of bone. Thus, a senescent fracture would be expected to show diminished signal on DWI and elevated diffusion coefficients (**Fig. 22**).

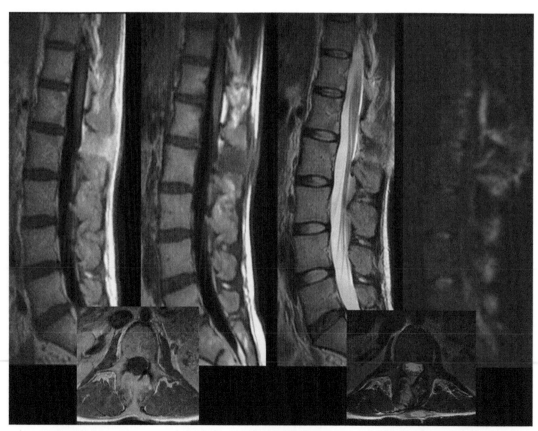

Fig. 27. Treated osteomyelitis. From left: T1 FLAIR, contrast-enhanced T1 FLAIR, T2, DWI. Inset: axial T1 postcontrast (*left*) and T2. Same case as previous figure. Note the absence of continued diffusion restricted after surgical and antibiotic therapy.

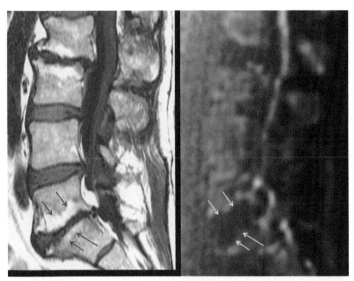

Fig. 28. Type II Modic changes. T1 FLAIR (*left*) and DWI. Note the characteristic fatty changes (*arrows*) on T1-weighted image that manifest as diminished signal on the (routinely) fat-suppressed DWI creating the appearance of a widened disc space.

A malignant compression fracture, in which tumor cells infiltrate bone, should show evidence of restricted diffusion compared with normal (and particularly edematous) marrow and show increased signal on DWI and restricted diffusion (**Fig. 23**). To date, consensus has not shown DWI to be a definitive tool for the challenging differentiation of benign senescent compression fractures from pathologic fractures (**Fig. 24**). Although some have reported excellent and characteristic results, others have described a wide spectrum of signal changes in pathologic fractures.[37–39]

This may be caused by the complexity and overlap of edema, hemorrhage, and bone fragmentation in both conditions and the varied expected associated appearance on DWI.

Infectious Disease

As in the brain, DWI can be helpful in the evaluation and detection of infectious disease (**Fig. 25**). Osteomyelitis, discitis, and abscess show characteristic hyperintensity, which can be critical to diagnosis (**Fig. 26**).[40] Diffusion can be useful in

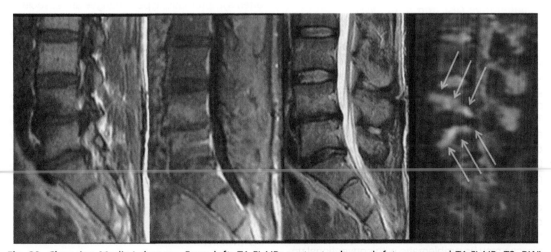

Fig. 29. Claw sign Modic I changes. From left: T1 FLAIR; contrast-enhanced, fat-suppressed T1 FLAIR; T2; DWI. Note the nonspecific signal changes about the L4-5 disc space on routine imaging sequences. The DWI reveals paired well-defined linear regions of increased signal (*arrows*) at the border zone between the abnormal and normal marrow mitigating against the likelihood of infection.

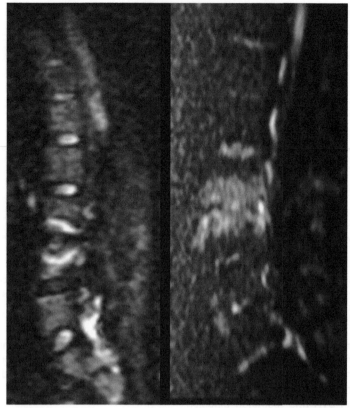

Fig. 30. Modic I degenerative changes and osteomyelitis. DW images show a well-defined high signal claw (*left*) consistent with degenerative disease and amorphous increased signal (*right*) in a case of proven osteomyelitis.

following the course of treatment and may outperform routine scanning sequences in detecting response and recurrence (**Fig. 27**).

Degenerative Disc and Joint Disease

Degenerative disease of the spine has a spectrum of characteristic appearances on DWI, which correlate with those described by Modic and colleagues.[41] To avoid ghosting caused by the precession frequency differences between fat and water, all EPI images are fat suppressed. This leads to a characteristic widened disc space appearance in patients who manifest type II fatty changes in marrow adjacent to the endplates (**Fig. 28**). The endplate sclerosis of the type III pattern will manifest as diminished signal on conventional and DW sequences. Despite the broad clinical utility of MR imaging in the spine, definitive differentiation between degenerative changes of the vertebral bodies and inflammatory disease may be problematic with conventional unenhanced and contrast-enhanced MR imaging sequences.[42] The appearance of type I degenerative signal changes in the spine can, not

uncommonly, overlap with and raise the concern for osteomyelitis and discitis using routine imaging sequences. The granulation tissue and edema about the vertebral endplates in patients with, often symptomatic, type I changes are associated with a claw of increased signal and diffusion restriction at the advancing border of the proliferative process (**Fig. 29**). When present, the claw mitigates against the likelihood of infection. In a recently presented trial including cases of known infection, in cases in which infection was suggested based on routine MR imaging and cases with routine symptomatic type I findings, the claw sign had a high sensitivity, specificity, and positive and negative predictive value with respect to the possibility of infection and was much more useful than the presence or absence of contrast enhancement or high T2 disc signal[43] images of infection and the claw (**Fig. 30**).

SUMMARY

DWI is one of the most powerful tools used in clinical MR imaging. This universally available technique is a valuable complement to the array of routine spine MR imaging and offers a valuable boost in sensitivity and improved lesion characterization.

REFERENCES

1. Koh DM, Collins DJ. Diffusion-weighted MRI in the body: applications and challenges in oncology. AJR Am J Roentgenol 2007;188(6):1622–35.
2. Shimofusa R, Fujimoto H, Akamata H, et al. Diffusion-weighted imaging of prostate cancer. J Comput Assist Tomogr 2005;29(2):149–53.
3. Park MJ, Cha ES, Kang BJ, et al. The role of diffusion-weighted imaging and the apparent diffusion coefficient (ADC) values for breast tumors. Korean J Radiol 2007;8(5):390–6.
4. Le Bihan D. Molecular diffusion nuclear magnetic resonance imaging. Magn Reson Q 1991;7(1):1–30.
5. Thomsen C, Henriksen O, Ring P. In vivo measurement of water self diffusion in the human brain by magnetic resonance imaging. Acta Radiol 1987; 28(3):353–61.
6. Mulkern RV, Spencer RG. Diffusion imaging with paired CPMG sequences. Magn Reson Imaging 1988;6(6):623–31.
7. Gudbjartsson H, Maier SE, Mulkern RV, et al. Line scan diffusion imaging. Magn Reson Med 1996; 36(4):509–19.
8. Xu D, Henry RG, Mukherjee P, et al. Single-shot fast spin-echo diffusion tensor imaging of the brain and spine with head and phased array coils at 1.5 T and 3.0 T. Magn Reson Imaging 2004; 22(6):751–9.
9. Saritas EU, Cunningham CH, Lee JH, et al. DWI of the spinal cord with reduced FOV single-shot EPI. Magn Reson Med 2008;60:468–73.
10. Atkinson D, Counsell SJ, Larkman DJ, et al. Navigated Multi-Shot EPI Diffusion Imaging of the Spine [abstract 1038]. Proceedings ISMRM. Seattle (WA): 2006.
11. Castillo M, Arbelaez A, Smith JK, et al. Diffusion-weighted MR imaging offers no advantage over routine non-contrast MR imaging in the detection of vertebral metastases. AJNR Am J Neuroradiol 2000;21(5):948–53.
12. Castillo M. Diffusion-weighted imaging of the spine: is it reliable? AJNR Am J Neuroradiol 2003;24(6): 1251–3.
13. Le Bihan D, Mangin JF, Poupon C, et al. Diffusion tensor imaging: concepts and applications. J Magn Reson Imaging 2001;13:534–46.
14. Hesseltine SM, Ge Y, Law M. Applications of diffusion tensor imaging and fiber tractography. Appl Radiol 2007;36(5):8–13.
15. Clark CA, Werring DJ. Diffusion tensor imaging in spinal cord: methods and applications – a review. NMR Biomed 2002;15(7–8):578–86.
16. Bammer R, Fazekas F, Augustin M, et al. Diffusion-weighted MR imaging of the spinal cord. AJNR Am J Neuroradiol 2000;21:587–91.
17. Quencer RM, Pattany PM. Diffusion-weighted imaging of the spinal cord: is there a future? AJNR Am J Neuroradiol 2000;21:1181–2.
18. Lowe GM. Magnetic resonance imaging of intramedullary spinal cord tumors. J Neurooncol 2000;47(3): 195–210.
19. Küker W, Weller M, Klose U, et al. Diffusion-weighted MRI of spinal cord infarction-high resolution imaging and time course of diffusion abnormality. J Neurol 2004;251(7):818–24.
20. Zhang J, Huan Y, Qian Y, et al. Multishot diffusion-weighted imaging features in spinal cord infarction. J Spinal Disord Tech 2005;18(3):277–82.
21. Larsson HB, Thomsen C, Frederiksen J, et al. In vivo magnetic resonance diffusion measurement in the brain of patients with multiple sclerosis. Magn Reson Imaging 1992;10(1):7–12.
22. Filippi M, Iannucci G, Cercignani M, et al. A quantitative study of water diffusion in multiple sclerosis lesions and normal-appearing white matter using echo-planar imaging. Arch Neurol 2000;57: 1017–21.
23. Roychowdhury S, Maldjian JA, Grossman RI. Multiple sclerosis: comparison of trace apparent diffusion coefficients with MR enhancement pattern of lesions. AJNR Am J Neuroradiol 2000; 21:869–74.
24. Werring DJ, Clark CA, Barker GJ, et al. Diffusion tensor imaging of lesions and normal-appearing white matter in multiple sclerosis. Neurology 1999; 52(8):1626–32.
25. Facon D, Ozanne A, Fillard P, et al. MR diffusion tensor imaging and fiber tracking in spinal cord compression. AJNR Am J Neuroradiol 2005;26: 1587–94.
26. Shanmuganathan K, Gullapalli RP, Zhuo J, et al. Diffusion tensor MR imaging in cervical spine trauma. AJNR Am J Neuroradiol 2008;29:655–9.
27. Demir A, Ries M, Moonen CT, et al. Diffusion-weighted MR imaging with apparent diffusion coefficient and apparent diffusion tensor maps in cervical spondylotic myelopathy. Radiology 2003;229:37–43.
28. Ducreux D, Lepeintre JF, Fillard P, et al. MR diffusion tensor imaging and fiber tracking in 5 spinal cord astrocytomas. AJNR Am J Neuroradiol 2006;27: 214–6.
29. Herneth AM, Friedrich K, Weidekamm C, et al. Diffusion weighted imaging of bone marrow pathologies. Eur J Radiol 2005;55(1):74–83.
30. Luboldt W, Küfer R, Blumstein N, et al. Prostrate carcinoma: diffusion-weighted imaging as potential alternative to conventional MR and C-choline PET/CT for detection of bone metastases. Radiology 2008;249:1017–25.

31. Parag Y, Delman B, Pawha P, et al. Diffusion weighted imaging facilitates detection of spinal metastases and assists in the diagnosis of equivocal lesions. Proceedings American Society of Spine Radiology Annual Meeting 2010, American Society of Neuroradiology Annual Meeting 2010, European College of Radiology Annual Meeting. 2010.

32. Kessler J, Pawha P, Shpilberg K, et al. Diffusion weighted imaging facilitates detection of spinal multiple myeloma and assists in diagnosing equivocal lesions. Proceedings American Society of Spine Radiology Annual Meeting 2011, American Society of Neuroradiology Annual Meeting 2011, European College of Radiology Annual Meeting. 2011.

33. Frager D, Elkin C, Swerdlow M, et al. Subacute osteoporotic compression fracture: misleading magnetic resonance appearance. Skeletal Radiol 1988;17(2): 123–6.

34. Rupp RE, Ebraheim NA, Coombs RJ. Magnetic resonance imaging differentiation of compression spine fractures or vertebral lesions caused by osteoporosis or tumor. Spine (Phila Pa 1976) 1995; 20(23):2499–503 [discussion: 2504].

35. Yuh WT, Zachar CK, Barloon TJ, et al. Vertebral compression fractures: distinction between benign and malignant causes with MR imaging. Radiology 1989;172(1):215–8.

36. Baker LL, Goodman SB, Perkash I, et al. Benign versus pathologic compression fractures of vertebral bodies: assessment with conventional spin-echo, chemical-shift, and STIR MR imaging. Radiology 1990;174(2):495–502.

37. Dietrich O, Biffar A, Reiser MF, et al. Diffusion-weighted imaging of bone marrow. Semin Musculoskelet Radiol 2009;13(2):134–44.

38. Karchevsky M, Babb JS, Schweitzer ME. Can diffusion-weighted imaging be used to differentiate benign from pathologic fractures? A meta-analysis. Skeletal Radiol 2008;37(9):791–5.

39. Park SW, Lee JH, Ehara S, et al. Single shot fast spin echo diffusion-weighted MR imaging of the spine; is it useful in differentiating malignant metastatic tumor infiltration from benign fracture edema? Clin Imaging 2004;28(2):102–8.

40. Dunbar JA, Sandoe JA, Rao AS, et al. The MRI appearances of early vertebral osteomyelitis and discitis. Clin Radiol 2010;65(12):974–81.

41. Modic MT, Steinberg PM, Ross JS, et al. Degenerative disk disease: assessment of changes in vertebral body marrow with MR imaging. Radiology 1988;166:193–9.

42. Eguchi Y, Ohtori S, Yamashita M, et al. Diffusion magnetic resonance imaging to differentiate degenerative from infectious endplate abnormalities in the lumbar spine. Spine (Phila Pa 1976) 2011;36(3): E198–202.

43. Poplawski MM, Pawha P, Naidich TP, et al. Diffusion-weighted MRI (DWI) "claw sign" is useful in differentiation of infectious from degenerative Modic I signal changes of the spine. Proceedings of the American Society of Neuroradiology. 50th Annual Meeting. New York; April 2012.

Breast Magnetic Resonance Imaging: Diffusion-Weighted Imaging

Alice C. Brandão, MD[a],*, Constance D. Lehman, MD, PhD[b],
Savannah C. Partridge, PhD[b]

KEYWORDS

- Breast MR imaging • MRI • Functional breast MRI • Breast diseases • Breast cancer diffusion
- Apparent diffusion coefficient (ADC)

KEY POINTS

- Magnetic resonance (MR) imaging is becoming a first-line radiological modality in the management of breast cancer.
- The main advantages of breast MR imaging are lack of ionizing radiation, high sensitivity, and a high negative predictive value.
- Diffusion-weighted MR imaging has been introduced for cancer imaging, and it can be used for differentiating benign and malignant breast lesions.
- Diffusion-weighted imaging can help to correctly classify as benign many false-positive cases seen on dynamic contrast-enhanced (DCE)-MR imaging, such as fibroadenomas.
- Malignant lesions show restricted diffusion, with high signal intensity on DWI and low apparent diffusion coefficient (ADC) values, mostly related to increased cellularity and decreased extracellular space.
- Mucinous cancer shows a very high ADC value because of low tumor cell density and a large amount of mucin around the tumor cells.
- The choice of b values directly affects quantitative analysis of the ADC, because the signal intensity at DWI is influenced by the b value.
- DWI may be a viable noncontrast alternative method for breast MR imaging screening.
- DWI may be able to offer earlier and more precise information on response to neoadjuvant treatment than DCE-MR imaging.

INTRODUCTION

Breast magnetic resonance (MR) imaging is the most sensitive imaging modality for the detection of breast cancer, and it has become a valuable breast screening technique in select patient populations.[1] Standard breast MR imaging protocols incorporate evaluation by dynamic contrast-enhanced (DCE) MR imaging, which shows tissue vascularity and vascular permeability. Alterations in tissue vascular properties are characteristic to breast malignancies, enabling their detection by DCE-MR imaging. Although DCE-MR imaging has extremely high sensitivity in the diagnosis of breast cancer, as high as 89% to 100% for invasive cancers, the specificity is moderate (ranging widely from 21% to 100% across 44 studies, with an average of 72%).[2,3]

Breast MR imaging is an area of intense research, and over the past decade, new MR techniques and

[a] Department of Radiology, Clínica Felippe Mattoso, Avenida das Américas 700, 319, Rio De Janeiro 30112011, Brazil; [b] Department of Radiology, University of Washington School of Medicine, Seattle Cancer Care Alliance, 825 Eastlake Avenue East, G2-600, Seattle, WA 98109-1023, USA
* Corresponding author.
E-mail address: brandaosalomao@gmail.com

Magn Reson Imaging Clin N Am 21 (2013) 321–336
http://dx.doi.org/10.1016/j.mric.2013.01.002
1064-9689/13/$ – see front matter © 2013 Elsevier Inc. All rights reserved.

interpretation strategies have been developed to increase its specificity and positive predictive value (PPV). Recommended techniques for image acquisition include high spatial and temporal resolution for careful assessment of both morphologic and kinetic features of lesions. In recent publications, using more current approaches, the reported increased specificities ranged between 67% and 92%.[4]

However, despite improvements in DCE-MR imaging acquisition techniques, overlap in morphologic characteristics and kinetic features of some malignant and benign lesions still causes improper classifications. MR imaging false-positive results may be influenced by patient factors such as phase of menstrual cycle, hormone replacement therapy, and patient age. In addition, false-positive results may occur with lesions that share MR features of breast malignancy, such as papilloma, proliferative disease, and fibroadenoma. Thus, there is interest in studying new techniques that can be implemented into the standard breast MR imaging practice to reduce false-positive results and increase specificity, and consequently reduce morbidity, and economic and psychosocial costs associated with unnecessary biopsies.

Diffusion-weighted imaging (DWI) is one such MR imaging technique that is showing promise for improving diagnostic accuracy as an adjunct to DCE-MR imaging. DWI is a short scan available on most commercial MR scanners that does not require any exogenous contrast and can be added to breast MR imaging examinations to provide additional complementary information on tissue microstructural properties. Recent MR imaging technological advances, including echo planar imaging (EPI), high-amplitude gradients, multichannel coils, and parallel imaging, have been instrumental in extending the use and applications of DWI outside the brain. DWI provides a quantitative evaluation, and studies have shown that the apparent diffusion coefficient (ADC) values derived from DWI can facilitate in differentiating benign and malignant breast tumors as well as identifying early response in tumors undergoing preoperative treatment. Furthermore, DWI may provide a useful alternative to gadolinium-enhanced sequences for MR imaging evaluation of patients at risk for nephrogenic systemic fibrosis.

DWI
Principles of DWI

DWI is a noninvasive technique that measures the random motion of free water protons (Brownian motion) and characterizes different tissue properties from conventional MR parameters, such as T1 and T2 relaxation. In contrast to freely diffusing water, the movement of water molecules in biological tissues is restricted by interactions with cell membranes and macromolecules.[5]

In vivo, the degree to which water diffusion is restricted is inversely proportional to the tissue cellularity and the cell membrane integrity. In tissues with a high cell density and intact cell membranes (such as tumor), diffusion is more restricted because the lipophilic cell membranes act as barriers to motion of water molecules. Conversely, in tissues with low cellularity or compromised cellular membranes, water diffusion is less restricted due to the larger extracellular space and ability of diffusing water molecules to move freely across cell membranes.

DWI Acquisition

Stejskal and Tanner[7] described an experimental quantification of water diffusion in vivo that is now the basis of many DWI sequences in clinical use. Their approach was to apply a symmetric pair of diffusion-sensitizing (bi-polar) gradients around the 180° refocusing pulse of a standard T2-weighted spin-echo sequence, thereby attenuating the resulting signal in proportion to water movement. Diffusion can be expressed as the following monoexponential equation:

$SDW = SSE \cdot \exp(-b \cdot ADC)$, with $b = \gamma^2 G^2 \delta^2 (\Delta - \delta/3)$, where SDW is the attenuated spin-echo signal, SSE is the full T2-weighted spin-echo signal without diffusion attenuation, ADC is the apparent diffusion coefficient (mm^2/s), b is the diffusion sensitization factor (s/mm^2), γ is the proton gyromagnetic ratio, G is the gradient strength, δ is the duration of G, and Δ is the time delay between the leading edges of the 2 diffusion-sensitizing gradients.[5] The sequence generates 2 sets of images: the first set, in which the diffusion gradients are turned off (SSE; T2-weighted images), and the second set, with the diffusion gradients turned on (SDW; index diffusion-weighted (DW) images).

The faster the water molecules diffuse, the greater the attenuation and the weaker the corresponding signal intensity (SDW). Thus, signal intensity is usually higher in a region with restricted diffusion, such as tumor, than in a region with fast diffusion, such as free extracellular water in normal breast tissue (Fig. 1).[5] However, visual assessment of index DW images (SDW) is complicated by the fact signal intensity depends on both water diffusion and the T2 relaxation time. Thus, tissues with long T2 relaxation times, such as a fluid-filled cyst, may retain significant signal on DWI and be misinterpreted as having restricted diffusion. This phenomenon is known as the T2 shine-through effect

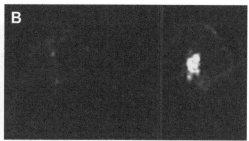
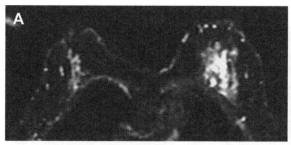

Fig. 1. DWI. (*A*) T2-weighted image (SSE). (*B*) The index DW image with the diffusion gradient turned on (SDW), with DW and T2-weighted information. Left breast ductal invasive carcinoma.

(Fig. 2). However, in this case, the conventional images are typically very clear, showing well-defined nonenhancing T2 bright lesions. The greater the strength of the diffusion sensitization (b value), the lower the impact of the T2 effect on the DW images.

DW images without T2 weighted information can be obtained by creating the exponential image, which is the ratio of the DW image divided by the corresponding unweighted reference image (SDW/SSE) at the same slice position (Fig. 3A, B).[5] Also, the quantitative ADC map can overcome the effects of T2 shine-through. ADC is calculated by:

ADC = −ln(SDW/SSE)/b, for each pixel of the image and is shown as a parametric map, performed on the scanner or work station (see Fig. 3C). Simple cysts can easily be differentiated from cellular tumors on ADC maps based on differences in water diffusion rates (Fig. 4).

Technical Aspects of DWI

There are challenges to obtaining good-quality breast DWI images and accurate ADC measures. Typical EPI-based DWI sequences can result in image distortion during data acquisition, because of eddy currents, susceptibility effects, and ghosting artifacts. These issues are particularly challenging for breast imaging because of the off-isocenter imaging and significant fat content in the breast. To reduce artifacts and optimize data quality, good shimming and suppression of lipid signal are essential. The optimal technique for fat suppression (eg, spectral attenuated inversion recovery [SPAIR], short-tau inversion recovery [STIR]) may vary between scanners. Parallel imaging techniques also help to reduce susceptibility-based distortions and ghosting artifacts through shortened imaging times. Protocols also must be optimized for adequate signal-to-noise ratio (SNR) by balancing spatial resolution and appropriate diffusion sensitizations or b values.

Influence of b value

The choice of b values may vary according to the protocol and directly affects quantitative analysis of the ADC, because the signal intensity at DWI is influenced by the b value. At lower b values, T2-weighted signal is emphasized (T2 shine-through effect). Lower b values also generate higher ADC values in vivo, because of the contribution of intravoxel incoherent motion effects other than diffusion. Microperfusion, defined as microcirculation within the capillary network, is an important potential influence on diffusion measures. In vivo, the measured ADC value includes the factors of both water diffusion and perfusion effect; hence the term apparent diffusion coefficient, and can be expressed in the equation:

$$\text{ADC value} \approx D + (f/b),$$ where D is the diffusion coefficient and f is the perfusion factor.[8]

At lower b values (b <400 s/mm^2 for breast tissue), the DWI signal is more influenced by attenuations caused by perfusion or flow, thus increasing the net ADC value. Conversely, higher b values emphasize the contribution from the diffusion coefficient alone and can improve contrast resolution between various diseases and normal breast tissue (Fig. 5).[5] Therefore, high b values (b >500 s/mm^2) are recommended for breast DWI.

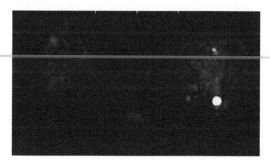

Fig. 2. T2 shine-through effect on DWI. A cyst in the left breast remains high signal at DWI.

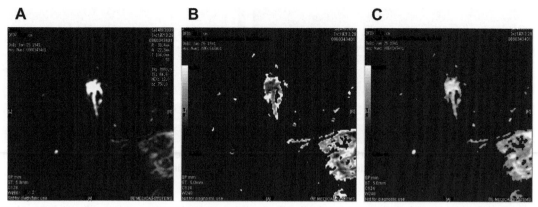

Fig. 3. DWI parametric maps. (*A*) T2-weighted image. (*B*) Exponential DW image, without T2-weighted information. (*C*) ADC map. Mucinous carcinoma.

However, the optimal maximum b value for breast imaging has not yet been established and there is no consensus. The b value has varied between 500 and 1500 s/mm^2 in the literature.

For lesion conspicuity and detection purposes, a very high b value may be preferred. Kuroki and Nasu reported that optimal contrast between cancer and normal mammary tissue was achieved at a b value of 1000 s/mm^2.[9] However, the use of higher b values may reduce sensitivity for the evaluation of small lesions, such as ductal carcinoma in situ (DCIS), because of more rapid signal decay (ie, lower SNR).

For differentiation between benign and malignant lesions, choice of b value may be less important. Several studies comparing DWI acquired at different b values showed that the mean ADC values of malignant lesions were in general lower than those of benign lesions and normal breast tissue and that diagnostic accuracy was not significantly increased by using higher b values.[10–12] However, specific optimal ADC cutoffs for lesion characterization are directly influenced by the choice of b value. Thus, the same ADC threshold or cutoff for lesions evaluated with DWI obtained using b values of 1500 s/mm^2 would not be used for lesions evaluated with DWI obtained using b values of 800 s/mm^2.

In theory, DWI acquisition using multiple b values should provide a more accurate sampling of signal decay for calculation of ADC. However, studies of multiple b value acquisitions in the breast found no improvement in the ability to discriminate benign and malignant lesions over standard 2 b value acquisitions.[11,12] Given the time constraints of clinical practice, ADC calculation using 2 b values may be considered reasonable and acceptable.[10]

Although standard DW sequences use b = 0 s/mm^2 as the reference for calculating ADC, a nonzero b value reference image may be preferable in vivo to obtain ADC measures free from perfusion and flow contamination. However, a diagnostic advantage was not clearly shown in one study investigating this approach.[12]

Determination of optimal b values for breast imaging and lesion characterization remain areas of active research.

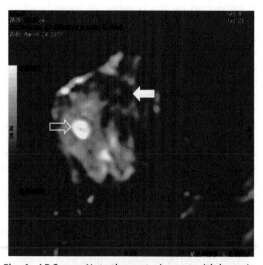

Fig. 4. ADC map. Note the posterior cyst with hyperintense signal (*open arrow*) and an anterior breast carcinoma with low signal (*solid arrow*). The cyst represents a less cellular environment, where the motion of water molecules is less restricted. In contrast, the breast carcinoma restricts the motion of water molecules, because of its highly cellular environment.

DWI Interpretation

The principle that underlies in vivo DWI is that the motion of the water molecules in the extracellular fluid enables the acquisition of an image that reflects both histologic structure and cellularity. Factors responsible for restriction of movement

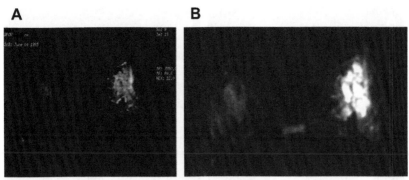

Fig. 5. Differentiation of breast tissues based on DWI. (*A*) Baseline T2-weighted image (b = 0 s/mm^2). (*B*) DW image with a high b value. Lobular carcinoma in the left breast.

of extracellular water molecules include high cellularity, intracellular edema, swelling, and extracellular medium with high viscosity (which is observed in the case of abscess and hematoma).[13]

The pathogenesis of the restriction of diffusion in breast cancer is cell proliferation. Tumor growth causes higher cellularity, tissue disorganization, and increased tortuosity of the extracellular space, which result in disruption or restriction of motion of the extracellular water within the tissue. These changes in the diffusion of water result in changes in the signal intensity on the DWI.[10] An inverse relationship between tumor cellularity and ADC measurements has been previously reported.[6,14] In breast lesions ranging from high cellularity (tumors) to low cellularity (cysts), Hatakenaka and colleagues[14] found that the greater the number of cells per area, the lower the ADC value.

DWI can be interpreted both qualitatively and quantitatively. Qualitatively, areas of restricted diffusion appear as higher signal intensity on the index DW images and lower signal intensity on the ADC map, which may be enhanced using color representation. Quantitative ADC analysis is typically performed by drawing a region of interest (ROI) on the ADC map and calculating the mean value for all pixels within the ROI. Tumor visibility is typically better on DCE-MR imaging because of the reduced spatial resolution of DWI. Therefore, lesions can be identified on the DCE-MR images and the ROI positioned in the lesion at the corresponding location on the DWI series and ADC map (**Fig. 6**).[15,16]

Diffusion interpretation must be taken in context with other imaging information to ensure an accurate diagnosis. In general, the clinical implication of ADC value depends on the tissue under investigation; an anomalous increase in ADC can indicate increased edema, cystic changes, and necrosis, whereas an anomalous reduction in ADC might indicate bleeding (hematoma, bleeding cyst) (**Fig. 7**), infection (abscess), or tumor. For example, the presence of blood or thick content in dilated ducts leads to restriction of diffusion, similar to ductal cancer. However, in the conventional images, ductal content can typically be identified with hyperintense signal on T1 and hypointense on T2 and no enhancement.

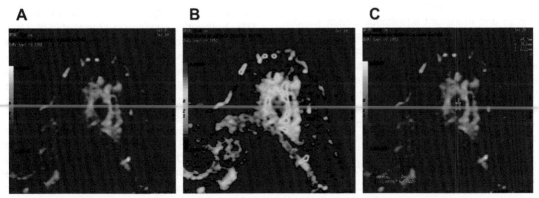

Fig. 6. DWI interpretation strategies. (*A*) Qualitative analysis involves assessing differences in signal intensity on the ADC map. (*B*) Differences in ADC are highlighted using color representation. (*C*) Quantitative analysis is performed by drawing an ROI on tissues of interest on the ADC map.

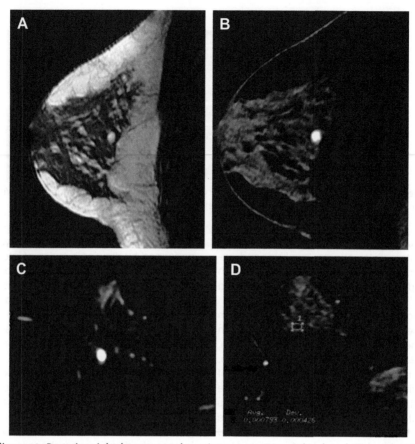

Fig. 7. Bleeding cyst. Posterior right breast cyst, hyperintense on T1-weighted and T2-weighted image, with restricted diffusion and low ADC value. (*A*) Sagittal T1-weighted image. (*B*) Sagittal T1-weighted image with fat saturation. (*C*) Axial T2-weighted image. (*D*) ADC map.

CLINICAL APPLICATIONS OF DIFFUSION

Although DWI is not required for clinical breast imaging, numerous recent studies have shown the usefulness of DWI to detect and characterize breast tumors. Areas in which DWI may add value to current clinical techniques are in differentiating benign and malignant suspicious breast tumors, as an alternate noncontrast breast MR imaging screening method for detecting cancer, and for identifying early changes in breast tumor cellularity in response to therapy. Tumors differ in their cellularity and microstructural characteristics, which may reflect their histologic composition and biological aggressiveness. These applications are actively being investigated.

Differentiation of Benign and Malignant Suspicious Breast Lesions

Several previous research studies have reported differences in the ADC of benign and malignant breast lesions.[6,14,17–19] The ADC of malignant breast lesions is usually lower than that of benign lesions, indicating restricted water diffusion and increased cellularity (**Fig. 8**). A meta-analysis of 12 articles regarding breast DWI on 1.5-T scanners confirmed the usefulness of ADC to distinguish between benign and malignant lesions. The meta-analysis showed a sensitivity of 89% and a specificity of 77%, both with a confidence interval of 95%. Using the ADC value allowed an adequate differentiation between benign and malignant lesions.[20]

Recent studies further show that incorporating DWI into the clinical breast MR imaging assessment can help to improve DCE-MR imaging diagnostic performance. Partridge and colleagues[18] reported that suspicious breast lesions detected initially by MR imaging and recommended for biopsy (BI-RADS [Breast Imaging-Reporting and Data System] 4 or 5) showed significantly lower mean ADC values compared with benign lesions. Increased PPV was achieved by incorporating an ADC threshold into the breast MR imaging assessment and it could have prevented biopsy for 33% of

A   **B**   **C**

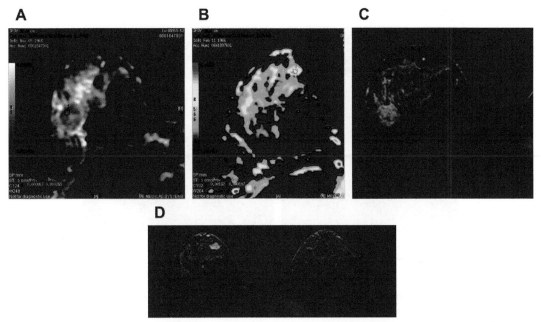

D

Fig. 8. Comparison of ADC values of benign and malignant masses, obtained with a b value of 750 s/mm^2. (*A*) Invasive ductal carcinoma shows an ADC value of 0.86×10^{-3} mm^2/s. (*B*) Fibroadenoma with an ADC value of 1.82×10^{-3} mm^2/s. (*C, D*) Corresponding DCE images for the invasive ductal carcinoma and fibroadenoma, respectively.

benign lesions. Moreover, the improvement in PPV by DWI was not limited by lesion type or size.

Several groups have determined that ADC measured by DWI provides distinct and complementary information to DCE-MR imaging morphology and kinetics for characterizing breast lesions and in combination may improve diagnostic accuracy.[17,21,22] Similar results were reported using both 1.5-T and 3.0-T field strengths. In diagnosing suspicious breast lesions based on 3.0-T MR characteristics, El Khouli and colleagues[17] found that adding normalized ADC measures to the diagnostic model reduced the false-positive rate from 36% to 24%. Similarly, Kul and colleagues[22] reported that the addition of DWI to standard DCE-MR imaging provided a 13.5% increase in the specificity of breast MR imaging at 1.5 T. In this study, the specificity of MR imaging improved from 75.7% to 89.2% ($P = .063$) with the combination of DCE-MR imaging morphology and kinetics and ADC criteria, without a significant decrease ($P = 1.000$) in sensitivity.

Yabuuchi and colleagues[23] also reported high diagnostic accuracy using a combined DWI and DCE breast MR imaging approach, with a reported 92% sensitivity and 86% specificity in the characterization of breast masses. These investigators found that malignant masses show lower ADC values than malignant nonmasslike lesions and optimal diagnostic performance was achieved using separate criteria for mass and nonmasslike lesions.[23,24]

False-positive and false-negative results
Overlap exists in the literature between benign and malignant diseases on DWI. Some benign breast tumors may have high cellularity and, consequently, a low ADC value (**Fig. 9**). On the other hand, malignant disease with low cellularity (such as intraductal carcinoma) may show higher ADC on DW images (**Fig. 10**).

A frequently encountered histology reported among false-positive lesions on DWI was intraductal papilloma.[10,19,25] One study showed that ADC values of intraductal papilloma were significantly lower than those of fibroadenoma and were comparable with those of mass-forming DCIS (**Fig. 11**).[25] A recent study of 175 DCE-MR imaging false-positive lesions showed that the high-risk subtype atypical ductal hyperplasia was the most common false-positive result on DWI after implementing a diagnostic ADC threshold.[26] Intramammary lymph nodes showed the lowest mean ADC of all nonmalignant lesion subtypes in that study.

Other causes of false-positive results on DWI, with low ADC values that can mimic malignancies, are bleeding (hematoma, bleeding cyst) (see **Fig. 7**) and infection (mastitis, abscess) (**Fig. 12**). However, clinical findings and conventional images can help with diagnosis. The presence of blood or thick content in dilated ducts also leads to restriction of diffusion, similar in appearance to ductal cancer.

A   B

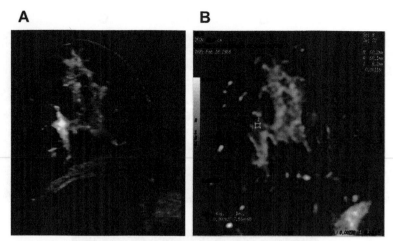

Fig. 9. Right irregular enhancing mass with an ADC value of 0.9×10^{-3} mm^2/s. Fibrocystic changes found in the percutaneous biopsy. (*A*) Axial postcontrast T1-weighted image. (*B*) ADC map.

Nonmass lesions, including intraductal carcinoma, fibrocystic disease, and lobular carcinoma, may contain interspersed normal fibroglandular tissue or fat tissue, which can affect the measured ADC value (**Fig. 13**).

High ADC values are usually associated with well-differentiated tumors or benign conditions. However, some invasive ductal carcinomas showed high ADC values, higher than the diagnostic threshold for a malignancy.[10,19] Mucinous carcinomas, which represent 1% to 7% of cases of breast cancer, are typically false-negative results by ADC (**Fig. 14**). In this rare type of breast cancer, the presence of both low cellularity and mucin-rich compartments has been shown to be responsible for markedly high ADC values. One DWI study of 15 mucinous tumors showed a mean ADC of 1.8×10^{-3} mm^2/s), which was substantially higher than other malignant breast lesions (mean, 0.9×10^{-3} mm^2/s) and even benign lesions (mean, 1.3×10^{-3} mm^2/s) in the study.[27]

Correlating the findings on conventional T2 and T1 precontrast and postcontrast images with the DWI information can reduce false-negative results of mucinous carcinomas.

Tumor Detection

Previous studies have identified an inverse relationship between ADC and tumor cellularity.[6,14]

Malignant tumors are frequently more cellular than the tissue from which they originate and, as a consequence, appear hyperintense to surrounding tissues on DWI, because of more restricted motion of the water molecules (**Fig. 15**). For this reason, DWI holds potential as a viable method of breast MR screening without the administration of a contrast agent.

Previous studies have shown that many breast cancers are detectable on DWI, including mammographically and clinically occult breast cancers.[16] In a study of 70 women with breast malignancies,

A

B

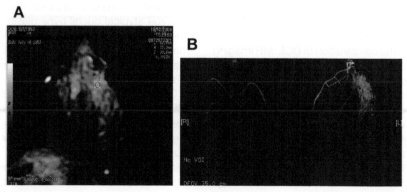

Fig. 10. Intraductal carcinoma false-negative result on DWI. (*A*) ADC map shows high ADC value (2.08×10^{-3} mm^2/s). (*B*) Axial postcontrast MIP.

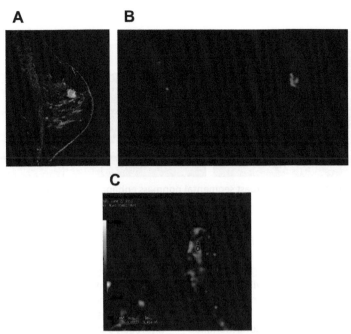

Fig. 11. Intraductal papilloma. Left breast irregular mass. (*A*) Sagittal postcontrast image. (*B*) DW image. (*C*) ADC map, with an ADC value of 1.29×10^{-3} mm^2/s.

noncontrast MR imaging using DWI in combination with STIR imaging showed similar sensitivity compared with DCE breast MR imaging for detecting cancers. Accurate detection of breast cancer was possible based on combined DWI and STIR criteria, regardless of the tumor size or background density of mammary gland (**Fig. 16**).[28] Another study[29] investigating women with suspicious breast masses reported comparable sensitivity and specificity between standard breast MR imaging (including DCE-MR imaging) and unenhanced MR imaging (T2-weighted and DWI) for detection of breast cancer based on specific diagnostic criteria.

Furthermore, in a reader study[30] of asymptomatic women, noncontrast DWI provided higher accuracy for detection of breast malignancies than screening radiograph mammography. Another reader study[31] in women with breast cancer also reported higher detection sensitivity using DWI compared with

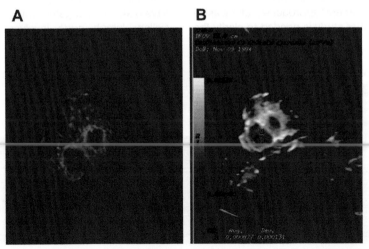

Fig. 12. Granulomatous mastitis. Two irregular masses in the right breast, with peripheral enhancement and central restricted diffusion with low ADC value (0.87×10^{-3} mm^2/s). (*A*) Axial postcontrast image. (*B*) ADC map.

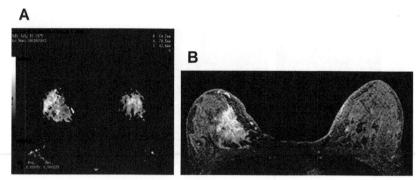

Fig. 13. Intraductal carcinoma. Right breast segmental nonmass enhancement with restricted diffusion. (*A*) Axial postcontrast image. (*B*) ADC map, with ADC value of 1.05×10^{-3} mm²/s.

radiograph mammography. These findings suggest DWI could provide a valuable adjunct to mammography for enhanced breast screening without the costs and toxicity associated with DCE-MR imaging, which may be particularly useful in younger women with dense breasts.

However, DWI cannot detect all lesions identified by conventional DCE-MR imaging. In a blinded reader study comparing the techniques,[30] 20% of malignant breast lesions identified on DCE-MR imaging were not visible on noncontrast MR imaging with DWI. Similarly, Tozaki and Fukuma found that 32% of nonmass intraductal carcinomas could not be visually detected on DWI, indicating that intraductal carcinomas may be misinterpreted as false-negative results on DWI and may limit the sensitivity of the method (see **Fig. 10**).[25] Both of the previous studies were performed at 1.5 T, and more data are needed to determine whether sensitivity can be improved with higher field strengths to increase SNR or spatial resolution. It may be that the DCIS lesions that are missed by DWI are low-grade lesions, which may not need intervention, or the same treatment approaches of invasive carcinomas. Further study is needed to clarify the

biological behavior of DCIS lesions, which are not evident on DWI. This information may be helpful in identifying in situ and invasive tumors with a high potential for poor outcomes in patients and distinguishing those tumors from the low-grade malignancies, which may not require the same aggressive treatments.

Tumor Characterization

Accurate assessment of tumor biology is critical for planning treatment strategies. Tumors differ in their cellularity, and this difference may reflect their histologic composition and biological aggressiveness. DWI is highly sensitive to tissue microstructure, and the ADC is typically reduced in invasive breast cancers. There is also some evidence that quantitative ADC assessment may help to differentiate among tumor subtypes. Biological markers like hormone receptor expression, human epidermal growth factor receptor 2 (HER2) status, and proliferation, defined by the Ki67 labeling index or by the pathologic description of the frequency of mitoses, have been used, together with tumor diameter and axillary lymph node involvement, to estimate

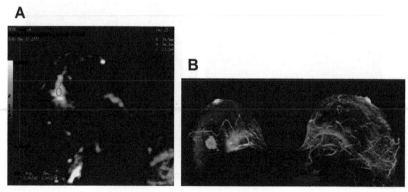

Fig. 14. Mucinous carcinoma. Irregular and heterogeneous enhancing mass, with a high ADC value (2.08×10^{-3} mm²/s). (*A*) ADC map. (*B*) Axial postcontrast MIP.

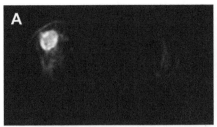 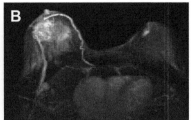

Fig. 15. Right breast malignant tumor. (*A*) DW image. Note high signal intensity on high b value image compared with noncancerous tissue. (*B*) Axial postcontrast MIP.

prognosis and to predict the efficacy of adjuvant postsurgical treatments. An imaging biomarker approach has the potential advantage of evaluating the whole lesion, especially important for characterizing heterogeneous tumors, in which biopsy may be prone to sampling error.

In the literature, several correlations between ADC values and tumor prognostic and predictive histologic features like tumor grade, diameter, and hormone receptor status have been reported in preliminary studies.

Razek and colleagues[32] observed that the mean ADC values of high-grade invasive breast cancers were significantly lower than those of intermediate-grade or low-grade. They also found that lower ADC values were associated with larger tumor size and presence of axillary lymph node metastasis. A statistically significant inverse correlation between ADC value and tumor grade was also reported in a series evaluating 136 women with malignancy.[33] The association between ADC and grade may be explained by the fact that histologic grading of breast cancer incorporates the number of mitoses, which is reflective of cellularity.

In 107 women with invasive ductal cancer, Jeh and colleagues[34] found significant correlations between ADC and estrogen receptor and HER2 status. Martincich and colleagues[35] observed similar associations between tumor ADC values and estrogen receptor status. Furthermore, within the luminal B/HER2-negative subtype, which includes estrogen receptor-positive, highly proliferating tumors, higher histopathologic grade was associated with lower ADC values.

Also, triple-negative invasive breast cancer shows higher ADC values than other sybtypes.[36] Uematsu and colleagues[37] previously reported that very high intratumoral signal intensity on T2-weighted MR images was significantly associated with triple-negative breast cancer and intratumoral necrosis. Areas of tumor necrosis show a decrease in cellularity with an associated increase in diffusion, loss of signal, and higher ADC value on DWI (**Fig. 17**).

Improved risk stratification of DCIS would help with better customizing treatment of this preinvasive disease. Intraductal carcinoma shows higher ADC than that of invasive ductal carcinoma.[19,38,39] Lima and colleagues found a significant negative correlation between ADC and intraductal carcinoma grade. Furthermore, an ADC threshold $(1.3 \times 10^{-3}$ mm^2/s) was established to help identify low-grade intraductal carcinoma with very high specificity. Rahbar and colleagues[39] similarly developed a predictive model incorporating DWI and DCE-MR imaging features that was able to significantly distinguish high-grade from non–high-grade DCIS lesions. Both groups propose that DWI could potentially help decrease the distress of women with low-risk intraductal carcinoma, because they would be offered lighter treatment options than those treated for invasive breast cancer.[38]

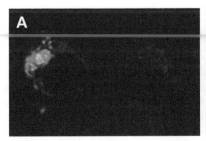 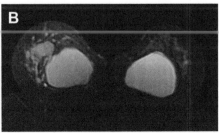

Fig. 16. Comparison of DW and STIR images. Right breast multifocal disease. Note multiple irregular masses with high signal intensity on DWI, isointense on STIR imaging. (*A*) DW image. (*B*) STIR.

A   B

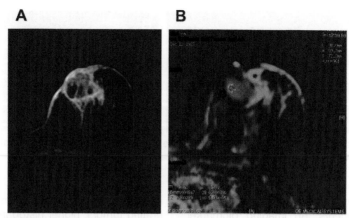

Fig. 17. Triple-negative invasive breast cancer with intratumoral necrosis. Note nonenhancing irregular central area of the tumor, with higher ADC value on DWI (ADC value 2.9×10^{-3} mm^2/s). There is enhancement and restricted diffusion at the periphery of the tumor (ADC value 0.8×10^{-3} mm^2/s). (*A*) Axial postcontrast image. (*B*) ADC map.

Predicting and Monitoring Therapeutic Response

Tumor response is typically assessed via tumor size measurements during the course of a treatment, such as the RECIST (response evaluation criteria in solid tumors) approach. However, changes in morphologically based measures occur late in the course of a treatment. Alternative biomarkers are being evaluated to enable an earlier assessment of treatment response to facilitate individualized and more effective therapies. One of the hallmarks of cancer is unregulated cell replication, which can lead to increased cellularity and reduced extracellular volume in tumors compared with healthy tissue. Based on the association between ADC and tumor cellularity, DWI may be able to offer earlier and more precise information on response to neoadjuvant treatment than DCE-MR imaging and analysis of tumor size.[40] Effective anticancer treatment results in tumor lysis, loss of cell membrane integrity, increased extracellular space, and, therefore, an increase in water diffusion and tumor ADC.[15]

Studies in both cerebral gliomas and breast carcinomas have found that the ADC in tumors increases in response to treatment earlier than detectable changes in tumor size or vascularity measured by DCE-MR imaging.[15,41–43] Furthermore, a growing number of studies in breast tumors have found change in ADC with treatment to be significantly greater in responders,[44,45] even after the first cycle of chemotherapy.[43,46] In prediction of pathologic response, Fangberget and colleagues[47] further showed that midtreatment ADC was higher in patients who achieved a pathologic complete response compared with those with residual disease (**Fig. 18**).

Although effective therapy results in an increase in tumor water diffusion, transient reductions in ADC have been observed at the beginning of chemotherapy (within the first 24 hours) because of cellular edema induced by the treatment. In chemosensitive tumors, this acute response was followed by necrosis, apoptosis, reducing edema and, subsequently, normalization of the value of the ADC.[5]

Several clinical DWI studies have shown that cellular breast tumors with low baseline pretreatment ADC values respond better to chemotherapy than tumors that show high pretreatment ADC values.[44–46] One possible explanation is that tumors with high pretreatment ADC values are likely to be more necrotic than those with low values. Necrotic tumors frequently are hypoxic, acidotic, and poorly perfused, leading to diminished sensitivity to chemotherapy.

On the other hand, ADC was not predictive of clinical response in several other studies, whether measured before therapy or midtreatment.[48–50] These disparate findings may be attributable to differences in DWI methods, analysis approaches, or study populations. Further larger studies are needed to validate the use of ADC as a predictive biomarker.

LIMITATIONS

Considerable strides have been made to translate DWI from an experimental tool to a valuable and routinely used breast imaging technique. However, there are limitations to this technique that can delay its widespread use.

The lack of consensus on an accepted range of b values for DWI of the breast has prevented determination of generalizable recommendations

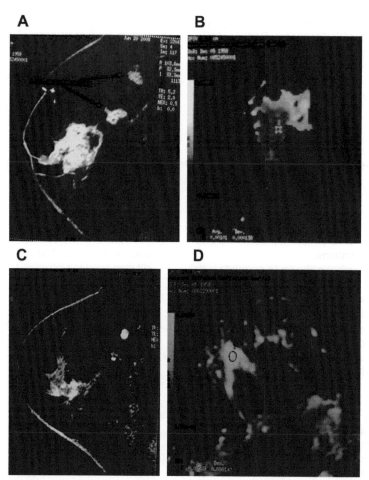

Fig. 18. DWI in a patient undergoing neoadjuvant chemotherapy. Right irregular, spiculated, and enhancing mass and 2 enlarged lymph nodes. (*A, C*) Sagittal postcontrast images before and after chemotherapy, respectively. (*B, D*) ADC maps before and after chemotherapy, respectively. Note an increase in the tumor ADC value (from 1.01×10^{-3} mm²/s before treatment to 2.29×10^{-3} mm²/s after chemotherapy) as well as volumetric reduction.

on diagnostic ADC cutoff values. ADC values are highly dependent on the imaging acquisition and analysis methods used, and wide variations in approach are reported in the literature. As a consequence, the reported mean ADC of malignant lesions ranges from 0.90 to 1.61×10^{-3} mm²/s and that of benign lesions from 1.41 to 2.01×10^{-3} mm²/s. These distributions have resulted in recommended ADC cutoff values between malignant and benign lesions ranging from 1.1 to 1.6×10^{-3} mm²/s.[20] Thus, there is a need for standardization of acquisition and postprocessing methods, which requires testing and validation across platforms and institutions.

Others factors can affect ADC values, including those related to pathophysiologic features (cellular density, tissue composition) of the lesions and hormonal status, with a 5.5% variation in normal breast ADC throughout the menstrual cycle.[51]

However, El Khouli and colleagues[17] did not detect a significant difference in lesion ADC values between the patients imaged during different portions of the menstrual cycle or between premenopausal and postmenopausal women.

There are challenges to identifying lesions on DW images. Artifacts such as susceptibility, chemical shift, or distortion, for which DW EPI is very sensitive, can impair lesion visibility and ADC measurements. Ongoing technical innovations can possibly help to further optimize breast DWI. Advanced radiofrequency coil design, parallel imaging, and improved shimming techniques can help to overcome some of the technical limitations to achieving high-quality breast DW images, particularly at higher field strengths. However, there is more work to be undertaken in this area.

Also, low spatial resolution is a primary limitation of DWI that can preclude detection of small cancer foci, including intraductal carcinoma and scattered foci of invasive lobular cancer. Partial volume effects caused by low resolution may also hinder evaluation of lesion morphologic characteristics, such as margin spiculations.[38,52,53] The higher SNR afforded by higher magnetic field strength can be used to increase the spatial resolution, thereby allowing the detection and characterization of smaller lesions. Matsuoka and colleagues[54] found that small lesions were more clearly visible on DWI at 3.0 T than at 1.5 T.

T2 shine-through effects, hemorrhage, necrosis, cystic lesions, or proteinaceous fluid components may also affect signal intensity and lesion appearance on DW images.[38] More studies are necessary to better understand the effects of these factors on breast DWI interpretations.

Although ADC has been shown to correlate with cellular density in breast cancer in several studies,[6,14,27] there have been varying findings in the literature, with some studies reporting no correlation.[55] The differences in study findings may be explained by the wide variation in image acquisition and analysis approaches, but more validation is needed to confirm this association.

SUMMARY

DWI represents a noninvasive technique that has great potential to provide tumor microstructural information, which may be helpful in detection, diagnosis, and therapeutic response of breast cancer.

Based on promising single-center studies, there is a strong drive in the research community to use DWI to help improve diagnostic specificity as an adjunct to breast DCE-MR in the distinction of benign from malignant lesions, and DWI is being integrated into the standard breast MR imaging examination at many institutions.

However, lack of standardization in the imaging approach makes it difficult to define recommendations for interpretation of breast DWI scans and reliably assess the usefulness of the technique. Therefore, more work must be carried out to validate single-center findings across platforms in multi-institutional trials and to define standardized diagnostic criteria. Regardless, the exciting potential of this new modality for breast imaging warrants continued research and clinical validation for a variety of applications.

REFERENCES

1. Siegmann KC, Krämer B, Claussena C. Current status and new developments in breast MRI. Breast Care (Basel) 2011;6(2):87–92.

2. Warren RM, Pointon L, Thompson D, et al. Reading protocol for dynamic contrast-enhanced MR images of the breast: sensitivity and specificity analysis. Radiology 2005;236:779–88.

3. Peters NH, Borel Rinkes IH, Zuithoff NP, et al. Meta-analysis of MR imaging in the diagnosis of breast lesions. Radiology 2008;246:116–24.

4. Wiener JI, Schilling KJ, Adami C, et al. Assessment of suspected breast cancer by MRI: a prospective clinical trial using a combined kinetic and morphologic analysis. AJR Am J Roentgenol 2005;184:878–86.

5. Koh DM, Collins DJ. Diffusion-weighted MRI in the body: applications and challenges in oncology. AJR Am J Roentgenol 2007;188(6):1622–35.

6. Guo Y, Cai YQ, Cai ZL, et al. Differentiation of clinically benign and malignant breast lesions using diffusion-weighted imaging. J Magn Reson Imaging 2002;16:172–8.

7. Stejskal EO, Tanner JE. Spin diffusion measurements: spin-echo in the presence of a time dependent field gradient. J Chem Phys 1965;42:288–92.

8. Le Bihan D, Breton E, Lallemand D, et al. Separation of diffusion and perfusion in intravoxel incoherent motion MR imaging. Radiology 1988;168:497–505.

9. Kuroki Y, Nasu K. Advances in breast MRI: diffusion-weighted imaging of the breast. Breast Cancer 2008;15(3):212–7.

10. Jin G, An N, Jacobs MA, et al. The role of parallel diffusion-weighted imaging and apparent diffusion coefficient (ADC) map values for evaluating breast lesions: preliminary results. Acad Radiol 2010;17(4):456–63.

11. Pereira FP, Martins G, Figueiredo E, et al. Assessment of breast lesions with diffusion-weighted MRI: comparing the use of different b values. AJR Am J Roentgenol 2009;193(4):1030–5.

12. Peters NH, Vincken KL, van den Bosch MA, et al. Quantitative diffusion weighted imaging for differentiation of benign and malignant breast lesions: the influence of the choice of b-values. J Magn Reson Imaging 2010;31(5):1100–5.

13. Brandão A. Ressonância magnética da mama. Editora Revinter; 2010 [in Portuguese].

14. Hatakenaka M, Soeda H, Yabuuchi H, et al. Apparent diffusion coefficients of breast tumors: clinical application. Magn Reson Med Sci 2008;7(1):23–9.

15. Pickles MD, Gibbs P, Lowry M, et al. Diffusion changes precede size reduction in neoadjuvant treatment of breast cancer. Magn Reson Imaging 2006;24(7):843–7.

16. Partridge SC, Demartini WB, Kurland BF, et al. Differential diagnosis of mammographically and clinically occult breast lesions on diffusion-weighted MRI. J Magn Reson Imaging 2010;31(3):562–70.

17. Ei Khouli RH, Jacobs MA, Mezban SD, et al. Diffusion-weighted imaging improves the diagnostic accuracy of conventional 3.0-T breast MR imaging. Radiology 2010;256(1):64–73.

18. Partridge SC, DeMartini WB, Kurland BF, et al. Quantitative diffusion-weighted imaging as an adjunct to conventional breast MRI for improved positive predictive value. AJR Am J Roentgenol 2009; 193(6):1716–22.

19. Woodhams R, Matsunaga K, Kan S, et al. ADC mapping of benign and malignant breast tumors. Magn Reson Med Sci 2005;4:35–42.

20. Tsushima Y, Takahashi-Taketomi A, Endo K. Magnetic resonance (MR) differential diagnosis of breast tumors using apparent diffusion coefficient (ADC) on 1.5-T. J Magn Reson Imaging 2009;30(2):249–55.

21. Partridge SC, Rahbar H, Murthy R, et al. Improved diagnostic accuracy of breast MRI through combined apparent diffusion coefficients and dynamic contrast-enhanced kinetics. Magn Reson Med 2011;65(6): 1759–67.

22. Kul S, Cansu A, Alhan E, et al. Contribution of diffusion-weighted imaging to dynamic contrast-enhanced MRI in the characterization of breast tumors. AJR Am J Roentgenol 2011;196:210–7.

23. Yabuuchi H, Matsuo Y, Okafuji T, et al. Enhanced mass on contrast-enhanced breast MR imaging: lesion characterization using combination of dynamic contrast-enhanced and diffusion-weighted MR images. J Magn Reson Imaging 2008;28(5):1157–65.

24. Yabuuchi H, Matsuo Y, Kamitani T, et al. Non-mass-like enhancement on contrast-enhanced breast MR imaging: lesion characterization using combination of dynamic contrast-enhanced and diffusion-weighted MR images. Eur J Radiol 2010;75(1):e126–32.

25. Tozaki M, Fukuma E. 1H MR spectroscopy and diffusion-weighted imaging of the breast: are they useful tools for characterizing breast lesions before biopsy? AJR Am J Roentgenol 2009;193:840–9.

26. Parsian S, Rahbar H, Allison KH, et al. Nonmalignant breast lesions: ADCs of benign and high-risk subtypes assessed as false-positive at dynamic enhanced MR imaging. Radiology 2012;265(3):696–706.

27. Woodhams R, Kakita S, Hata H, et al. Diffusion-weighted imaging of mucinous carcinoma of the breast: evaluation of apparent diffusion coefficient and signal intensity in correlation with histologic findings. AJR Am J Roentgenol 2009;193(1):260–6.

28. Kuroki-Suzuki S, Kuroki Y, Nasu K, et al. Detecting breast cancer with non-contrast MR imaging: combining diffusion-weighted and STIR imaging. Magn Reson Med Sci 2007;6(1):21–7.

29. Baltzer PA, Benndorf M, Dietzel M, et al. Sensitivity and specificity of unenhanced MR mammography (DWI combined with T2-weighted TSE imaging, ueMRM) for the differentiation of mass lesions. Eur Radiol 2010;20(5):1101–10.

30. Yabuuchi H, Matsuo Y, Sunami S, et al. Detection of non-palpable breast cancer in asymptomatic women by using unenhanced diffusion-weighted and T2-weighted MR imaging: comparison with mammography and dynamic contrast-enhanced MR imaging. Eur Radiol 2011;21(1):11–7.

31. Yoshikawa MI, Ohsumi S, Sugata S, et al. Comparison of breast cancer detection by diffusion-weighted magnetic resonance imaging and mammography. Radiat Med 2007;25:218–23.

32. Razek AA, Gaballa G, Denewer A, et al. Invasive ductal carcinoma: correlation of apparent diffusion coefficient value with pathological prognostic factors. NMR Biomed 2010;23:619–23.

33. Costantini M, Belli P, Rinaldi P, et al. Diffusion-weighted imaging in breast cancer: relationship between apparent diffusion coefficient and tumour aggressiveness. Clin Radiol 2010;65:1005–12.

34. Jeh SK, Kim SH, Kim HS, et al. Correlation of the apparent diffusion coefficient value and dynamic magnetic resonance imaging findings with prognostic factors in invasive ductal carcinoma. J Magn Reson Imaging 2011;33:102–9.

35. Martincich L, Aglietta M, Regge D, et al. Correlations between diffusion-weighted imaging and breast cancer biomarkers. Eur Radiol 2012;22(7): 1519–28.

36. Youk JH, Son EJ, Chung J, et al. Triple-negative invasive breast cancer on dynamic contrast-enhanced and diffusion-weighted MR imaging: comparison with other breast cancer subtypes. Eur Radiol 2012; 22(8):1724–34.

37. Uematsu T, Kasami M, Yuen S. Triple-negative breast cancer: correlation between MR imaging and pathologic findings. Radiology 2009;250:638–47.

38. Iima M, Le Bihan D, Okumura S, et al. Apparent diffusion coefficient as an MR imaging biomarker of low-risk ductal carcinoma in situ: a pilot study. Radiology 2011;260(2):364–72.

39. Rahbar H, Partridge SC, Demartini WB, et al. In vivo assessment of ductal carcinoma in situ grade: a model incorporating dynamic contrast-enhanced and diffusion-weighted breast MR imaging parameters. Radiology 2012;263(2):374–82.

40. Sinha S, Sinha U. Recent advances in breast MRI and MRS. NMR Biomed 2009;22(1):3–16.

41. Chenevert TL, Stegman LD, Taylor JM, et al. Diffusion magnetic resonance imaging: an early surrogate marker of therapeutic efficacy in brain tumors. J Natl Cancer Inst 2000;92:2029–36.

42. Theilmann RJ, Borders R, Trouard TP, et al. Changes in water mobility measured by diffusion MRI predict response of metastatic breast cancer to chemotherapy. Neoplasia 2004;6:831–7.

43. Sharma U, Danishad KK, Seenu V, et al. Longitudinal study of the assessment by MRI and diffusion-weighted imaging of tumor response in patients

with locally advanced breast cancer undergoing neoadjuvant chemotherapy. NMR Biomed 2009;22: 104–13.

44. Iacconi C, Giannelli M, Marini C, et al. The role of mean diffusivity (MD) as a predictive index of the response to chemotherapy in locally advanced breast cancer: a preliminary study. Eur Radiol 2010;20(2):303–8.

45. Park SH, Moon WK, Cho N, et al. Diffusion-weighted MR imaging: pretreatment prediction of response to neoadjuvant chemotherapy in patients with breast cancer. Radiology 2010;257(1):56–63.

46. Li XR, Cheng LQ, Liu M, et al. DW-MRI ADC values can predict treatment response in patients with locally advanced breast cancer undergoing neoadjuvant chemotherapy. Med Oncol 2012;29(2): 425–31.

47. Fangberget A, Nilsen LB, Hole KH, et al. Neoadjuvant chemotherapy in breast cancer-response evaluation and prediction of response to treatment using dynamic contrast-enhanced and diffusion-weighted MR imaging. Eur Radiol 2010;21(6):1188–99.

48. Manton DJ, Chaturvedi A, Hubbard A, et al. Neoadjuvant chemotherapy in breast cancer: early response prediction with quantitative MR imaging and spectroscopy [Erratum appears in Br J Cancer 2006;94(10):1544]. Br J Cancer 2006;94(3):427–35.

49. Nilsen L, Fangberget A, Geier O, et al. Diffusion-weighted magnetic resonance imaging for pretreatment prediction and monitoring of treatment response of patients with locally advanced breast cancer undergoing neoadjuvant chemotherapy. Acta Oncol 2010;49(3):354–60.

50. Woodhams R, Kakita S, Hata H, et al. Identification of residual breast carcinoma following neoadjuvant chemotherapy: diffusion-weighted imaging–comparison with contrast-enhanced MR imaging and pathologic findings. Radiology 2010;254(2):357–66.

51. Partridge SC, McKinnon GC, Henry RG, et al. Menstrual cycle variation of apparent diffusion coefficients measured in the normal breast using MRI. J Magn Reson Imaging 2001;14(4):433–8.

52. Park MJ, Cha ES, Kang BJ, et al. The role of diffusion-weighted imaging and the apparent diffusion coefficient (ADC) values for breast tumors. Korean J Radiol 2007;8(5):390–6.

53. Chen X, Zhao X, Kang H, et al. Conspicuity of breast lesions at different b values on diffusion-weighted imaging. BMC Cancer 2012;12:334.

54. Matsuoka A, Minato M, Harada M, et al. Comparison of 3.0- and 1.5-tesla diffusion- weighted imaging in the visibility of breast cancer. Radiat Med 2008; 26(1):15–20.

55. Yoshikawa MI, Ohsumi S, Sugata S, et al. Relation between cancer cellularity and apparent diffusion coefficient values using diffusion-weighted magnetic resonance imaging in breast cancer. Radiat Med 2008;26(4):222–6.

Modern Imaging Evaluation of the Liver
Emerging MR Imaging Techniques and Indications

Daniel Andrade Tinoco de Souza, MD[a],*,
Daniella Braz Parente, MD, PhD[b],
Antonio Luis Eiras de Araújo, MD[c,d],
Koenraad J. Mortelé, MD[e]

KEYWORDS

- Liver • Hepatic MRI • Diffusion-weighted imaging • Liver fibrosis • Hepatic steatosis
- MR elastography • MR spectroscopy • Hepatocellular contrast

KEY POINTS

- Modern MR imaging evaluation of the liver includes a comprehensive morphologic and functional assessment of the liver parenchyma, hepatic vessels, and biliary tree and thus aids in the diagnosis of both focal and diffuse liver diseases.
- Diffusion-weighted imaging (DWI) provides useful and additional information for the evaluation of the liver, in the identification and characterization of both focal and diffuse diseases, and should be integrated into routine MR imaging protocol.
- MR elastography (MRE) is a promising and emerging technique that has become widely accepted for the evaluation of liver fibrosis. Potential indications that are undergoing active research include evaluation of inflammation (hepatitis), differentiation between benign and malignant focal liver lesions, and assessment of portal hypertension.
- MR imaging is an accurate and reproducible noninvasive technique for the quantification of liver fat and iron deposition and may limit the use of liver biopsy in the diagnosis and follow-up of patients with steatosis and iron overload.
- Newer combined contrast agents combine the extracellular properties of traditional contrast agents with hepatobiliary-specific information and have become a key component of the standard work-up of focal liver lesions. Understanding of their unique pharmacologic properties and the MR imaging technique is fundamental, however, to achieve optimal performance. There is also a potential role for the use of these contrast agents in the anatomic and functional evaluation of the liver.

The authors have no disclosures.
[a] PET/CT and Nuclear Medicine, Dana-Farber Cancer Institute, Harvard Medical School, 400 Brookline Avenue, Boston, MA 02215, USA; [b] D'Or Institute for Research and Education, Labs D'Or Network – Fleury Group, Rua General Garzon 100/1002, RJ 22470-010, Brazil; [c] Department of Radiology, Universidade Federal do Rio de Janeiro, Rua Rodolpho Paulo Rocco, 255 Cidade Universitária, Ilha do Fundão, RJ 21941-913, Brazil; [d] Labs D'Or Network – Fleury Group, Rua Diniz Cordeiro, 39 Botafogo, RJ 22281-100, Brazil; [e] Division of Clinical MRI, Abdominal Imaging and Body MRI, Beth Israel Deaconess Medical Center, Harvard Medical School, 330 Brookline Avenue, Boston, MA 02215, USA
* Corresponding author.
E-mail address: daniel.radiology@gmail.com

Magn Reson Imaging Clin N Am 21 (2013) 337–363
http://dx.doi.org/10.1016/j.mric.2013.01.001

INTRODUCTION

During the past decade, there has been growing excitement and optimism regarding new technologic advances in the field of MR imaging, as well as emerging MR imaging applications, and new contrast agents that have been developed and approved for the evaluation of the liver. Although the superiority of MR imaging has long been acclaimed over other imaging techniques, particularly with regard to its lack of ionizing radiation and its higher sensitivity and specificity for detection and characterization of a broad range of hepatic conditions, it has become even more accessible and more widely available. Hepatic MR imaging allows for a comprehensive morphologic and functional assessment of the liver parenchyma, hepatic vessels, and biliary tree and thus aids in the diagnosis of both focal and diffuse liver diseases.

This article reviews some of these techniques and advances, including accepted and potential applications of DWI, MRE, and MR spectroscopy (MRS), as well as, in more detail, the evaluation of fat and iron deposition in the liver. Finally, the recently approved hepatospecific contrast agent, gadoxetate disodium (Eovist), and its clinical applications are discussed.

DIFFUSION-WEIGHTED IMAGING

DWI is an MR technique that exploits the normal brownian movement of the water molecules, or lack thereof. In pure water, molecules undergo free diffusion[1–3] whereas in tissues, water molecule movement is modified by interactions with cell membranes and macromolecules. DWI derives its contrast based on the difference in mobility of water molecules between tissues. Pathologic processes that alter the volume ratio of the physical nature of the intracellular and extracellular spaces affect the diffusion of water molecules. In highly cellular tissues (eg, tumors), abscesses, and cytotoxic edema, there is restricted diffusion due to the tortuosity of the extracellular space and higher density of cell membranes. In contrast, there is free diffusion of water molecules in cystic or necrotic tissues,[4] where cell membranes have been disrupted. Recent advances in hardware and software of the new-generation magnets (gradients, parallel and echo-planar imaging, coils with multiple channels, and movement-correction solutions) allowed the use of DWI in routine clinical evaluation of the abdomen.[3] Currently, DWI is used for detection and characterization of focal lesions, combined with conventional sequences. Emerging DWI applications include post-therapy tumor assessment

(thermal ablation and CyberKnife), evaluation of inflammatory conditions, as well as in the diagnosis and quantification of liver fibrosis and cirrhosis.[5,6]

Technique

DWI can be performed as a breath-hold or a free-breathing sequence. In breath-hold DWI, the whole abdomen can be evaluated in 2 apneas of only approximately 20 to 30 seconds each. The main disadvantages of the breath-hold acquisition, however, are (1) low signal-to-noise ratio (SNR), (2) lower spatial resolution, (3) wider section thickness, (4) distortion and ghosting artifacts, and (5) limited number of b values. Conversely, in free-breathing DWI, the liver is evaluated in 3 to 6 minutes. The main advantages of the free-breathing technique include (1) improved SNR, (2) higher spatial resolution, (3) thinner image sections, and (4) the possibility to use more b values. Besides the longer acquisition time, other disadvantages include slight image blurring, breathing artifacts, and volume averaging. Free breathing may be combined with respiratory triggering, either by placing a 2D navigator at the level of the liver dome on free-breathing sagittal and coronal scout images, or placement of respiratory sensor device over the area of greatest abdominal wall motion. In the left lobe of the liver, cardiac motion usually causes artifacts, which can be minimized by using pulse or cardiac triggering. In summary, respiratory-triggered DWI improves liver lesion detection, image quality, SNR, and apparent diffusion coefficient (ADC) quantification compared with the breath-hold technique but significantly increases the acquisition time and, therefore, is more prone to artifacts.[5]

Interpretation of DWIs requires the generation of ADC maps. The calculation from the native b-value images is a semiautomated process on most commercial MR imagers or workstations. The assessment can be qualitative, by visual assessment, or quantitative, by drawing regions of interest (ROIs) to record the mean ADC values in the tissue of interest. A major limitation for the widespread use of quantitative measurements is the variability in the results as a consequence of varying hardware and human and biologic factors. DWI standardization is needed, to allow comparison of the results and facilitate multicenter studies.

At the authors' institution, DWI of the liver is used routinely in all patients. Although there are different possible protocols, a suggested image acquisition scheme using breath-hold and respiratory-triggered techniques, as performed at the authors' institution, is summarized in **Table 1**.

Table 1
Proposed acquisition schemes for performing diffusion-weighted MR imaging of the liver

Parameter	Respiratory-Triggered Acquisition[a]	Breath-hold Acquisition[a]
Field of view	360	360
Matrix size	144 × 192	164 × 164
Repetition time	2500–6000	≥1600–2000
Echo time[b]	Minimum	Minimum
Echo-planar imaging factor	144	144
Phase-encoding direction	Anteroposterior	Anteroposterior
Parallel imaging acceleration factor	2	2
Number of signals acquired	5	1
Section thickness (mm)	6	8
Number of sections	20–25	10
Fat-suppression	Yes	Yes
B values (s/mm^2)	0, 50–100, 500, 700–1000	0, 50–100, 500, 700–1000
Comments	Improved SNR and spatial resolution, thinner image sections, more b values, longer acquisition time	Lower SNR and spatial resolution, wider section thickness, distortion and ghosting artifacts, limited number of b values, shorter acquisition time

[a] As it is performed at the author's institution.
[b] Minimum echo time depends on the system and the b values used and should be kept fixed for all b values.

Clinical Applications

DWI is used in the evaluation of focal and diffuse liver disease with increasing frequency. DWI obtained with low b values (10–200 s/mm^2) suppresses the signal from vessels and bile ducts, creating black-blood images, with high contrast-to-noise ratio, that highlights focal lesions similar to fat-suppressed fast spin-echo (FSE) T2-weighted images (**Fig. 1**). Low b-value images maintain reasonable quality with high SNR and still with significant reduction of blurring artifact. The improved focal liver detection rate of low b-value DWI compared with other MR imaging techniques, such as half-Fourier turbo spin-echo,[7] FSE T2,[8] T2

fat-saturated FSE,[9–11] and short-tau inversion recovery (STIR)[9] has been demonstrated (**Fig. 2**). Some investigators have suggested that low b-value DWI could replace the routine fat-saturated T2-weighted sequence.[8,12–14]

Differentiation between benign and malignant liver lesions

Benign hepatic lesions have generally higher ADC values compared with malignant lesions, but unfortunately there is considerable overlap in individual cases. Different ADC cutoff values have been described in the literature for the differentiation between benign and malignant lesions. Cutoff

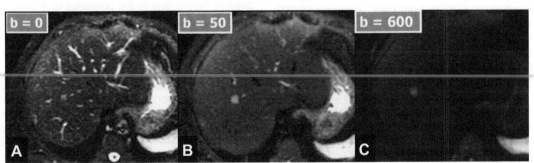

Fig. 1. Detection and characterization of focal liver lesion using DWI. Impact of increasing b values in the signal intensity of liver structures and resulting higher conspicuity of focal liver lesions. (*A*) b value = 0. (*B*) b value = 50. (*C*) b value = 600.

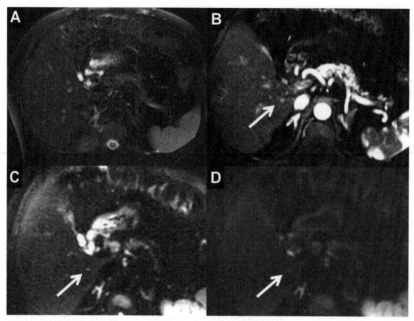

Fig. 2. Comparison between DWI and FSE T2-weighted images for the detection of focal liver lesions. A 44-year-old man with small liver metastasis in the right lobe. (*A*) Fat-suppressed T2-weighted MR image appears unremarkable. (*B*) Contrast-enhanced T1-weighted image shows focus of arterial enhancement in hepatic segment V (*arrow*), suspicious for metastatic disease. (*C, D*) DWIs show hyperintense focus at the same location (*arrows*) on the lower (b=50) and higher (b=600) b-values, consistent with metastatic disease.

values between 1.4×10^{-3} and 1.6×10^{-3} mm/s^2 have been shown to provide high sensitivity (74%–100%) and specificity (77%–100%).[10,15–19] These findings, however, have not been validated by other studies, which have found a much wider range of ADC values for metastatic disease (0.94×10^{-3} to 2.85×10^{-3} mm/s^2) and normal hepatic parenchyma (0.69×10^{-3} to 2.8×10^{-3} mm/s^2).[5,8,19–23]

Liver metastases

The added value of DWI for the detection of liver metastases has been demonstrated by several investigators.[8,20,24] Low b-value respiratory-triggered DWI has been shown to increase the conspicuity of hemangiomas and metastases in comparison with conventional unenhanced MR images (see **Fig. 1**).[8] Bruegel and colleagues[9] have found better results in DWI compared with turbo spin-echo T2 in the detection of liver metastases larger than 10 mm, with sensitivities of 88% and 91% and specificities of 45% and 62%, respectively. For lesions smaller than 10 mm, DWI performed even better than turbo spin-echo T2, with sensitivity of 85% for ADC and 26% to 44% for turbo spin-echo T2.[25] Koh and colleagues[26] have shown that the combination of DWI and mangafodipir trisodium (MnDPDP) can provide higher diagnostic accuracy (0.94–0.96) than MnDPDP alone (0.88–0.92) or DWI alone (0.83–0.90) for the detection of colorectal liver metastases. DWI should be used in combination with conventional MR imaging, because it is a functional sequence that lacks anatomic information. In addition, DWI is susceptible to motion artifacts, particularly in the left hepatic lobe. Thus, reader experience has a greater impact on the final image interpretation.

Malignant lesions associated with cystic, necrotic, and/or mucinous contents can lead to false-negative results, because these components can increase the ADC values, particularly when analysis is solely performed on the basis of the DWI information (**Fig. 3**). Conversely, abscesses and inflammatory lesions can lead to false-positive results due to the presence of inflammatory cells and viscous material lowering the ADC values.[3]

Hepatocellular carcinoma

Hepatocellular carcinoma (HCC) can be diagnosed after demonstration of the classic imaging features of rapid and intense arterial enhancement, followed by contrast washout in the portal venous and late phases. Diagnosis of small HCCs and their differentiation from benign hepatic nodules in cirrhosis remains a major challenge.[27] Potential benefits of DWI include greater contrast-to-noise ratio and suppression of the

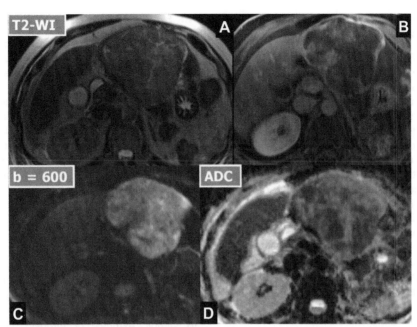

Fig. 3. DWI in the follow-up evaluation of liver lesion in 55-year-old man with metastatic colorectal cancer. (*A*) T2-weighted MR image shows large, exophytic mass in the left hepatic lobe, associated with heterogeneous signal intensity, consistent with metastatic disease. (*B*) Postcontrast T1-weighted image obtained in the portal venous phase shows heterogeneous enhancement, with several areas of reduced and/or absent enhancement. These necrotic and/or cystic areas correspond to T2-hyperintense regions, which correlate with regions of high signal intensity on the high b-value DWI (*C*), and relatively high signal intensity on the ADC map (*D*). These early changes are often seen as a result chemotherapy, particularly with the increasing use of antiangiogenic drugs (eg, VEGF inhibitors). DWI has been used as a surrogate marker of treatment response in the assessment of primary and secondary liver malignancy, with some studies showing that interval increase in ADC values after treatment can predict a more favorable response.

surrounding hepatic parenchyma, allowing for small HCCs to become more conspicuous, particularly those at the vicinity of vessels and bile ducts.[27] Some investigators have shown that ADC values are not useful in the context of cirrhosis due to considerable overlap.[24,28] Other investigators have shown that DWI can add value to the diagnosis of larger HCCs (>2 cm), with greater sensitivity, specificity, and positive predictive value than conventional MR imaging alone.[29] A recent publication by Kim and colleagues[30] has shown that DWI can be useful when used in combination with gadoxetic acid. Retrospecive evaluation of 214 nodules in 135 patients concluded that hyperintensity on DWI in hypovascular hypointense nodules seen on hepatobiliary phase is strongly associated with progression to hypervascular HCC.

Future Directions

Recent reports and ongoing research studies have explored other exciting and promising areas where DWI could prove useful.

Tumor response assessment

DWI has been used to predict treatment response in primary and secondary liver malignancy, based on the sensitivity of this technique to changes that occur in the tumor microenvironment after treatment. Some studies have demonstrated strong correlation between the mean pretreatment ADC values and the percentage of tumor reduction after chemotherapy and radiation treatment.[31,32] Cui and colleagues[32] studied 87 metastatic liver lesions arising from colorectal and gastric malignancies in 23 patients. Tumors that showed favorable responses to treatment were usually associated with significant increase in ADC values at the end of treatment, as opposed to those that did not respond, which typically showed no significant changes in ADC values.[32] There was weak correlation between tumor size reduction and ADC values before treatment.

DWI has been shown promise in monitoring the changes associated with radiofrequency ablation and transarterial chemoembolization, providing potential useful information and improving the detection of early local recurrence after thermal ablation, particularly in combination with conventional MR imaging.[27]

Liver fibrosis and inflammation

Liver biopsy is considered the gold standard in the diagnosis and monitoring of fibrosis and inflammation that occur in chronic and subacute conditions, such as cirrhosis and nonalcoholic fatty liver disease (NAFLD). It is believed that deposition of fat (hepatic steatosis), collagen, and fibrosis may lead to inflammation and consequent reduction in ADC values. DWI has the potential to provide noninvasive evaluation for detection and monitoring of these conditions, avoiding the risks associated with biopsy.[33] Some studies have demonstrated a reduction in ADC values in liver cirrhosis compared with normal liver, with initial results suggesting good performance of ADC calculation in distinguishing moderate and severe fibrosis (METAVIR score F2 and F3) from mild fibrosis (METAVIR score F0 and F1).[4,33,34] Nevertheless, further studies and technical improvements in DWI are still needed.

Summary

DWI is a relatively new imaging technique with enormous potential for the assessment of the liver. It provides additional useful information, and it should be integrated into the routine MR imaging protocol.

DWI has been demonstrated to be useful in the identification and characterization of focal hepatic lesions but should be used in conjunction with the conventional MR imaging information, particularly due to significant overlap of ADC values between benign and malignant lesions. DWI is also useful for the detection of small HCCs in cirrhotic patients, which is a common scenario in which conventional MR imaging shows severe limitations. Challenges in the implementation of DWI include more difficult interpretation, which requires a longer learning curve, and the susceptibility of this technique to different types of artifacts. Therefore, it is recommended that the DWI information be used altogether with the findings of the conventional MR imaging protocol. Method standardization is another challenge and prerequisite for the reproduction of findings from different services and equipment.

Other potential applications for DWI include post-treatment follow-up of primary and secondary liver malignancy, including early detection of local recurrence after thermal ablation and transarterial chemoembolization, assessment of tumor response, and diagnosis and quantification of fibrosis and inflammation that occur in chronic liver diseases.

MR ELASTOGRAPHY

MRE is another emerging technique that has become widely accepted for the evaluation of the liver. It is based on the biologic concept that physiologic states (eg, postprandial period) and disease processes, such as cancer, inflammation, and fibrosis, can dramatically affect liver stiffness.[35–39] The advantage over physical examination is that subtle changes can be detected, and diagnosis can be made at earlier stages, with potential positive impact on prognosis.[40]

Technique

Several modalities have been used for elastography, including optical imaging, ultrasound, and, more recently, MR imaging.[36,38,41–47] The ultimate goal in elastographic imaging of the liver is to provide noninvasive assessment of the mechanical tissue properties in vivo, evaluating the liver tissue response (internal displacement or stiffness) to stimuli, extrinsic or intrinsic, by generating images that express their mechanical properties: shear wave speed (velocity), which is equivalent to shear modulus (elastic Young modulus), or liver stiffness.[35,36,40,46,48]

Transient ultrasound elastography (FibroScan) has been proven effective in the detection and staging of liver fibrosis.[38,44,48–51] It is simple, fast, and inexpensive. MRE, however, is considered superior for several reasons.[40,41,52] It can be integrated into a comprehensive MR evaluation of the liver, it is less operator dependent, and its evaluation is not limited to a small fraction of the parenchyma, either due to limited depth and/or acoustic window within an intercostal space. As opposed to ultrasound, MRE also has been shown effective in obese patients and in patients with ascites.[35,40,41,43] Both MRE and ultrasound elastography express their results in units of kilopascals. Measurements are not directly interchangeable, however, because ultrasound-based transient elastography measures stiffness as Young elastic modulus and MRE measures stiffness as the shear modulus.[35,36] Potential disadvantages of MR imaging include longer examination time and cost.[37]

A detailed description of the technique involved in elastographic imaging is beyond the scope of this review. Three fundamental steps can be described, however, to provide basic understanding of the technique (**Box 1**).[35,36] The first step is to apply stress or source of motion that deforms the tissue. The stimuli can be internal sources of motion, such as respiration or cardiac pulsation, or external sources. In MRE, a mechanical driver device consisting of electromechanical voice coils, piezoelectric bending elements, or pneumatically powered actuators is placed in contact with a patient's body wall. This device applies time-harmonic motion at 1 frequency or several acoustic frequencies, typically between 40 Hz and 120 Hz. The second step is to acquire synchronized gradient-echo sequences that image the tissue response (displacement or velocity), using motion-sensitizing gradients similar to those used in phase-contrast MR angiography and DWI as the waves propagate throughout the liver. The wave propagation depends on the stiffness of the tissue; both wave velocity and wavelength increase with greater liver stiffness. The third step is to image the response and postprocess corresponding stiffness maps. The resulting phase-contrast images express the true vector tissue motion or propagating mechanical waves. Elastograms, or quantitative stiffness maps, are then generated, after complex postprocessing of the raw data, including temporal and spatial characteristics of the wave field (**Fig. 4**).[36,41,53] These maps can depict the tissue stiffness as the wave speed itself, or it can report effective shear stiffness on a per-pixel basis, in units of kilopascals, which represents the shear modulus of a purely elastic material that exhibits the observed wave speed. The liver stiffness can be typically assessed by placing ROIs in appropriate locations on the elastograms (**Fig. 4**).

Clinical Applications

In addition to regeneration, severe hepatic fibrosis is the hallmark of cirrhosis and the ultimate outcome of multiple types of chronic liver injury, including viral infection, alcoholism, NAFLD, and several autoimmune conditions.[41,47,54–56] Liver biopsy is currently considered the only validated

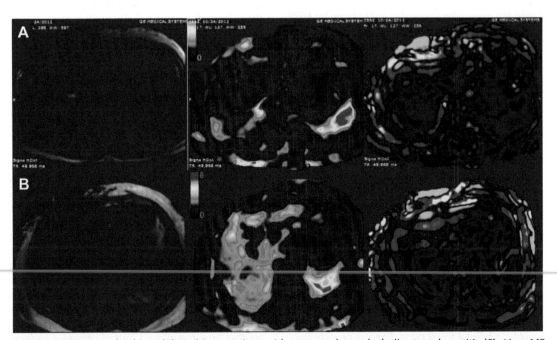

Fig. 4. MRE in normal subject (*A*) and in a patient with suspected nonalcoholic steatohepatitis (*B*). Liver MR imaging (*left*), color-coded elastograms (*center*), and MR elastographic wave images (*right*) of normal volunteer (*A*) demonstrate normal propagation of shear waves through the liver, with liver stiffness of 2.0 kPa (normal threshold approximately 2.7 kPa). In diabetic patients with suspected nonalcoholic steatohepatitis (*B*), elastogram demonstrates overall higher liver stiffness (3.5 kPa), most likely secondary to inflammation.

and universally accepted clinical method that enables the detection and staging of fibrosis.[41,57,58] However, it is an invasive procedure that carries the risk of serious complications, including procedure-related death. Similar to what has been shown with ultrasound-based transient elastography, MRE has the potential to replace biopsy for noninvasive quantitative assessment of hepatic fibrosis.[58] In a study by Rouvière and colleagues,[40] all patients with chronic liver disease had MR elastographic liver stiffness measurements that were higher than those of healthy volunteers. MRE has been shown by Huwart and colleagues[52] to be superior to aspartate aminotransferase–to-platelet ratio index method, one of the biochemical tests often used for grading of liver fibrosis.[59] It was able to differentiate patients with no (stage F0), minimal (stage F1), intermediate (stage F2), or advanced fibrosis (stage F3) and patients with cirrhosis (stage F4). A more recent study by Wang and colleagues[60] in 67 patients with chronic liver disease has demonstrated that MRE has a greater predictive ability in distinguishing the stages of liver fibrosis than DWI. In addition, MRE potentially can be used in the assessment of treatment response in patients undergoing antiviral treatment, in which patient serial biopsies would not be a feasible task.[60]

Future Directions

There are many other potential indications for MRE that need validation but are under active research, including the detection of inflammation.[36,51] MRE has been shown by Chen and colleagues[61] to identify steatohepatitis in patients with NAFLD, even before the onset of fibrosis. In this study, NAFLD patients with inflammation (and no fibrosis) had greater liver stiffness than those with simple steatosis and lower mean stiffness than those with fibrosis. Another promising potential application of MRE could include the differentiation of malignant and benign focal liver tumors.[45] A study by Venkatesh and colleagues[45] with 44 liver tumors showed that malignant liver tumors had significantly higher mean shear stiffness than benign tumors, fibrotic liver, and normal liver. Fibrotic livers, however, had stiffness values that were overlapping with both the benign and malignant tumors. Cutoff values of 5 kPa accurately differentiated malignant tumors from benign tumors and normal liver parenchyma.[45]

Noninvasive assessment of portal hypertension would be helpful to monitor disease progression, and to evaluate response to treatment.[62] The hepatic stiffness is a dynamic process that is impacted by changes in central venous pressure and presence of significant portal hypertension.

MRE has been used to demonstrate an increase in liver stiffness during the postprandial period in patients with advanced liver disease, which typically have an abnormal regulation of portal blood flow.[62]

Summary

MRE is an advanced and promising tool that can be integrated into a comprehensive MR evaluation of the liver, providing accurate and reproducible assessment of liver fibrosis and potentially many other liver conditions, such as steatohepatitis and portal hypertension.

HEPATIC STEATOSIS

Hepatic steatosis or fatty liver is a major cause of chronic liver disease in the world and, because of the rising obesity epidemic, it will remain an important cause of chronic liver disease in the future.[63–68] Currently, the only method for diagnosing and staging steatosis is liver biopsy, which is invasive, may be related to complications, and is subject to sampling errors and to significant intraobserver and interobserver variability.[69–72] Due to the limitations of liver biopsy and the need for staging of fatty liver, with early detection of inflammation and fibrosis, noninvasive methods are under development. Several MR imaging–based techniques are in clinical use and others are in development.

Technique

MR imaging is considered the best imaging technique for the detection and quantification of liver fat. Several MR imaging techniques allow the detection and quantification of fat, based on the difference of the precession frequency of the hydrogen protons present in water and fat.[43,73–78]

Chemical Shift Imaging

Hepatic steatosis as low as 10% to 15% can be diagnosed by chemical shift imaging.[79–81] This sequence has many advantages, including whole-liver evaluation, breath-hold acquisition, wide availability, high sensitivity for fat detection, and relative stability for magnetic field heterogeneity. Hydrogen protons of water and fat have different precessional frequencies. After the radiofrequency pulse, their magnetization vectors alternate positions, being at one time aligned (in-phase) and at another time misaligned (out of phase). Gradient-echo sequence with varied echo times generates images that reflect those characteristics.[73,82]

The echo time where water and fat are in phase or out of phase depends on the magnetic field strength. For example, at 1.5 T, out-of-phase images are acquired at echo times of 2.3 ms, in-phase images at echo times of 4.6 ms, and so forth. At 3.0 T, out-of-phase images are acquired at echo times of 1.15 ms, in-phase images at echo times of 2.3 ms, and so forth. When protons of water and fat are in phase, the magnetization vectors are added and when hydrogen protons are out of phase, the magnetization vectors cancel each other, thus reducing the image signal.[73,77–79,83,84] The intensity of the signal loss depends on the proportion of water and fat in each voxel and is highest when there is 50% water and 50% fat at the same voxel.

The signal loss due to T2* effect (loss of phase coherence of proton spin-spin interactions and magnetic field heterogeneities) is another relevant issue. The higher the TE, the more signal loss due to T2* effect. The out-of-phase images should always precede in-phase images, so the signal drop observed from the first echo (out of phase) to the second echo (in phase), due to T2* effects, appears as signal loss at in-phase images and is not confused with fatty change that causes signal loss in out-of-phase images (**Fig. 5**).[85] Thus, the signal loss that occurs in the out-of-phase images

(first echo − shortest TE) is always due to fatty change.[73,77,79,85,86]

There are two common formulas to calculate the percentage of hepatic fat using the dual-echo technique. The first formula uses liver signal intensity at in-phase and out-of-phase images, as follows: $(SIP − SOP)/2 (SIP) \times 100$, where *SIP* is the liver signal intensity at in-phase image and *SOP* is the liver signal intensity at out-of-phase image. The second formula uses the spleen normalization factor as $[(SIIP-SIOP)/2(SIIP) \times 100]$, where *SIIP* is the ratio between the liver and spleen signal intensity on the in-phase image and *SIOP* is the ratio between the liver and spleen signal intensity on the out-of-phase image.[73,82]

T2* effects may interfere with fat quantification and should be corrected whenever possible, especially in the presence of siderosis, when T2* effects are significant. More sophisticated sequences, such as triple-echo (**Fig. 6**) and multiecho acquisition, can be performed for this correction.[77,85–87] However, T1 effects can also interfere with fat evaluation but can be minimized by using a low flip angle (eg, 10°).[73] Heavily T1-weighted sequences tend to overestimate fat quantity and are best suited for the detection of

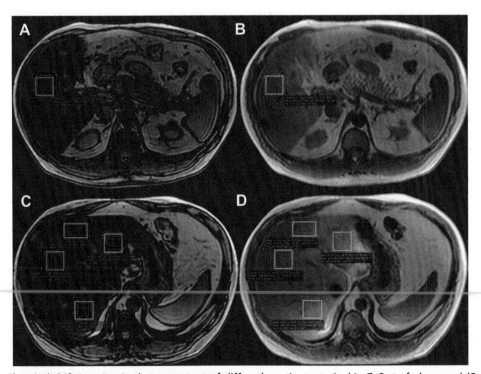

Fig. 5. Chemical shift imaging in the assessment of diffuse hepatic steatosis. (*A, C*) Out-of-phase and (*B, D*) in-phase breath-hold spoiled gradient-echo sequence images show diffuse fat deposition. The diagnosis is made by characterizing diffuse hepatic signal intensity loss on the out-of-phase images, which is due to cancellation of fat and water signals. Various regions of interest (squares) are placed over different locations within the liver.

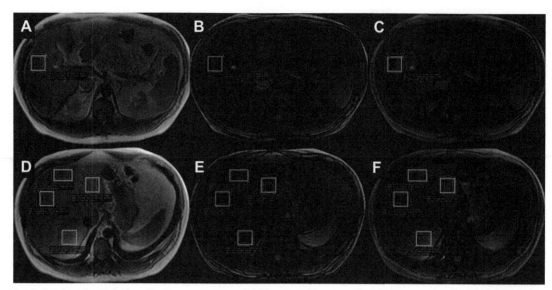

Fig. 6. Triple-echo technique in the assessment of diffuse hepatic steatosis. MR images obtained from the triple-echo breath-hold spoiled gradient-echo sequence include sequential in-phase (*A, D*), out-of-phase (*B, E*), and in-phase (*C, F*) images with increasing echo times and show diffuse fat deposition. Multiple ROIs (*squares*) are placed over different locations within the fatty liver. The cancellation of fat and water signals causes diffuse signal intensity loss on the out-of-phase images.

small amounts of fat. In contrast, low T1 weighting (long repetition time or low flip angle) causes the T1 terms of the fat and water to be more balanced and reduces the relative amplification of the fat signal.[73]

Frequency-Selective MR Imaging

In fat-saturation techniques, two sets of MR images are obtained: one with and one without a fat-saturation pulse, with identical imaging parameters, except for application of the presaturation pulse. The non–fat-saturated image shows the signal intensity of the water signal plus fat signal, whereas the fat-saturated image shows only the water signal. Fat fraction can be calculated by subtracting the fat-saturated image (water signal only) from the non–fat-saturated image (water signal plus fat signal). Spectral separation is proportional to B0 and more effective in high-field scanners. These sequences are theoretically less susceptible to T2* effects than chemical-shift imaging but require a complete and homogeneous magnetic field that is almost impossible to reliably achieve throughout the liver. This technique is not commonly used because of frequent fat-fraction miscalculation due to incomplete fat saturation and inadvertent water suppression.[73,82]

IDEAL Technique

The iterative decomposition of water and fat with echo asymmetry and least-squares estimation

(IDEAL) technique is a chemical-shift water-fat separation method that improves the accuracy of hepatic steatosis quantification through accurate modeling of the multiple spectral peaks of fat. It is a complex technique that allows reliable fat quantification in the presence of moderate heterogeneities of the magnetic field. Some limitations include noise bias and longitudinal relaxation effects that can be partially overcome by small-flip or dual-flip angle approaches, magnitude discrimination, and phase-constrained methods.[88–90]

MR Spectroscopy

MRS analyzes tissue chemical composition present in the voxel of interest to generate a spectral curve, where each metabolite is detected at a specific parts per million. Water is located at 4.7 ppm, lipids at 0.9 to 1.4 ppm, and choline at 3.0 ppm. Currently, the main clinical application for liver MRS is to detect and quantify liver fat. It is a complex imaging method that demands long postprocessing times and is discussed later.[73,91]

HEPATIC IRON OVERLOAD

Hepatic iron overload can be classified as primary hemochromatosis or hemosiderosis. Primary hemochromatosis is a recessive autosomal genetic disorder that alters a protein involved in the regulation of iron absorption in the gut. Primary hemochromatosis is the most common genetic disease in the white population, with 0.2% to 0.5% incidence for homozygous disease and 10% for heterozygous disease. Hemosiderosis is caused by increased iron absorption, abnormal red blood cell breakdown with resultant iron release related to ineffective erythropoiesis, and exogenous increase by multiple transfusions. Liver biopsy is the reference standard for the diagnosis, staging, and quantification of iron overload. However, because of its invasiveness, potential risks, and possible sampling errors, noninvasive methods are under development.[92,93]

Technique

MR imaging is an accurate, precise, and reproducible noninvasive method for diagnosis and quantification of iron deposition in the liver, useful for monitoring the disease and treatment response. The accumulation of iron in the organs causes magnetic field distortion, which results in T1, T2, and T2* shortening in sequences using longer echo times, with signal loss proportional to the iron deposition. All organs darken with increasing echo time, but those containing iron darken more rapidly (Fig. 7).[92–94]

Iron quantification with MR imaging has high correlation to liver biopsy results and can be performed using the method described by Gandon and colleagues,[95] available at the Web site of the University of Rennes (http://www.radio.univ-rennes1.fr/Sources/EN/Hemo.html) and also published in the Lancet.[96] Their technique uses gradient-echo sequences with T2* weighting and progressively longer echo times (Fig. 8). Patients with no iron overload have higher liver signal intensity than that of the paraspinal musculature in all sequences. In patients with slight to moderate iron overload, a decrease in liver signal intensity is seen on the gradient-echo images obtained with longer echo times. The accuracy of

quantification of iron by MR imaging is low in patients with severe iron overload, because of the complete liver signal loss. Castiella and colleagues[97] assessed the accuracy of the University of Rennes model and found it reliable for ruling out iron overload when values less than 60 μmol Fe/g were present and to confirm severe iron overload estimated to be greater than 170 μmol Fe/g. Technical advances allow new estimation models with T2 relaxometry methods using breath-hold or free-breathing acquisitions at various echo times. T2* is the necessary echo time for a tissue to become twice as dark. R2* represents the rate of darkening. R2* values are 1000/T2*; thus, both can be used for iron quantification. Ferritin aggregates and their breakdown product, hemosiderin, determine tissue R2 and R2* (or T2 and T2*). R2* values are almost entirely determined by hemosiderin concentration, whereas R2 retains some sensitivity to the amount of soluble ferritin. Either liver R2 or liver R2* can be used to estimate liver iron concentration. Liver R2* images are the easiest and quickest to collect. Image analysis and iron quantification are similar whether using R2 or R2* images. Postprocessing with commercial or locally developed software is required for R2 and R2* and both values should be converted to liver biopsy equivalents using established calibration curves. The upper limit of liver iron that can be reliably estimated depends on scanner specifications but is generally 30 mg/g to 40 mg/g dry weight at 1.5 T.[93,98,99]

In conclusion, MR imaging is an accurate and reproducible noninvasive technique for the quantification of liver iron deposition that may limit the use of liver biopsy in the diagnosis and follow-up of patients with iron overload. These techniques will become the standard of care with future implementation of simple postprocessing methods.

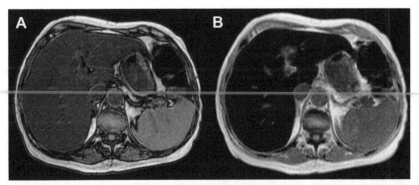

Fig. 7. Chemical shift imaging in the assessment of hepatic iron deposition. (A) Out-of-phase and (B) in-phase breath-hold spoiled gradient-echo images show diffuse iron deposition. The diagnosis is made by observing diffuse hepatic signal intensity loss on the in-phase images, because of signal loss due to T2* effect (higher TE).

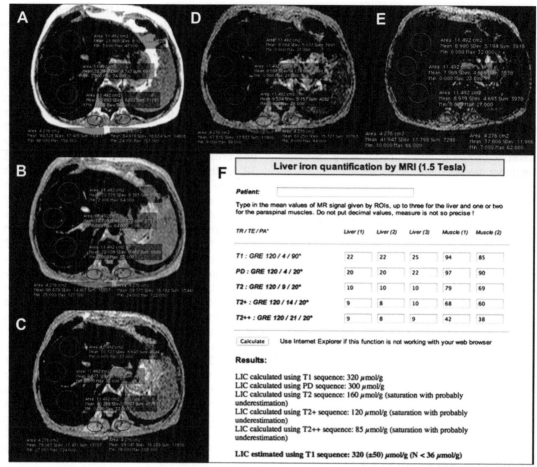

Fig. 8. University of Rennes Web site with suggested MR imaging protocol for the assessment of hepatic iron deposition. Severe hepatic iron overload. Example of suggested University of Rennes MR imaging protocol for the assessment of iron deposition in patient with severe hepatic iron overload. (*A–E*) The mean values of MR signal given by multiple ROIs placed in the liver and paraspinal muscles are required for calculation using multiple MR pulse sequences, as shown. (*F*) This algorithm calculates liver iron concentration from every sequence and selects the most appropriate result. In this patient, the liver iron concentration was estimated using the T1 sequence, and consistent with severe hepatic iron overload (above 300 mmol Fe/g).

MR SPECTROSCOPY

MRS analyzes tissue chemical composition using the precession frequency of different molecules present in the voxel of interest to generate a spectral curve, where the X axis represents the molecules precession frequency in parts per million and the Y axis represents the signal intensity of each peak in arbitrary units. Each metabolite is detected at a specific parts per million. Water, the dominant peak in the liver, usually used as the reference standard, is located at 4.7 ppm. Lipids are located at 0.9 ppm to 1.4 ppm, and choline, a tumor marker, is located at 3.0 ppm (**Fig. 9**). The area under the metabolite peak is used to quantify the amount of the metabolite within the sampled voxel. MRS reliably detects quantities as

small as 0.5% of fat deposition and is sensitive to fat variations after treatment. Spectral curve quality depends on magnetic field homogeneity, which is often technically difficult.[73,78,85,89,91,100–107] Several studies have shown that this is the most reliable imaging technique for liver fat quantification.[73,76,102,104,108] A long repetition time is important to minimize T1 effects and multiple-echo MRS is necessary for T2 correction. MRS can measure water and fat proton densities.[85] Fat fraction calculated from the proton densities determined by MRS has been shown to be equivalent to the concentration of triglycerides in the liver.[109,110]

Two MRS sequences can be used to evaluate the liver, point-resolved spectroscopy and stimulated echo acquisition mode. Point-resolved

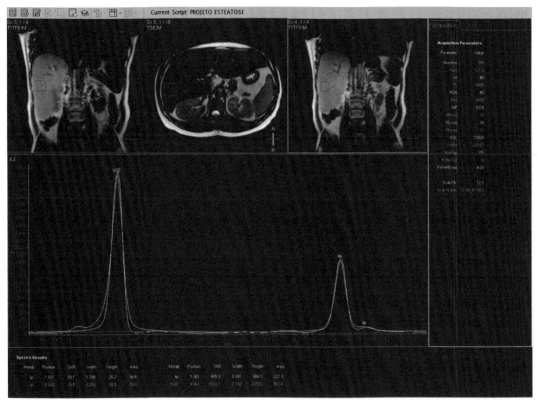

Fig. 9. Liver MRS. Characteristic frequencies of water and fat signal at MRS. A single voxel is positioned in right hepatic lobe, avoiding the biliary tract, vessels, and the liver margin. The graph shows peaks of 4.7 ppm and 1.3 ppm, which are characteristic frequencies of water and fat, respectively.

spectroscopy is a multiecho acquisition with long pulses of 90°–180°–180° that allow better visualization of metabolites with long TR and a higher SNR. Stimulated echo acquisition mode is similar to multiecho point-resolved spectroscopy, with pulses of 90°–90°–90°. A single voxel, 10 mm³ to 30 mm³, is positioned in right hepatic lobe, avoiding biliary tract, vessels, and the liver edge to avoid partial volume effects. Postprocessing is performed on commercially available software based on different algorithms. Fat quantification is obtained with peak areas of lipids summation in regions from 0.9 ppm to 3.0 ppm (**Fig. 10**).[77,82,91]

Future Directions

Future indications for MRS include the detection of inflammation and fibrosis in NAFLD, identification of fibrosis severity and cirrhosis secondary to chronic liver disease, characterization of focal liver lesions, and evaluation of tumor response after treatment.[91]

MRS of the liver is complex, susceptible to variations due to different methods of analysis, acquisition parameters, and MR imaging systems,

which demand large postprocessing time and has not been validated for clinical use.

COMBINED EXTRACELLULAR AND HEPATOBILIARY-SPECIFIC MR CONTRAST AGENTS

The vast majority of MR contrast agents used for routine liver imaging are gadolinium-based compounds, and they have been in clinical use for decades. After intravenous administration, these so-called traditional or extracellular agents are freely and rapidly distributed from the vascular to the extracellular space, providing optimal vascular and parenchymal evaluation.[111–115] In contrast, hepatobiliary-specific contrast agents are taken up to varying degrees by functioning hepatocytes and are excreted in the bile, providing dedicated anatomic (and functional) information about the liver and the biliary tree.[111,116,117]

Currently, there are only two available hepatobiliary-specific agents in the United States: gadobenate dimeglumine (MultiHance, Bracco Diagnostics, Princeton, NJ) and gadoxetate disodium (Gd-EOB-DTPA, gadoxetic acid, Eovist or

A

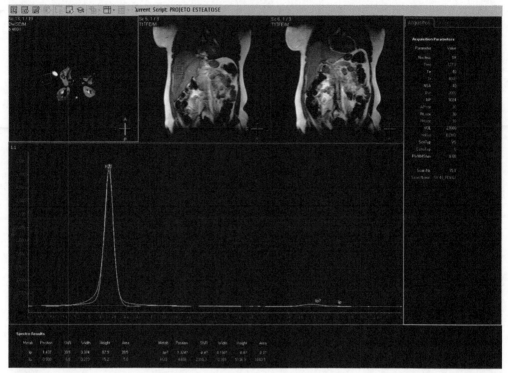

B

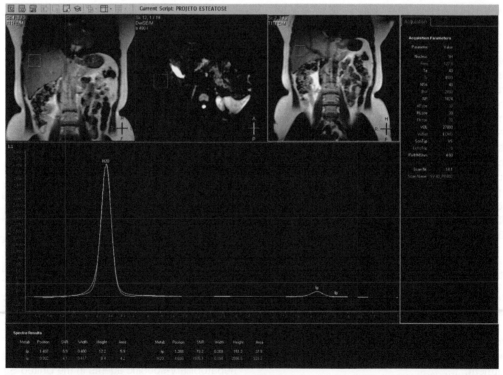

Fig. 10. MRS in the assessment of hepatic fat deposition. MRS in normal subject (*A*), and in patients with mild (*B*), moderate (*C*), and severe (*D*) hepatic fat deposition. Note the progressive elevation of lipid peaks (and resulting areas under the peak) located at 0.9–1.4 ppm, correlating with progressive increase in fat deposition. MRS can reliably detect quantities as small as 0.5% of fat deposition, and it is sensitive to fat variations after treatment.

C

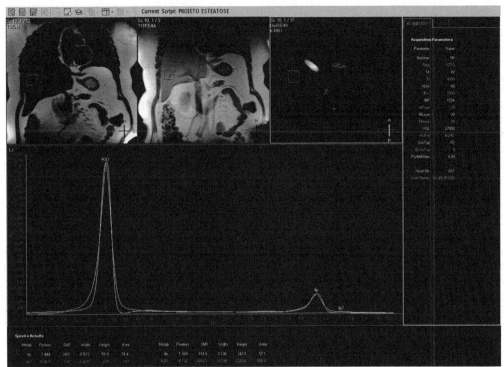

D

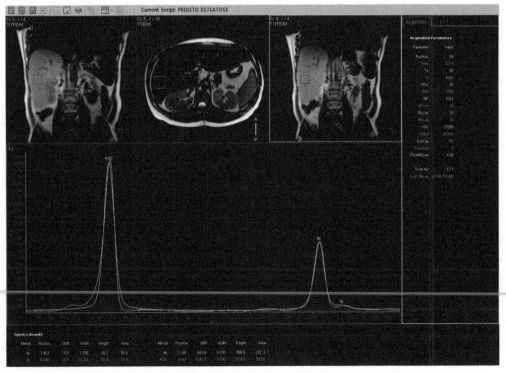

Fig. 10. (*continued*)

Primovist, Bayer HealthCare, Leverkusen, Germany). Their unique dual pharmacokinetic profile, with both extracellular and hepatobiliary-specific properties, allows them to provide both dynamic and hepatocyte imaging information. Although both agents are considered combined agents, there are significant differences between these agents. Gadoxetate disodium (Eovist) has been recently approved by the Food and Drug Administration (FDA) and has a few advantages over gadobenate dimeglumine (MultiHance), including higher rate of biliary excretion (50% vs 5%) , and shorter delay for the acquisition of the hepatocyte phase (20 minutes vs 2 hours).[111,118–120]

Technique

Radiologists should be familiar with the particular pharmacologic properties and technical challenges associated with gadoxetic acid. After intravenous injection and free distribution into the vascular and extracellular space, which allows for dynamic evaluation, approximately 50% of the gadoxetate disodium is taken up by hepatocytes, by means of the ATP-dependent organic anion transporting polypeptide (OATP1). It is subsequently excreted into the biliary system by the canalicular multispecific organic anion transporter (cMOAT), which also is responsible for bilirubin excretion. For that reason, hyperbilirubinemia in late-stage cirrhotic patients may affect the rate of excretion. In normal patients, approximately 50% of the administered dose is excreted via the hepatobiliary pathway, with the percentage of renal elimination increasing at higher doses, as opposed to gadobenate dimeglumine, which has lower biliary excretion rate (approximately 3%–5%).[111,118–120]

Gadoxetic acid has another particular property that might have an impact in the quality of the examination. Due to much higher plasma T1-relaxivity, the FDA-approved dose of gadoxetic acid is 0.025 mmol/kg of body weight, which is only 1/4 of the administered dose for traditional extracellular agents. This unique property, in association with its shorter plasma half-life, makes dynamic imaging more challenging, in particular proper bolus timing for the acquisition of the arterial phase. Strategies that have been used to overcome these obstacles include (1) decreasing the acquisition time, usually at the expense of spatial resolution, and/or (2) increasing the bolus time, by slowing the injection rate and thus diluting the contrast bolus.[111,118,120] Although gadoxetic acid can often be seen in the bile ducts as early as within 5 minutes after intravenous injection, optimal hepatocyte phase imaging is obtained at 20 minutes (Fig. 11). In contrast, gadobenate dimeglumine requires longer delay for hepatocyte imaging, typically of 1 to 2 hours.[120] This feature is considered one of the main advantages of gadoxetate disodium, because patient comfort is increased with shorter acquisition times, and throughput is improved. The workflow can be further ameliorated by acquiring FSE T2-weighted

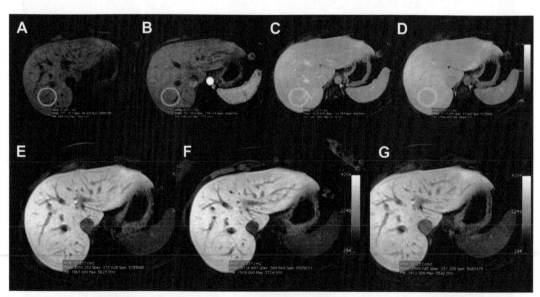

Fig. 11. Normal hepatic enhancement after the administration of gadoxetate disodium (Gd-EOB-DTPA, Eovist, Bayer HealthCare). (A–D). Dynamic axial T1-weighted fat-saturated MR images are obtained before (A) and after contrast administration in the arterial (B), portal venous (C), and late dynamic (D) images. (E–G). Hepatobiliary phase images obtained at 10 (E), 15 (F), and 20 (G) minutes demonstrate progressive parenchymal enhancement, qualitatively and quantitatively by the ROIs placed in the right hepatic lobe.

and DWI sequences after contrast administration during the time interval between the dynamic (5′) and the hepatocyte (20′) phases. This protocol allows for qualitative assessment of the DWI images, but the reader should proceed with caution if pursuing quantitative interpretation of ADC values. Conversely, there is an adverse effect in the acquisition of MR cholangiopancreatography images, both qualitatively and quantitatively, and these images should be obtained before intravenous contrast administration.[121] In uncooperative patients, multiple acquisitions can be obtained; and in selected cases, different acquisition planes (eg, coronal or sagittal) can be acquired within a reasonable time interval, until optimal breath-hold images are obtained. This unique biodistribution has led to discussion of the proper terminology that should be used in radiology reports. To avoid confusion, some authors argue that the term late dynamic phase should be preferred over equilibrium phase, when describing findings visible at 3–5 minutes after gadoxetic acid administration.[111,117,122–124]

Clinical Applications

Detection and characterization of focal liver lesions in noncirrhotic patients

The use of gadoxetate disodium has proved clinically helpful in the detection and characterization of focal liver lesions. The main role of HSCAs is to determine whether a lesion is of hepatocellular origin (eg, focal nodular hyperplasia [FNH] or adenoma) or not (eg, cyst, hemangioma, and others). One of the most common clinical applications is for the diagnosis of FNH.[117,125–131] Differentiation between FNH, the second most common benign liver tumor, from other premalignant (adenoma) or malignant conditions (metastases) is critical but sometimes challenging. FNH is considered a congenital vascular malformation, containing normal hepatocytes and abnormal bile ductules. Except in rare instances, FNH appears isointense or hyperintense relative to the surrounding hepatic parenchyma during the hepatocyte phase (**Fig. 12**). Other helpful discriminating imaging features include (1) nearly isointense T1 and T2 signal, (2) popcorn-like, avid homogeneous arterial enhancement with no contrast washout, and (3) the central stellate scar, containing disorganized vascular structures with radiating fibrous septa.[125,130] It should be noted that the typical delayed enhancement of the central scar, a helpful discriminating feature between FNH and fibrolamellar HCC, should not be expected with gadoxetic acid use. In fact, the central scar can appear hypointense on the hepatocyte phase in up to 47% of cases.[128–131] Another imaging pitfall with gadoxetic acid imaging includes the characterization of hepatic hemangiomas.[119] The typical enhancement pattern of hemangiomas described with extracellular agents, that of slow progressive centripetal enhancement with delayed washout, should not be expected, even during the dynamic phase. Instead, it is not uncommon for hemangiomas to appear isointense or hypointense in the late dynamic phase, and they always appear hypointense during the hepatocyte phase (**Fig. 13**). The underlying causes for this appearance include (1) relative increase in the signal intensity of the surrounding hepatic parenchyma (due to hepatocyte uptake), (2) low-contrast dose, and (3) shorter half-life in comparison to extracellular agents.[111,118,120] This feature can be particularly challenging in the diagnosis flash-filling hemangiomas, because differentiation from hypervascular metastases can be made extremely difficult.

The role of gadoxetic acid in the differentiation between FNH and other hepatocellular lesions, such as hepatocellular adenoma and carcinoma (HCC), has been described previously.[128,129,132,133] Although it could be presumed that hepatocellular tumors such as hepatic adenomas and HCCs should demonstrate the same enhancement pattern as FNH, they usually appear hypointense in the hepatocyte phase, due to the lack of bile ducts and/or (2) the membrane receptors OATP1 and cMOAT (**Figs. 14** and **15**).[134–136] Several investigators have described gadoxetic acid as valuable in the differentiation between FNH and adenoma.[117,126,128–131] Grazioli and colleagues[128] found a sensitivity of 92% and specificity of 91% in a cohort of 58 patients and 111 liver lesions. In this study, 91.2% of FNHs were isointense or hyperintense, and 93% of hepatocellular adenomas were hypointense to the surrounding liver parenchyma on hepatobiliary phase images.[129]

Detection and characterization of focal and diffuse liver disease in cirrhotic patients

The hallmark of cirrhosis is the presence of fibrosis.[41] Although biopsy remains the gold standard, the uptake of a liver-specific contrast agent has been described as a noninvasive alternative and could be used as a surrogate parameter of liver fibrosis.[56] In a study by Goshima and colleagues,[137] there was an inverse relationship between the uptake of gadoxetic acid in the liver parenchyma and the degree of fibrosis, with high diagnostic performance of the increase in liver-to-spleen ratio in differentiating the degree of liver fibrosis.

Cirrhosis is associated with an increased risk for the development of HCC. Early detection is

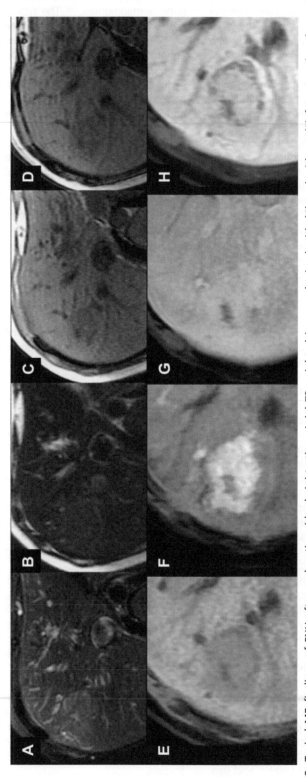

Fig. 12. Typical MR findings of FNH after gadoxetic acid administration. Axial T2-weighted images obtained with (*A*) and without (*B*) fat saturation demonstrate popcorn-like lesion that appears nearly isointense to the surrounding parenchyma, with T2-hyperintense central scar. In-phase (*C*) and out-of-phase (*D*) images show no signal drop to suggest microscopic fat. Dynamic images obtained before (*E*) and after administration of gadoxetic acid during the arterial (*F*) and portal venous (*G*) phases show typical enhancement pattern, consisting of intense and homogeneous arterial enhancement that fades during the portal venous phase. On the hepatocyte phase image (*H*), the FNH appears hyperintense relative to the surrounding liver. Because the central stellate scar contains malformed vascular structures, it shows enhancement characteristics similar to hemangiomas, appearing hyperintense on delayed images using the traditional extracellular agents but hypointense on hepatocyte phase.

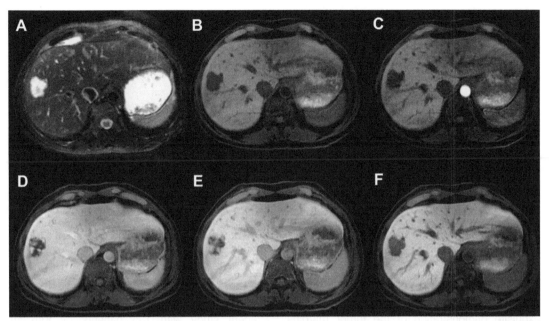

Fig. 13. Typical MR findings of hepatic hemangioma after gadoxetic acid administration. (*A*) Axial fat-suppressed T2-weighted image shows profoundly hyperintense lesion in the right hepatic lobe, with signal intensity similar to the CSF. Axial fat-suppressed T1-weighted images obtained before (*B*) and after administration of contrast in the arterial (*C*), portal venous (*D*), and late dynamic (*E*) phases show typical findings of progressive centripetal enhancement, similar to what is observed with traditional extracellular agents. (*F*) Hepatocyte phase image shows hypointensity of the lesion due to marked hepatocyte uptake of gadoxetic acid in the surrounding parenchyma, lower plasma half-life and overall administered dose. However, the signal intensity should still be similar to the portal venous branches.

crucial for improved survival. Typical MR features using traditional extracellular agents include hypervascular lesion that demonstrates rapid washout.[138] The same enhancement pattern should be expected with gadoxetic acid, but washout may appear even more rapid due to enhancement of the surrounding hepatic parenchyma. However, the pharmacokinetics and pharmacodynamics can be altered in patients with advanced or decompensated cirrhosis, with resulting diminished parenchymal enhancement in the hepatocyte phase, diminished (and delayed) biliary excretion, and prolonged blood pool enhancement.[118] Typical HCCs appear as well-delineated areas of low signal intensity in the hepatocyte phase, because they generally do not demonstrate contrast uptake. Liver-to-lesion contrast enhancement typically peaks during this

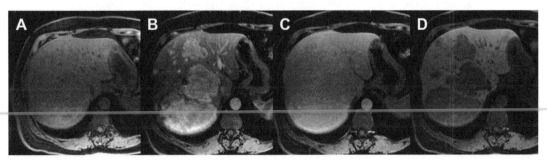

Fig. 14. Typical MR appearance of hepatocellular adenomas in 50-year-old woman with diagnosis of hepatic adenomatosis. Axial fat-suppressed T1-weighted images obtained before (*A*) and after administration of gadoxetic acid in the arterial (*B*), portal venous (*C*), and hepatocyte (*D*) phases show multiple heterogeneously hyperintense lesions that demonstrate intense, transient and heterogeneous arterial enhancement. On the hepatocyte phase (*D*), lesions appear hypointense because of the lack of biliary canaliculi, a main feature that allows for differentiation between adenomas from FNH.

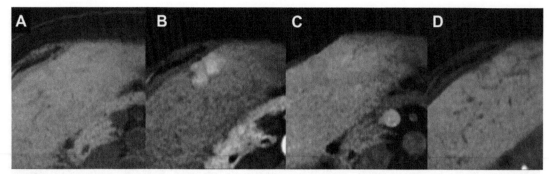

Fig. 15. Atypical MR findings in biopsy-proven moderately-differentiated HCC in patient with cirrhosis. Axial fat-suppressed T1-weighted images obtained before (*A*) and after administration of gadoxetic acid in the arterial (*B*), portal venous (*C*), and hepatocyte (*D*) phase show T1-isointense lesion in subcapsular location, with transient, intense, and heterogeneous arterial enhancement. On the hepatocyte phase (*D*), the lesion appears isointense to hyperintense compared with the surrounding parenchyma. HCC usually has hypointense signal relative to the background liver in the hepatocyte phase. Although still controversial, it has been shown that a minority of HCCs, particularly more well-differentiated tumors, can demonstrate contrast uptake in the hepatocyte phase.

phase, allowing for improved detection and more exquisite demonstration of the tumor margins. Paradoxic uptake of contrast in the hepatocyte phase has been shown in a minority of cases, which has been attributed to the degree of differentiation and expression of OATP1 receptors, although it remains controversial.[118,139,140] A recent study with 135 patients by Kim and colleagues[30] has shown that diagnosis of HCC in cirrhotic patients can be improved with the combination of the hepatocyte phase findings with DWIs. They concluded that restricted diffusion in

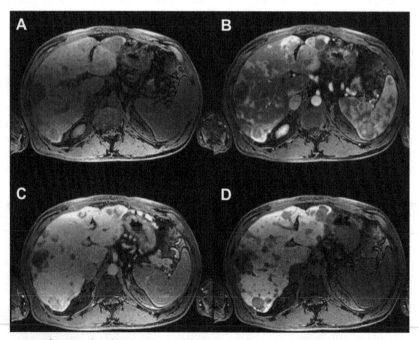

Fig. 16. Assessment of tumor burden in 42-year-old man with metastatic neuroendocrine tumor. Axial fat-suppressed T1-weighted images obtained before (*A*) and after administration of gadoxetic acid in the arterial (*B*), portal venous (*C*), and hepatocyte (*D*) phases show multiple hypervascular liver lesions distributed throughout the parenchyma, consistent with metastases. Note the greater conspicuity of the lesions in the hepatocyte phase (*D*). Another potential advantage of the hepatocyte phase in the follow-up of these patients is greater reproducibility, because multiple acquisitions can be obtained in uncooperative patients, until optimal breath-hold is obtained.

hypovascular, hypointense nodules on hepatobiliary phase was strongly associated with progression to hypervascular HCC.[30] In summary, although gadoxetic acid can be helpful in characterizing focal lesions in cirrhotic patients, its fundamental and less controversial role has been in the detection of these lesions and to assist in surgical planning.

Evaluation of metastatic disease

No contrast uptake should be seen in hepatic metastases on the hepatocyte phase, because they do not contain hepatocytes. There is a wide range of benign and malignant lesions, however, that demonstrates this same nonspecific pattern of enhancement in the hepatocyte phase.[141–145] For this reason, interpretation of the hepatocyte phase findings should be made in conjunction with the available clinical information and other imaging findings, including signal characteristics and degree of vascularization. Another important role for the use of gadoxetic acid in the oncologic setting is in the detection and evaluation of small hypervascular metastases, because it improves lesion conspicuity and ultimately increases reader confidence (**Fig. 16**). Increased lesion conspicuity is crucial in the serial evaluation of hepatic tumor burden, particularly in certain types of cancer (eg, breast, neuroendocrine), for accurate assessment of treatment response (**Fig. 17**).

Anatomic and functional evaluation

Gadoxetic acid can be useful for anatomic evaluation of the biliary tree.[117] It has been shown useful in the preoperative evaluation of the liver, during which it can be integrated as part of a more comprehensive MR imaging evaluation, providing information about the hepatic vasculature and parenchyma, and for the assessment of postoperative complications.[146,147] In a study by Salvolini and colleagues,[146] with a total of 142 postoperative patients, gadoxetic acid–enhanced MR cholangiopancreatography was able to allow definitive diagnosis, including the diagnosis of anastomotic stenosis and biliary leakage, in

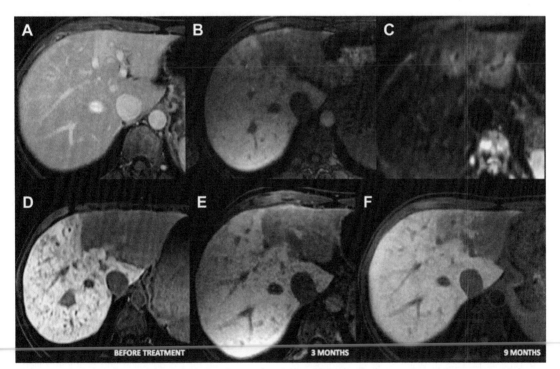

Fig. 17. Evaluation of metastatic tumor burden and serial assessment of tumor response in 42-year-old woman with metastatic breast cancer. Axial fat-suppressed T1-weighted images obtained after administration of gadoxetic acid in the portal venous phase (*A*) show unremarkable appearance of the liver. Hepatocyte phase (*B*) and DWI (*C*) show to better extent the infiltrative appearance of the biopsy-proved metastatic lesions, which appear hypointense in the hepatocyte phase (*B*) and hyperintense in the high b-value DWI (*C*). Serial axial MR images obtained in the hepatocyte phase (*D–F*) demonstrate decrease in tumor burden after treatment, with the progressive appearance of areas of hepatocyte uptake within the known sites of metastatic disease. The findings are suggestive of interval response to treatment.

100% of cases. A more controversial use of gadoxetic acid would be for the functional evaluation
of cystic duct patency as an alternative to HIDA
scans in the diagnosis of acute cholecystitis.[148]

SUMMARY

Modern MR imaging evaluation of the liver allows
for a comprehensive morphologic and functional
assessment of the liver parenchyma, hepatic
vessels, and biliary tree and thus aids in the diagnosis of both focal and diffuse liver diseases.

REFERENCES

1. Stejskal EO, Tanner J. Spin diffusion measurements: spin echoes in the presence of a time-
dependent field gradient. J Chem Phys 1965;
42(1):288.

2. Le Bihan D, Breton E, Lallemand D, et al. MR
imaging of intravoxel incoherent motions: application to diffusion and perfusion in neurologic disorders. Radiology 1986;161(2):401–7.

3. Bittencourt LK, Matos C, Coutinho AC Jr. Diffusion-
weighted magnetic resonance imaging in the
upper abdomen: technical issues and clinical
applications. Magn Reson Imaging Clin N Am
2011;19(1):111–31.

4. Taouli B, Tolia AJ, Losada M, et al. Diffusion-
weighted MRI for quantification of liver fibrosis:
preliminary experience. AJR Am J Roentgenol
2007;189(4):799–806.

5. Taouli B, Koh DM. Diffusion-weighted MR imaging
of the liver. Radiology 2010;254(1):47–66.

6. Thoeny HC, De Keyzer F. Extracranial applications
of diffusion-weighted magnetic resonance imaging.
Eur Radiol 2007;17(6):1385–93.

7. Hussain SM, De Becker J, Hop WC, et al. Can
a single-shot black-blood T2-weighted spin-echo
echo-planar imaging sequence with sensitivity
encoding replace the respiratory-triggered turbo
spin-echo sequence for the liver? An optimization
and feasibility study. J Magn Reson Imaging
2005;21(3):219–29.

8. Coenegrachts K, Delanote J, Ter Beek L, et al.
Improved focal liver lesion detection: comparison
of single-shot diffusion-weighted echoplanar and
single-shot T2 weighted turbo spin echo techniques. Br J Radiol 2007;80(955):524–31.

9. Bruegel M, Gaa J, Waldt S, et al. Diagnosis of
hepatic metastasis: comparison of respiration-
triggered diffusion-weighted echo-planar MRI and
five t2-weighted turbo spin-echo sequences. AJR
Am J Roentgenol 2008;191(5):1421–9.

10. Parikh T, Drew SJ, Lee VS, et al. Focal liver lesion
detection and characterization with diffusion-
weighted MR imaging: comparison with standard

breath-hold T2-weighted imaging. Radiology
2008;246(3):812–22.

11. Zech CJ, Herrmann KA, Dietrich O, et al. Black-
blood diffusion-weighted EPI acquisition of the liver
with parallel imaging: comparison with a standard
T2-weighted sequence for detection of focal liver
lesions. Invest Radiol 2008;43(4):261–6.

12. Okada Y, Ohtomo K, Kiryu S, et al. Breath-hold
T2-weighted MRI of hepatic tumors: value of echo
planar imaging with diffusion-sensitizing gradient.
J Comput Assist Tomogr 1998;22(3):364–71.

13. Moteki T, Sekine T. Echo planar MR imaging of the
liver: comparison of images with and without
motion probing gradients. J Magn Reson Imaging
2004;19(1):82–90.

14. Nasu K, Kuroki Y, Nawano S, et al. Hepatic metastases: diffusion-weighted sensitivity-encoding versus SPIO-enhanced MR imaging. Radiology 2006;
239(1):122–30.

15. Namimoto T, Yamashita Y, Sumi S, et al. Focal liver
masses: characterization with diffusion-weighted
echo-planar MR imaging. Radiology 1997;204(3):
739–44.

16. Kim T, Murakami T, Takahashi S, et al. Diffusion-
weighted single-shot echoplanar MR imaging for
liver disease. AJR Am J Roentgenol 1999;173(2):
393–8.

17. Yamada I, Aung W, Himeno Y, et al. Diffusion coefficients in abdominal organs and hepatic lesions:
evaluation with intravoxel incoherent motion
echo-planar MR imaging. Radiology 1999;210(3):
617–23.

18. Taouli B, Vilgrain V, Dumont E, et al. Evaluation of
liver diffusion isotropy and characterization of focal
hepatic lesions with two single-shot echo-planar
MR imaging sequences: prospective study in 66
patients. Radiology 2003;226(1):71–8.

19. Bruegel M, Holzapfel K, Gaa J, et al. Characterization of focal liver lesions by ADC measurements
using a respiratory triggered diffusion-weighted
single-shot echo-planar MR imaging technique.
Eur Radiol 2008;18(3):477–85.

20. Low RN, Gurney J. Diffusion-weighted MRI (DWI)
in the oncology patient: value of breathhold DWI
compared to unenhanced and gadolinium-
enhanced MRI. J Magn Reson Imaging 2007;
25(4):848–58.

21. Goshima S, Kanematsu M, Kondo H, et al. Diffusion-weighted imaging of the liver: optimizing
b value for the detection and characterization of
benign and malignant hepatic lesions. J Magn Reson Imaging 2008;28(3):691–7.

22. Holzapfel K, Bruegel M, Eiber M, et al. Characterization of small (≤10 mm) focal liver lesions: value
of respiratory-triggered echo-planar diffusion-
weighted MR imaging. Eur J Radiol 2010;76(1):
89–95.

23. Kandpal H, Sharma R, Madhusudhan KS, et al. Respiratory-triggered versus breath-hold diffusion-weighted MRI of liver lesions: comparison of image quality and apparent diffusion coefficient values. AJR Am J Roentgenol 2009;192(4):915–22.

24. Xu PJ, Yan FH, Wang JH, et al. Added value of breathhold diffusion-weighted MRI in detection of small hepatocellular carcinoma lesions compared with dynamic contrast-enhanced MRI alone using receiver operating characteristic curve analysis. J Magn Reson Imaging 2009;29(2):341–9.

25. Bruegel M, Rummeny EJ. Hepatic metastases: use of diffusion-weighted echo-planar imaging. Abdom Imaging 2010;35(4):454–61.

26. Koh DM, Brown G, Riddell AM, et al. Detection of colorectal hepatic metastases using MnDPDP MR imaging and diffusion-weighted imaging (DWI) alone and in combination. Eur Radiol 2008;18(5):903–10.

27. Kele PG, van der Jagt EJ. Diffusion weighted imaging in the liver. World J Gastroenterol 2010;16(13):1567–76.

28. Xu H, Li X, Xie JX, et al. Diffusion-weighted magnetic resonance imaging of focal hepatic nodules in an experimental hepatocellular carcinoma rat model. Acad Radiol 2007;14(3):279–86.

29. Vandecaveye V, De Keyzer F, Verslype C, et al. Diffusion-weighted MRI provides additional value to conventional dynamic contrast-enhanced MRI for detection of hepatocellular carcinoma. Eur Radiol 2009;19(10):2456–66.

30. Kim YK, Lee WJ, Park MJ, et al. Hypovascular hypointense nodules on hepatobiliary phase gadoxetic acid-enhanced MR images in patients with cirrhosis: potential of DW imaging in predicting progression to hypervascular HCC. Radiology 2012;265(1):104–14.

31. Koh DM, Scurr E, Collins D, et al. Predicting response of colorectal hepatic metastasis: value of pretreatment apparent diffusion coefficients. AJR Am J Roentgenol 2007;188(4):1001–8.

32. Cui Y, Zhang XP, Sun YS, et al. Apparent diffusion coefficient: potential imaging biomarker for prediction and early detection of response to chemotherapy in hepatic metastases. Radiology 2008;248(3):894–900.

33. Qayyum A. Diffusion-weighted imaging in the abdomen and pelvis: concepts and applications. Radiographics 2009;29(6):1797–810.

34. Koinuma M, Ohashi I, Hanafusa K, et al. Apparent diffusion coefficient measurements with diffusion-weighted magnetic resonance imaging for evaluation of hepatic fibrosis. J Magn Reson Imaging 2005;22(1):80–5.

35. Glaser KJ, Manduca A, Ehman RL. Review of MR elastography applications and recent developments. J Magn Reson Imaging 2012;36(4):spcone.

36. Mariappan YK, Glaser KJ, Ehman RL. Magnetic resonance elastography: a review. Clin Anat 2010;23(5):497–511.

37. Talwalkar JA, Yin M, Fidler JL, et al. Magnetic resonance imaging of hepatic fibrosis: emerging clinical applications. Hepatology 2008;47(1):332–42.

38. Talwalkar JA. Elastography for detecting hepatic fibrosis: options and considerations. Gastroenterology 2008;135(1):299–302.

39. Manduca A, Oliphant TE, Dresner MA, et al. Magnetic resonance elastography: non-invasive mapping of tissue elasticity. Med Image Anal 2001;5(4):237–54.

40. Rouvière O, Yin M, Dresner MA, et al. MR elastography of the liver: preliminary results. Radiology 2006;240(2):440–8.

41. Faria SC, Ganesan K, Mwangi I, et al. MR imaging of liver fibrosis: current state of the art. Radiographics 2009;29(6):1615–35.

42. Glaser KJ, Manduca A, Ehman RL. Review of MR elastography applications and recent developments. J Magn Reson Imaging 2012;36(4):757–74.

43. Schwenzer NF, Springer F, Schraml C, et al. Non-invasive assessment and quantification of liver steatosis by ultrasound, computed tomography and magnetic resonance. J Hepatol 2009;51(3):433–45.

44. Talwalkar JA, Kurtz DM, Schoenleber SJ, et al. Ultrasound-based transient elastography for the detection of hepatic fibrosis: systematic review and meta-analysis. Clin Gastroenterol Hepatol 2007;5(10):1214–20.

45. Venkatesh SK, Yin M, Glockner JF, et al. MR elastography of liver tumors: preliminary results. AJR Am J Roentgenol 2008;190(6):1534–40.

46. Xu L, Gao PY. "Palpation by imaging": magnetic resonance elastography. Chin Med Sci J 2006;21(4):281–6.

47. Yin M, Talwalkar JA, Glaser KJ, et al. Assessment of hepatic fibrosis with magnetic resonance elastography. Clin Gastroenterol Hepatol 2007;5(10):1207–1213.e2.

48. Adebajo CO, Talwalkar JA, Poterucha JJ, et al. Ultrasound-based transient elastography for the detection of hepatic fibrosis in patients with recurrent hepatitis C virus after liver transplantation: a systematic review and meta-analysis. Liver Transpl 2012;18(3):323–31.

49. Enomoto M, Mori M, Ogawa T, et al. Usefulness of transient elastography for assessment of liver fibrosis in chronic hepatitis B: regression of liver stiffness during entecavir therapy. Hepatol Res 2010;40(9):853–61.

50. Ferraioli G, Lissandrin R, Zicchetti M, et al. Assessment of liver stiffness with transient elastography by using S and M probes in healthy children. Eur J Pediatr 2012;171(9):1415.

51. Vigano M, Massironi S, Lampertico P, et al. Transient elastography assessment of the liver stiffness dynamics during acute hepatitis B. Eur J Gastroenterol Hepatol 2010;22(2):180–4.

52. Huwart L, Sempoux C, Salameh N, et al. Liver fibrosis: noninvasive assessment with MR elastography versus aspartate aminotransferase-to-platelet ratio index. Radiology 2007;245(2):458–66.

53. Huwart L, Sempoux C, Vicaut E, et al. Magnetic resonance elastography for the noninvasive staging of liver fibrosis. Gastroenterology 2008;135(1):32–40.

54. Brancatelli G, Federle MP, Ambrosini R, et al. Cirrhosis: CT and MR imaging evaluation. Eur J Radiol 2007;61(1):57–69.

55. Talwalkar JA. Current and emerging surrogate markers of hepatic fibrosis in primary biliary cirrhosis. Liver Int 2008;28(6):761–3.

56. Watanabe H, Kanematsu M, Goshima S, et al. Staging hepatic fibrosis: comparison of gadoxetate disodium-enhanced and diffusion-weighted MR imaging–preliminary observations. Radiology 2011;259(1):142–50.

57. Regev A, Berho M, Jeffers LJ, et al. Sampling error and intraobserver variation in liver biopsy in patients with chronic HCV infection. Am J Gastroenterol 2002;97(10):2614–8.

58. Schmeltzer PA, Talwalkar JA. Noninvasive tools to assess hepatic fibrosis: ready for prime time? Gastroenterol Clin North Am 2011;40(3):507–21.

59. Huwart L, Salameh N, ter Beek L, et al. MR elastography of liver fibrosis: preliminary results comparing spin-echo and echo-planar imaging. Eur Radiol 2008;18(11):2535–41.

60. Wang Y, Ganger DR, Levitsky J, et al. Assessment of chronic hepatitis and fibrosis: comparison of MR elastography and diffusion-weighted imaging. AJR Am J Roentgenol 2011;196(3):553–61.

61. Chen J, Talwalkar JA, Yin M, et al. Early detection of nonalcoholic steatohepatitis in patients with nonalcoholic fatty liver disease by using MR elastography. Radiology 2011;259(3):749–56.

62. Vizzutti F, Arena U, Romanelli RG, et al. Liver stiffness measurement predicts severe portal hypertension in patients with HCV-related cirrhosis. Hepatology 2007;45(5):1290–7.

63. Angulo P. Nonalcoholic fatty liver disease. N Engl J Med 2002;346(16):1221–31.

64. Browning JD, Szczepaniak LS, Dobbins R, et al. Prevalence of hepatic steatosis in an urban population in the United States: impact of ethnicity. Hepatology 2004;40(6):1387–95.

65. Farrell GC, Larter CZ. Nonalcoholic fatty liver disease: from steatosis to cirrhosis. Hepatology 2006;43(2 Suppl 1):S99–112.

66. Lavine JE, Schwimmer JB. Nonalcoholic fatty liver disease in the pediatric population. Clin Liver Dis 2004;8(3):549–58, viii–ix.

67. Szczepaniak LS, Nurenberg P, Leonard D, et al. Magnetic resonance spectroscopy to measure hepatic triglyceride content: prevalence of hepatic steatosis in the general population. Am J Physiol Endocrinol Metab 2005;288(2):E462–8.

68. Wang Y, Beydoun MA, Liang L, et al. Will all Americans become overweight or obese? estimating the progression and cost of the US obesity epidemic. Obesity (Silver Spring) 2008;16(10):2323–30.

69. Arun J, Jhala N, Lazenby AJ, et al. Influence of liver biopsy heterogeneity and diagnosis of nonalcoholic steatohepatitis in subjects undergoing gastric bypass. Obes Surg 2007;17(2):155–61.

70. Brunt EM, Tiniakos DG. Histopathology of nonalcoholic fatty liver disease. World J Gastroenterol 2010;16(42):5286–96.

71. Ratziu V, Charlotte F, Heurtier A, et al. Sampling variability of liver biopsy in nonalcoholic fatty liver disease. Gastroenterology 2005;128(7):1898–906.

72. Tiniakos DG, Vos MB, Brunt EM. Nonalcoholic fatty liver disease: pathology and pathogenesis. Annu Rev Pathol 2010;5:145–71.

73. Cassidy FH, Yokoo T, Aganovic L, et al. Fatty liver disease: MR imaging techniques for the detection and quantification of liver steatosis. Radiographics 2009;29(1):231–60.

74. Cho CS, Curran S, Schwartz LH, et al. Preoperative radiographic assessment of hepatic steatosis with histologic correlation. J Am Coll Surg 2008;206(3):480–8.

75. Machann J, Stefan N, Schick F. (1)H MR spectroscopy of skeletal muscle, liver and bone marrow. Eur J Radiol 2008;67(2):275–84.

76. Mehta SR, Thomas EL, Bell JD, et al. Non-invasive means of measuring hepatic fat content. World J Gastroenterol 2008;14(22):3476–83.

77. Reeder SB, Cruite I, Hamilton G, et al. Quantitative assessment of liver fat with magnetic resonance imaging and spectroscopy. J Magn Reson Imaging 2011;34(4):spcone.

78. Valls C, Iannacconne R, Alba E, et al. Fat in the liver: diagnosis and characterization. Eur Radiol 2006;16(10):2292–308.

79. Hussain HK, Chenevert TL, Londy FJ, et al. Hepatic fat fraction: MR imaging for quantitative measurement and display–early experience. Radiology 2005;237(3):1048–55.

80. Rinella ME, McCarthy R, Thakrar K, et al. Dual-echo, chemical shift gradient-echo magnetic resonance imaging to quantify hepatic steatosis: Implications for living liver donation. Liver Transpl 2003;9(8):851–6.

81. Schuchmann S, Weigel C, Albrecht L, et al. Non-invasive quantification of hepatic fat fraction by fast 1.0, 1.5 and 3.0 T MR imaging. Eur J Radiol 2007;62(3):416–22.

82. Ma X, Holalkere NS, Kambadakone RA, et al. Imaging-based quantification of hepatic fat: methods and clinical applications. Radiographics 2009;29(5): 1253–77.

83. Bahl M, Qayyum A, Westphalen AC, et al. Liver steatosis: investigation of opposed-phase T1-weighted liver MR signal intensity loss and visceral fat measurement as biomarkers. Radiology 2008; 249(1):160–6.

84. Borra RJ, Salo S, Dean K, et al. Nonalcoholic fatty liver disease: rapid evaluation of liver fat content with in-phase and out-of-phase MR imaging. Radiology 2009;250(1):130–6.

85. Yokoo T, Bydder M, Hamilton G, et al. Nonalcoholic fatty liver disease: diagnostic and fat-grading accuracy of low-flip-angle multiecho gradient-recalled-echo MR imaging at 1.5 T. Radiology 2009;251(1): 67–76.

86. Westphalen AC, Qayyum A, Yeh BM, et al. Liver fat: effect of hepatic iron deposition on evaluation with opposed-phase MR imaging. Radiology 2007; 242(2):450–5.

87. Alustiza JM, Castiella A. Liver fat and iron at in-phase and opposed-phase MR imaging. Radiology 2008;246(2):641.

88. Springer F, Machann J, Claussen CD, et al. Liver fat content determined by magnetic resonance imaging and spectroscopy. World J Gastroenterol 2010;16(13):1560–6.

89. Reeder SB, Robson PM, Yu H, et al. Quantification of hepatic steatosis with MRI: the effects of accurate fat spectral modeling. J Magn Reson Imaging 2009;29(6):1332–9.

90. Reeder SB, Pineda AR, Wen Z, et al. Iterative decomposition of water and fat with echo asymmetry and least-squares estimation (IDEAL): application with fast spin-echo imaging. Magn Reson Med 2005;54(3):636–44.

91. Qayyum A. MR spectroscopy of the liver: principles and clinical applications. Radiographics 2009; 29(6):1653–64.

92. Queiroz-Andrade M, Blasbalg R, Ortega CD, et al. MR imaging findings of iron overload. Radiographics 2009;29(6):1575–89.

93. Wood JC. Impact of iron assessment by MRI. Hematology Am Soc Hematol Educ Program 2011;2011: 443–50.

94. Beddy P, McCann J, Ahern M, et al. MRI assessment of changes in liver iron deposition post-venesection. Eur J Radiol 2011;80(2):204–7.

95. Gandon Y, Guyader D, Heautot JF, et al. Hemochromatosis: diagnosis and quantification of liver iron with gradient-echo MR imaging. Radiology 1994;193(2):533–8.

96. Gandon Y, Olivie D, Guyader D, et al. Non-invasive assessment of hepatic iron stores by MRI. Lancet 2004;363(9406):357–62.

97. Castiella A, Alustiza JM, Emparanza JI, et al. Liver iron concentration quantification by MRI: are recommended protocols accurate enough for clinical practice? Eur Radiol 2011;21(1):137–41.

98. Hankins JS, McCarville MB, Loeffler RB, et al. R2* magnetic resonance imaging of the liver in patients with iron overload. Blood 2009;113(20): 4853–5.

99. Wood JC. Magnetic resonance imaging measurement of iron overload. Curr Opin Hematol 2007; 14(3):183–90.

100. Chang JS, Taouli B, Salibi N, et al. Opposed-phase MRI for fat quantification in fat-water phantoms with 1H MR spectroscopy to resolve ambiguity of fat or water dominance. AJR Am J Roentgenol 2006; 187(1):W103–6.

101. Cotler SJ, Guzman G, Layden-Almer J, et al. Measurement of liver fat content using selective saturation at 3.0 T. J Magn Reson Imaging 2007; 25(4):743–8.

102. Fischbach F, Bruhn H. Assessment of in vivo 1H magnetic resonance spectroscopy in the liver: a review. Liver Int 2008;28(3):297–307.

103. Hamilton G, Middleton MS, Bydder M, et al. Effect of PRESS and STEAM sequences on magnetic resonance spectroscopic liver fat quantification. J Magn Reson Imaging 2009;30(1):145–52.

104. Irwan R, Edens MA, Sijens PE. Assessment of the variations in fat content in normal liver using a fast MR imaging method in comparison with results obtained by spectroscopic imaging. Eur Radiol 2008;18(4):806–13.

105. Longo R, Ricci C, Masutti F, et al. Fatty infiltration of the liver. Quantification by 1H localized magnetic resonance spectroscopy and comparison with computed tomography. Invest Radiol 1993;28(4): 297–302.

106. Machann J, Thamer C, Schnoedt B, et al. Hepatic lipid accumulation in healthy subjects: a comparative study using spectral fat-selective MRI and volume-localized 1H-MR spectroscopy. Magn Reson Med 2006;55(4):913–7.

107. Thomsen C, Becker U, Winkler K, et al. Quantification of liver fat using magnetic resonance spectroscopy. Magn Reson Imaging 1994;12(3):487–95.

108. Johnson NA, Walton DW, Sachinwalla T, et al. Noninvasive assessment of hepatic lipid composition: advancing understanding and management of fatty liver disorders. Hepatology 2008;47(5):1513–23.

109. Longo R, Pollesello P, Ricci C, et al. Proton MR spectroscopy in quantitative in vivo determination

of fat content in human liver steatosis. J Magn Reson Imaging 1995;5(3):281–5.

110. Szczepaniak LS, Babcock EE, Schick F, et al. Measurement of intracellular triglyceride stores by H spectroscopy: validation in vivo. Am J Physiol 1999;276(5 Pt 1):E977–89.

111. Gandhi SN, Brown MA, Wong JG, et al. MR contrast agents for liver imaging: what, when, how. Radiographics 2006;26(6):1621–36.

112. Karabulut N, Elmas N. Contrast agents used in MR imaging of the liver. Diagn Interv Radiol 2006;12(1):22–30.

113. Low RN. Contrast agents for MR imaging of the liver. J Magn Reson Imaging 1997;7(1):56–67.

114. Mahfouz AE, Hamm B. MR imaging of the liver. Contrast agents. Magn Reson Imaging Clin N Am 1997;5(2):223–40.

115. Semelka RC, Helmberger TK. Contrast agents for MR imaging of the liver. Radiology 2001;218(1):27–38.

116. Hammerstingl R, Zangos S, Schwarz W, et al. Contrast-enhanced MRI of focal liver tumors using a hepatobiliary MR contrast agent: detection and differential diagnosis using Gd-EOB-DTPA-enhanced versus Gd-DTPA-enhanced MRI in the same patient. Acad Radiol 2002;9(Suppl 1):S119–20.

117. Seale MK, Catalano OA, Saini S, et al. Hepatobiliary-specific MR contrast agents: role in imaging the liver and biliary tree. Radiographics 2009;29(6):1725–48.

118. Cruite I, Schroeder M, Merkle EM, et al. Gadoxetate disodium-enhanced MRI of the liver: part 2, protocol optimization and lesion appearance in the cirrhotic liver. AJR Am J Roentgenol 2010;195(1):29–41.

119. Goodwin MD, Dobson JE, Sirlin CB, et al. Diagnostic challenges and pitfalls in MR imaging with hepatocyte-specific contrast agents. Radiographics 2011;31(6):1547–68.

120. Ringe KI, Husarik DB, Sirlin CB, et al. Gadoxetate disodium-enhanced MRI of the liver: part 1, protocol optimization and lesion appearance in the noncirrhotic liver. AJR Am J Roentgenol 2010;195(1):13–28.

121. Kim KA, Kim MJ, Park MS, et al. Optimal T2-weighted MR cholangiopancreatographic images can be obtained after administration of gadoxetic acid. Radiology 2010;256(2):475–84.

122. Frydrychowicz A, Lubner MG, Brown JJ, et al. Hepatobiliary MR imaging with gadolinium-based contrast agents. J Magn Reson Imaging 2012;35(3):492–511.

123. Tamada T, Ito K, Higaki A, et al. Gd-EOB-DTPA-enhanced MR imaging: evaluation of hepatic enhancement effects in normal and cirrhotic livers. Eur J Radiol 2011;80(3):e311–6.

124. Tamada T, Ito K, Sone T, et al. Gd-EOB-DTPA enhanced MR imaging: evaluation of biliary and renal excretion in normal and cirrhotic livers. Eur J Radiol 2011;80(3):e207–11.

125. Ba-Ssalamah A, Schima W, Schmook MT, et al. Atypical focal nodular hyperplasia of the liver: imaging features of nonspecific and liver-specific MR contrast agents. AJR Am J Roentgenol 2002;179(6):1447–56.

126. Fidler J, Hough D. Hepatocyte-specific magnetic resonance imaging contrast agents. Hepatology 2011;53(2):678–82.

127. Fujiwara H, Sekine S, Onaya H, et al. Ring-like enhancement of focal nodular hyperplasia with hepatobiliary-phase Gd-EOB-DTPA-enhanced magnetic resonance imaging: radiological-pathological correlation. Jpn J Radiol 2011;29(10):739–43.

128. Grazioli L, Bondioni MP, Haradome H, et al. Hepatocellular adenoma and focal nodular hyperplasia: value of gadoxetic acid-enhanced MR imaging in differential diagnosis. Radiology 2012;262(2):520–9.

129. Grazioli L, Morana G, Kirchin MA, et al. Accurate differentiation of focal nodular hyperplasia from hepatic adenoma at gadobenate dimeglumine-enhanced MR imaging: prospective study. Radiology 2005;236(1):166–77.

130. Karam AR, Shankar S, Surapaneni P, et al. Focal nodular hyperplasia: central scar enhancement pattern using Gadoxetate Disodium. J Magn Reson Imaging 2010;32(2):341–4.

131. Morana G, Grazioli L, Kirchin MA, et al. Solid hypervascular liver lesions: accurate identification of true benign lesions on enhanced dynamic and hepatobiliary phase magnetic resonance imaging after gadobenate dimeglumine administration. Invest Radiol 2011;46(4):225–39.

132. Fowler KJ, Brown JJ, Narra VR. Magnetic resonance imaging of focal liver lesions: approach to imaging diagnosis. Hepatology 2011;54(6):2227–37.

133. Takara K, Saito K, Kusama H, et al. Gd-EOB-DTPA-enhanced MR imaging findings of hepatocellular adenoma: correlation with pathological findings. Magn Reson Med Sci 2011;10(4):245–9.

134. Zucman-Rossi J, Jeannot E, Nhieu JT, et al. Genotype-phenotype correlation in hepatocellular adenoma: new classification and relationship with HCC. Hepatology 2006;43(3):515–24.

135. Katabathina VS, Menias CO, Shanbhogue AK, et al. Genetics and imaging of hepatocellular adenomas: 2011 update. Radiographics 2011;31(6):1529–43.

136. van Aalten SM, Thomeer MG, Terkivatan T, et al. Hepatocellular adenomas: correlation of MR imaging findings with pathologic subtype classification. Radiology 2011;261(1):172–81.

137. Goshima S, Kanematsu M, Watanabe H, et al. Gd-EOB-DTPA-enhanced MR imaging: Prediction of hepatic fibrosis stages using liver contrast enhancement index and liver-to-spleen volumetric ratio. J Magn Reson Imaging 2012;36:1148–53.

138. Bolog N, Andreisek G, Oancea I, et al. CT and MR imaging of hepatocellular carcinoma. J Gastrointestin Liver Dis 2011;20(2):181–9.

139. Goshima S, Kanematsu M, Watanabe H, et al. Gadoxetate disodium-enhanced MR imaging: differentiation between early-enhancing non-tumorous lesions and hypervascular hepatocellular carcinomas. Eur J Radiol 2011;79(2):e108–12.

140. Onishi H, Kim T, Imai Y, et al. Hypervascular hepatocellular carcinomas: detection with gadoxetate disodium-enhanced MR imaging and multiphasic multidetector CT. Eur Radiol 2012;22:845–54.

141. Hahn PF, Saini S. Liver-specific MR imaging contrast agents. Radiol Clin North Am 1998;36(2):287–97.

142. Goshima S, Kanematsu M, Watanabe H, et al. Hepatic hemangioma and metastasis: differentiation with gadoxetate disodium-enhanced 3-T MRI. AJR Am J Roentgenol 2010;195(4):941–6.

143. Jeong HT, Kim MJ, Park MS, et al. Detection of liver metastases using gadoxetic-enhanced dynamic and 10- and 20-minute delayed phase MR imaging. J Magn Reson Imaging 2012;35:635–43.

144. Sofue K, Tsurusaki M, Tokue H, et al. Gd-EOB-DTPA-enhanced 3.0 T MR imaging: quantitative and qualitative comparison of hepatocyte-phase images obtained 10 min and 20 min after injection for the detection of liver metastases from colorectal carcinoma. Eur Radiol 2011;21(11):2336–43.

145. Tajima T, Akahane M, Takao H, et al. Detection of liver metastasis: is diffusion-weighted imaging needed in Gd-EOB-DTPA-enhanced MR imaging for evaluation of colorectal liver metastases? Jpn J Radiol 2012;30:648–58.

146. Salvolini L, Urbinati C, Valeri G, et al. Contrast-enhanced MR cholangiography (MRCP) with GD-EOB-DTPA in evaluating biliary complications after surgery. Radiol Med 2012;117:354–68.

147. Tamrazi A, Vasanawala SS. Functional hepatobiliary MR imaging in children. Pediatr Radiol 2011;41(10):1250–8.

148. Krishnan P, Gupta RT, Boll DT, et al. Functional evaluation of cystic duct patency with Gd-EOB-DTPA MR imaging: an alternative to hepatobiliary scintigraphy for diagnosis of acute cholecystitis? Abdom Imaging 2012;37:457–64.

MR Enterography for the Assessment of Small Bowel Diseases

Luciana Costa-Silva, MD, MSc[a],*, Alice C. Brandão, MD[b]

KEYWORDS

- MR enterography • MR imaging • Crohn disease • Small bowel diseases
- Inflammatory bowel diseases

KEY POINTS

- MR enterography is rapidly becoming the first-line radiological modality to evaluate patients with Crohn disease in whom multiple serial examinations may be needed to assess progression of the disease, detect complications, and monitor response to therapy.
- MR enterography is a useful technique for the evaluation of intraluminal and extraluminal small bowel disease, particularly in adolescent and young adults with Crohn disease.
- The main advantages of MR enterography and MR enteroclysis are lack of ionizing radiation, the ability to provide dynamic information regarding bowel distention and motility, and the relatively safe intravenous contrast agent profile.
- Mural hyperenhancement is the most sensitive finding in patients diagnosed with Crohn disease presenting with active inflammation. This finding is significantly correlated to histology as well as to the clinical findings of active disease.
- One of the most important roles of MR enterography is to assess disease activity and differentiate fibrotic stenosis from active inflammation, which has a different treatment.
- Beyond Crohn disease, MR enterography can play a role in the evaluation of small bowel neoplasms and celiac disease.

INTRODUCTION

The small bowel has always been considered a structure of difficult propedeutic evaluation, mainly because of its length and position in the digestive tube between the stomach and the large bowel. Traditionally, the radiological evaluation of the small bowel disorders has always been performed by means of barium examinations, such as conventional enteroclysis and small bowel follow-through (SBFT) (Fig. 1). The latter was, for many years, considered the standard imaging method.[1–3]

However, cross-sectional techniques, especially CT scans and MR imaging, optimized for small bowel imaging are currently replacing these conventional techniques and playing an increasing role in the noninvasive evaluation of small bowel disorders. These methods have several advantages over traditional barium examinations because of improvements in spatial and temporal resolution combined with improved bowel distending agents (Fig. 2). They allow the evaluation of the lumen and the mucosal surface and the intestinal wall, as well as identification of associated mesenteric and extra enteric findings.[4] Furthermore, CT scans and MR imaging allow the visualization of the entire bowel without overlapping loops.

[a] Department of Anatomy and Imaging, Federal University of Minas Gerais, Av. Prof. Alfredo Balena 190, Belo Horizonte 30130-100, Brazil; [b] Department of Radiology, Clínica Felippe Mattoso, Av. Das Américas 700, 319, Barra da Tijuca, Rio de Janeiro 30112011, Brazil.
* Corresponding author. Rua Antonio de Albuquerque 1021/901, Belo Horizonte 30112-011, Brazil.
E-mail address: costaluciana@ufmg.br

Magn Reson Imaging Clin N Am 21 (2013) 365–383
http://dx.doi.org/10.1016/j.mric.2013.01.005
1064-9689/13/$ – see front matter © 2013 Elsevier Inc. All rights reserved.

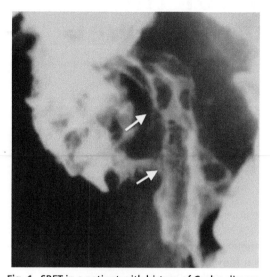

Fig. 1. SBFT in a patient with history of Crohn disease. Spot view of the ileocecal region demonstrates the cobblestone pattern (*white arrows*), with nodular aspect of the mucosa of the terminal ileum, ileocecal valve, and along the medial border of the cecum. This pattern is related to the presence of longitudinal and transverse ulcerations interspersed with areas of mucosal edema. This nonsectional method does not allow the visualization of the bowel wall itself and the mesentery.

CT enterography is widely used in the evaluation of small bowel diseases. However, recently, the knowledge of the risks of ionizing radiation has been increasing and there has been an emphasis on reducing patient exposure by using alternative imaging tests, including ultrasound and MR imaging. The use of ionizing radiation has received growing attention mainly in the setting of small bowel inflammatory disorders when these chronic conditions manifest early in life.[5] MR enterography is an alternative method, considering its lack of ionizing radiation. Both MR enterography and CT enterography, clearly demonstrate endoluminal, mural, and extramural enteric changes. In addition, they provide functional information on the peristalsis of the involved segment. The accuracy of the MR enterographic methods (MR enterography and MR enteroclysis) for the evaluation of Crohn disease is well described in the literature.[2,6–11]

CROSS-SECTIONAL METHODS: ENTEROGRAPHY VERSUS ENTEROCLYSIS

The optimal distention of small bowel loops plays a pivotal role in the correct evaluation of small bowel diseases at cross-sectional imaging. Collapsed loops may result in an apparently thickened wall, which can hide lesions or mimic disease.

The main difference between MR enteroclysis and MR enterography is the use of nasoduodenal intubation under fluoroscopic guidance in enteroclysis for optimal distension of the small bowel, whereas with enterography the contrast agent is given orally. Both technics involve the administration of a large volume of fluid to produce small bowel filling and distension. Enteroclysis is considered a method that yields a better distention, mainly of the proximal jejunal loops, but it has the main disadvantage of placing the nasoenteric tube that may cause patient discomfort and may also be related to various logistical and technical difficulties (**Fig. 3**). Moreover, this enterographic method uses ionizing radiation exposure (tube placement under fluoroscopic guidance) and is sometimes difficult to perform. There is a general preference among radiologists for performing MR enterography over MR enteroclysis because it is easier, less time consuming, and better tolerated by the patients.[6,9,12]

The advantages and disadvantages of MR enterography, MR enteroclysis and CT enterography are summarized in **Table 1**.

TECHNICAL CONSIDERATIONS

Although there is no consensus regarding the ideal technique, there are some trends in performing MR enterography: the use of hyperosmolar oral contrast, prone-position, acquisition of the images mainly in the coronal plane using fast sequences, evaluation of the motility of the small bowel with the cine dynamic sequences, and dynamic evaluation of the intravenous contrast uptake. The prone position is preferred because there is a thinner volume of tissue to image.[13] Most protocols require at least 4 to 6 hours of fasting before the procedure. The examination in the MR room takes between 25 and 30 minutes and the entire study, including the preparation at the radiology department takes about 90 minutes.

Evaluation of the small bowel with MR enterography faces one important obstacle: bowel motion that can result in blurring of the images. This is an issue mainly for the contrast-enhanced sequences, considering that the remaining pulse sequences used (single-shot fast spin echo and steady-state free precession) are sufficiently fast.[2] Therefore, most centers administer pharmacologic bowel paralytics to minimize small-bowel motion. Specific techniques vary between institutions; however, 1 mg of glucagon or 20 mg of a dose of hyoscine butylbromide is intravenously administered in a single dose or in split doses after the cine dynamic sequence, to reduce small-bowel peristalsis and related motion artifact.[2,10,14,15]

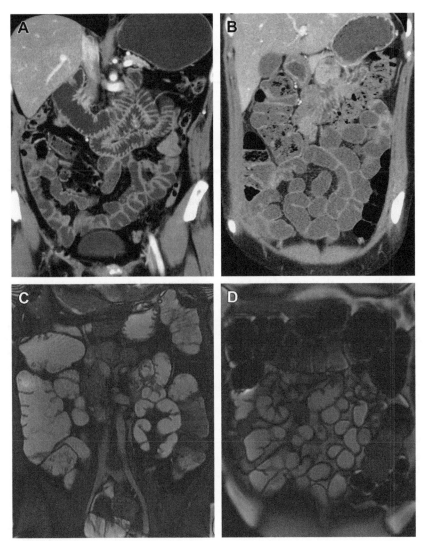

Fig. 2. CT enterography (*A, B*) and MR enterography (*C, D*). Comparison of spatial resolution between CT and MR enterography. Note the adequate small bowel loops filling and distention in both; the possibility of evaluation of the lumen, mucosal surface, and intestinal wall; and, eventually, associated mesenteric and extraenteric findings.

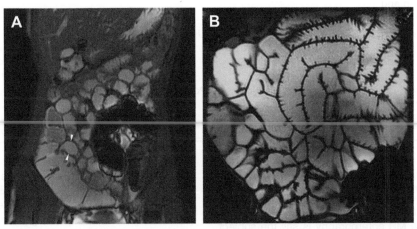

Fig. 3. MR enterography (*A*) and MR enteroclysis (*B*). Compare the better bowel distention achieved by MR enteroclysis, mainly of the proximal loops, but with the disadvantage of using a nasoenteric tube. *Arrows* in (*A*): terminal ileum.

Table 1
Advantages of MR enterography, MR enteroclysis, and CT enterography

	MR Enterography	MR Enteroclysis	CT Enterography
Availability	Less available	Less available	Widely available
Cost	Medium	Higher costs	Lower costs
Enteric contrast delivery	Oral administration	Administration through a nasoenteric tube	Oral administration
Length of examination	30 min	60 min, considering placement of nasoenteric tube	Fast examination time (scanning time <1 min)
Invasive nature	Noninvasive	Invasiveness related to the placement of a nasoenteric tube to administer the enteric contrast material	Noninvasive
Visualization of the small bowel wall	Displays the entire thickness of the bowel wall and perienteric tissues	Displays the entire thickness of the bowel wall and perienteric tissues	Displays the entire thickness of the bowel wall and perienteric tissues
Distention of the small bowel loops	Suboptimal distention and filling of the proximal small bowel (jejunal loops)	Yields the best distention, mainly of the jejunal loops	Suboptimal distention and filling of the proximal small bowel (jejunal loops)
Exposure to ionizing radiation	No	Needs of additional ionizing radiation exposure for duodenal intubation	Yes
Examination quality	Variable	Variable	Consistent
Multiplanar imaging capability	Yes	Yes	Yes
Soft-tissue contrast resolution	Excellent	Excellent	Medium
Spatial resolution	Lower	Lower	Higher, with submillimeter near-isotropic voxel
Temporal resolution	Lower	Lower	Higher
Dynamic information regarding bowel distention and motility	Yes	Yes	No
Intravenous contrast agent	Use of a relatively safe intravenous contrast agent (gadolinium-based agents)	Use of a relatively safe intravenous contrast agent (gadolinium-based agents)	Iodinated contrast agent with the risk of serious allergic reaction and nephrotoxicity
Multiphase postcontrast dynamic imaging	Possibility to perform	Possibility to perform	Limited ability to perform multiphasic examination due to radiation exposure

MR Enterography: Enteral Contrast Agents and Imaging Timing

The ideal protocol for small-bowel distention and filling before MR enterography is still the subject of investigation.[2,6,9,13,15-19] Luminal distention is critical for diagnosis of diseases of the small bowel because collapsed bowel may mimic thickened or segmentally hyperenhancing bowel. The most important features concerning enteric contrast agents include uniform and homogeneous filling of the bowel loops, adequate distention of the lumen, high contrast between the lumen and the small bowel, low cost, and absence of serious adverse side effects.

Several enteric contrast agents have been described: plain water, polyethylene glycol (PEG) solution, mannitol, low-concentration barium sulfate, methylcellulose, and gadolinium chelates. These agents are categorized according to their effects on T1-weighted and T2-weighted images: negative (low-signal intensity), positive (high-signal intensity), or biphasic (low-signal intensity on T1-weighted image and high-signal intensity on T2-weighted images).[6]

Biphasic contrast agents are the most commonly used contrast agents for both MR enteroclysis and MR enterography. The low-signal intensity on T1-weighted images observed after its administration improves contrast between the small bowel lumen and the hyperenhancing wall inflammation as well as the demonstration of masses.

On a T2-weighted image, an enhanced contrast between the bright lumen and the dark bowel wall will be observed after biphasic contrast agent administration, improving the detection of endoluminal abnormalities as well as allowing a more effective demonstration of transmural ulcers.

Some studies have demonstrated that low-concentration barium sulfate and PEG solution are better for achieving optimal small bowel filling and distention.[6,20,21] PEG solution is a high-osmolality, nonabsorbed contrast medium that has shown to provide excellent intraluminal contrast. Its main side effect is related to the high osmolality that may cause mild diarrhea, which often occurs within 1 hour of ingestion. All patients should be aware of this possibility before undergoing the procedure, so that they may better plan the timing and way to get home after the examination.[18] Moreover, PEG solution is inexpensive. Water is the preferred contrast agent among patients and is associated with the fewest side effects, but it is absorbed along the length of small bowel and currently not commonly used for MR enterography.

The volume and imaging timing of oral contrast administration vary among institutions. In most of them, the volume varies between 1 L and 2 L. In the authors' institution, we currently ask patients to drink a total of 1 L of PEG solution before the examination (500 mL over 20 minutes, beginning 50 minutes before imaging; then 500 mL more in the next 20 minutes; and, finally, 450 mL of water just before imaging begins). We prefer using plain water immediately before imaging because it is intended only to distend the proximal small bowel and we can, therefore, reduce the amount of hyperosmolar fluid administered and its subsequent side effects. The images should be acquired

when the enteric agent reaches the terminal ileum–right colon. Tolan and colleagues[17] advocate imaging 40 minutes after contrast administration and consider that this protocol is effective in terms of both patient compliance and efficient use of time at the MR.

MR Enterography Imaging Protocol

There is no consensus on the optimal imaging protocol used for MR enterography. We apply various pulse sequences in combination and the examinations are always performed at a 1.5-T MR imaging system (Signa HDxT; GE systems, Milwaukee, USA) with an eight-channel phased-array coil.

T2-weighted cholangiopancreatography-like sequence

The examination begins with thick-slab T2-weighted cholangiopancreatography-like sequence, to evaluate if enteric contrast has reached the terminal ileum and/or right colon area. If so, the examination continues (**Fig. 4**). If not, we consider further administration of 500 mL of enteric contrast agent and then we repeat the sequence 15 to 30 minutes later.

Coronal T2 nondynamic sequences

In our protocol, a coronal 5-mm Half-Fourier Single-Shot T2-weighted sequence (HASTE) is

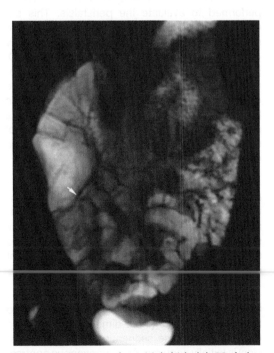

Fig. 4. MR enterography. Initial thick-slab T2-cholangiography-like sequence performed to be certain that the enteric contrast has reached the ileocecal region (*arrow*).

the next step, with and without fat saturation, followed by a 5-mm coronal T2-weigthed sequence steady-state free precession (TrueFISP). Various acronyms are used to describe these gradient-echo sequences, depending on the equipment manufacturer, including TrueFISP, Fast Imaging Employing Steady-state Acquisition (FIESTA), and Balanced Gradient-Echo (GE). Both HASTE and TrueFISP produce high contrast between the lumen and the bowel wall and are particularly effective as a means of obtaining information about extraintestinal abnormalities.[22] TrueFISP sequence eliminates phase shifts caused by motion, thus both fluid and blood appear bright. It is a fast acquisition in which each image is acquired in a few hundred milliseconds. It best depicts mesenteric adenopathy and the prominence of vasa recta in active Crohn disease (the comb sign).

HASTE is considered the best sequence to demonstrate focal wall thickening, fold pattern changes, and ulceration, but it is susceptible to intraluminal motion and often produces intraluminal low-signal-intensity artifacts.[9] Fat-saturated HASTE sequences are added to differentiate submucosal and mesenteric edema from fatty infiltration.

Coronal T2 cine dynamic sequences: evaluation of bowel motility

After these initial coronal fast sequences, dynamic cine true fast imaging with TrueFISP is performed to evaluate the peristalsis. This sequence uses an intermediate-weighted kinematic multiphase sequence (slice thickness 5 mm; FOV 480 × 360 mm; effective matrix 224 × 224; NEX [number of excitations] 1) performing 10 measurements of the same slice over an acquisition time of 9 seconds. It is becoming routinely used in MR enterography protocols and initial data suggest that a simple subjective assessment of motility may add value to conventional anatomic observations.[23–25]

Diffusion-weighted imaging

Diffusion-weighted imaging (DWI) has been investigated recently in the assessment of bowel inflammation in Crohn disease.[19,26,27] In our institution, we acquire a coronal DWI with b-values of 0 and 800 mm^2/s. It can be also useful in the assessment of small bowel malignancies.

Contrast-enhanced sequences

Coronal high-resolution precontrast T1-weighted LAVA sequence (three-dimensional spoiled gradient echo pulse sequence with fat suppression) is initially acquired. After intravenous contrast agent administration (gadolinium-based agents) at a dose of 0.1 mmol/kg, followed by a 20-mL saline flush (at the rate of 2.0 mL/s), the coronal LAVA sequence is again performed after 30-second and 70-second delays, followed by an entire abdomen axial volumetric sequence at 100-seconds. Coronal LAVA is obtained at the end. These sequences are helpful in the evaluation of neoplastic and inflammatory bowel disorders.

CLINICAL APPLICATIONS

The main clinical application of MR enterography is the evaluation of patients with suspected or confirmed Crohn disease. In these patients, MR enterography may provide information on disease activity and may demonstrate associated complications.

MR enterography has a less well documented developing clinical application, which consists of the evaluation of other small-bowel diseases, including various benign and malignant neoplasms arising in isolation or along with polyposis syndromes (**Box 1**).[9,14]

Crohn Disease: Initial Evaluation and Assessment of Inflammatory Activity

Crohn disease has a worldwide distribution; it is more prevalent in Europe and North America. The peak incidence is in adolescents and young adults between 15 and 25 years of age and a second peak is seen between 50 and 80 years of age.[28] The disease is characterized by bowel inflammation, which can affect any part of the gastrointestinal tract with relapses and remissions throughout its course.[29] Although the precise cause of Crohn disease is unknown, there is evidence that the disease is due to an abnormal mucosal response to an unknown antigen. Shanahan[29] suggests that there are genetically susceptible patients.

Crohn disease predominantly involves the terminal ileum and ileocecal region in 90% of the patients with small bowel compromise. In 40% to 55% of these patients, the ileum and the colon

---

Box 1
Evolving indications of MR enterography beyond Crohn disease

Evaluation of benign and malignant neoplasms

Polyposis syndromes (eg, Peutz-Jeghers syndrome)

Celiac disease

Inflammatory conditions (vasculitis, treatment-induced enteritis)

Meckel diverticulum

Intussusception

Postoperative adhesions

are both affected, whereas in a minority of patients (between 15% and 25%) the lesion affects only the colon.[30] Involvement of other parts of the gastrointestinal tract does occur but is rare.[31] Patients may present with vague abdominal symptoms, watery diarrhea, or complications such as perineal sinuses, anorectal fistulas, and abscesses.

Characteristic pathologic findings of Crohn disease in the gastrointestinal tract include transmural granulomatous inflammation with a discontinuous involvement. A pathognomonic feature of this disease is the presence of clearly defined normal segments between diseased segments known as skip lesions. The earliest macroscopic findings in Crohn disease are seen in the mucosa and submucosa and consist of aphthous ulceration, hyperemia, and edema. With increasing severity, transmural involvement is demonstrated, with the shallow ulcers becoming deeper and coalescent, resulting in linear and transversal large ulcerations. The presence of islands of normal mucosa interspersed between deep ulcers leads to the formation of a cobblestone pattern. Later, these extensive transmural ulcerations may be associated with luminal narrowing in the affected segment. This transmural ulceration can evolve to extramural abscesses or fistulas.

The edematous bowel with transmural involvement becomes aperistaltic, causing obstructive symptoms. In long-standing disease, chronic obstruction can develop secondary to scarring and stenosis. Extramural manifestations of Crohn disease are fistulas, abscesses, adhesions, creeping fat, and enlargement of lymph nodes. Extraintestinal manifestations are common and include arthritis; cholelithiasis; ocular manifestations; dermatologic abnormalities; and, in children, growth retardation.

The primary goal of radiology in the evaluation Crohn disease is to provide information that may allow the initial diagnosis of the inflammatory process, predict disease activity, and monitor therapeutic response.

The diagnosis of Crohn disease is based on a combination of clinical, laboratory, histologic, and imaging findings. The imaging characteristics and distribution of the disease give supportive evidence for the diagnosis. Traditionally, the SBFT has been the standard imaging method used to assess patients with Crohn disease.[32] However, some studies have demonstrated that this imaging method does not allow accurate detection of disease activity, mainly because it does not provide direct information with respect to the state of the bowel wall and extraluminal extension of the disease.[33,34] The accuracy may be limited by overlapping bowel loops.[35–37] In

this setting, the role of cross-sectional imaging has expanded with the recent advances in CT scan and MR imaging that have the main advantage of direct evaluation of the bowel wall and perienteric tissues. This means a complete change in the diagnostic approach: from the analysis of the bowel lumen to the direct evaluation of parietal thickness, as well as the assessment of the perienteric involvement.[37]

Then, with cross-sectional imaging, after confirmation of the diagnosis, it is important to evaluate the number, length, and locations of the segments involved. Later, the second requisite is to evaluate whether there is bowel stenosis and, if so, it needs to be classified in inflammatory or fibrous, because treatment will be different according to this classification. Furthermore, if active inflammation is identified, it is important to discriminate between mild, moderate, and severe inflammation, to establish appropriate medical or surgical treatment. The identification of mesenteric complications must be also reported, including abscesses and fistulas, because they influence the choice of treatment. Many new therapeutic strategies have been developed in the last decade, allowing the gastroenterologist and surgeons to treat almost all different presentations of Crohn disease.[38] The success of these strategies depends on accurate diagnosis of the nature and extent of disease. Thus, it is necessary, from now on, not only to diagnose Crohn disease but also to assess its location, subtype and severity.

CT enterography is an accurate technique to evaluate Crohn disease, providing details about the bowel wall and perienteric tissues, although superficial lesions cannot be accurately visualized.[10] This method can show clearly active Crohn disease and its complications because of its high spatial resolution. Although CT enterography is now widely used in the evaluation of Crohn disease, the exposure of adolescents and young adults to ionizing radiation is an important issue, specially because there is a frequent need for reassessment these patients, due the chronicity of the disease.

MR enterography is an alternative method for the evaluation of Crohn disease and it clearly demonstrates endoluminal, mural, and extramural enteric changes. In addition, it can provide functional information concerning peristalsis of the involved segment through the dynamic cine sequences and accurately display bowel wall changes in early Crohn disease.[39] Its accuracy in the diagnosis and depiction of Crohn disease extent is similar to CT enterography and superior to SBFT.[16] Lee and colleagues[16] demonstrated that sensitivities for the detection of extraenteric complications of Crohn disease were significantly higher for CT and MR enterography (100% for both) than for SBFT (32%–37%). They also demonstrated a high intraobserver and interobserver reproducibility of these cross-sectional methods. Another pivotal role of the cross-sectional imaging methods is to monitor disease activity and severity.[40]

MR enterography findings in Crohn disease

The main imaging findings on MR enterography are: mural thickening, mural hyperenhancement, parietal stratification, creeping fat, lymphadenomegaly, engorged of the vasa recta (the comb sign), fistulas or abscesses (**Box 2**).

A wall thickness greater than 3 mm is considered abnormal in a distended small bowel loop and has 83% to 91% sensitivity and 86% to 100% specificity for the diagnosis of Crohn disease (**Fig. 5**).[8,41] The wall thickness is better evaluated on HASTE sequences, which are insensitive to chemical shift artifacts, as seen on True-FISP sequences (a black border artifact is seen in these images).

Moderate to deep ulceration can be seen in Crohn disease, especially on HASTE sequences. Depiction of subtle wall ulcerations is highly dependent on the degree of luminal distention. An aphthous ulcer is seen on MR images as a nidus of high-signal intensity surrounded by a rim of moderate-signal intensity (**Fig. 6**). The disease progresses to longitudinal and horizontal transmural ulceration, resulting in sinuses, fistulas, and perienteric abscesses that are well demonstrated on MR enterography (**Fig. 7**).

Intravenous contrast agent administration is mandatory for patients with Crohn disease because it improves the detection of active inflammation and

helps to differentiate between active and inactive disease. Postcontrast mural enhancement is best evaluated by comparing normal to abnormal bowel segments. It is important to notice that inadequate small bowel distention can adversely affect the evaluation of mural enhancement. Mural stratification, with variable mucosal enhancement surrounded by relatively poor submucosal enhancement (reflecting edema), is seen in active disease (**Fig. 8A**). The target or halo sign representing this mural stratification on bowel loop axial sections is related to active inflammatory disease (see **Fig. 8B**). This should be differentiated from the halo produced by submucosal fat deposition seen in chronic disease.

Compared with CT enterography, MR enterography can add value to contrast-enhanced sequences by demonstrating the high T2-signal intensity of the submucosal edema (**Fig. 9**).

Intense diffuse enhancement of the entire wall thickness usually represents transmural inflammation. Mild heterogeneous enhancement can be seen in fibrosis.

Identification of an asymmetric segmental small bowel mural thickening and hyperenhancement with a discontinuous involvement is pathognomonic for Crohn disease (see **Fig. 6A, B**; **Fig. 10A–C**).[42] The sensitivity and specificity of this finding on MR imaging for the diagnosis of Crohn disease range from 88% to 98% and from 78% to 100%, respectively.[10]

On DWI, active inflammation of the small bowel in Crohn disease patients can be demonstrated by restricted diffusion (indicated by low apparent diffusion coefficient [ADC] values) when compared with normal bowel wall (see **Fig. 10D, E**). Oto and colleagues[26] showed that low ADC values provided a sensitivity of 94% for the detection of inflammation of the terminal ileum on patients with active Crohn disease.

Another cross-sectional imaging sign that indicates active Crohn disease is the prominent vasa recta (the comb sign) and mesenteric fat stranding. The comb sign represents the engorged vasa recta that penetrates the bowel wall perpendicularly.

The detection of any intraabdominal abscess is important because antitumor necrosis factor agents, such as infliximab, are not indicated in patients presenting with these abscesses.

In chronic phases of the disease, intestinal inflammation with associated to fatty infiltration of the submucosal bowel wall layer, sacculations (see **Fig. 9**), or dilated amorphous bowel loops, fibrofatty proliferation in adjacent mesenteric (**Fig. 11**), and strictures. Some investigators have demonstrated that the perienteric fat in subjects with Crohn disease is not simply a result of

---

Box 2
Active Crohn disease: MR enterography findings

Segmental mural thickness greater than 3 mm

Segmental mural hyperenhancement with layer stratification

Intense segmental wall full-thickness hyperenhancement

T2-weighted high-signal intensity of the submucosal bowel wall layer (edema)

Superficial or deep ulceration

Prominent vasa recta (the comb sign)

Fistulas

Abscesses

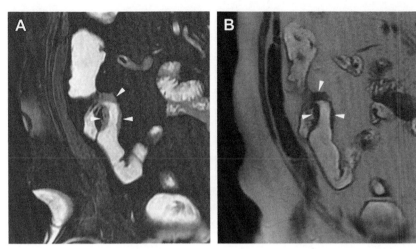

Fig. 5. MR enterography in a 53-year-old woman with biopsy-proven Crohn disease. Coronal TrueFISP image obtained with fat saturation (*A*) and coronal HASTE (*B*) demonstrates mural thickening of terminal ileum (*white arrowheads*).

inflammation but is actually hormonally active and may, in fact, help drive the inflammatory process.[43,44]

Acute and chronic changes may be simultaneously demonstrated within the same diseased segment. HASTE fat-saturated sequence can help differentiate fat infiltration from edema (**Box 3**).

Imaging-based classification of Crohn disease

In 2003, Maglinte and colleagues[3] proposed a radiologic-based classification of Crohn disease to overcome the limitations and subjective nature of the clinical inflammatory index. This classification provides useful information for the clinician and surgeon when used in combination with clinical and laboratory data. It is considered a reproducible classification that emphasizes morphologic features. The investigators classified Crohn disease into four broad groups: active inflammatory, perforating and fistulating, fibrostenotic, and reparative and regenerative subtypes (**Box 4**). The detection of ulceration, bowel edema, fistulas, stenosis, and extraintestinal abnormalities allows proper classification. MR enterography can demonstrate these pathologic changes and, consequently, can help in guiding decisions regarding medical and surgical therapy.

Active inflammatory disease In this subtype of disease, the classic MR enterography findings are focal inflammation (without fistulas or perforation) characterized by ulcers, mural thickening, hyperenhancement, and mural stratification, and engorgement of the vasa recta. Mucosal

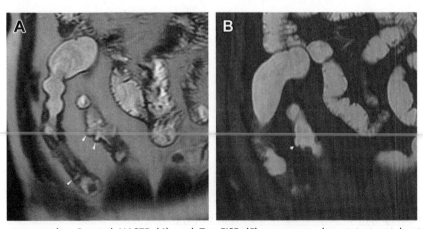

Fig. 6. MR enterography. Coronal HASTE (*A*) and TrueFISP (*B*) sequences demonstrate at least two bowel segments with thickened wall interspersed with normal segments—the skip lesions. Deep ulcerations in both sequences appear as a nidus filled with enteric contrast agent (*arrowheads*).

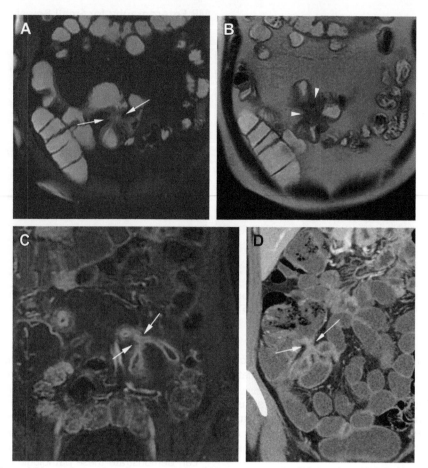

Fig. 7. A 36-year-old woman undergoing treatment of biopsy-proven Crohn disease. Coronal TrueFISP obtained with fat saturation (*A*), HASTE (*B*), and postcontrast LAVA (*C*) sequences showing an ileoileal fistula (*A* and *C*, *arrows*). Notice the mural high-signal intensity on the T2 (*B*, *arrowheads*) related to disease activity. There are also desmoplastic and/or fibrotic reactions in the mesentery around the fistula, creating a stellar appearance. Coronal CT enterography (*D*) of another patient with Crohn disease showing a similar appearance of the fistula (*arrows*).

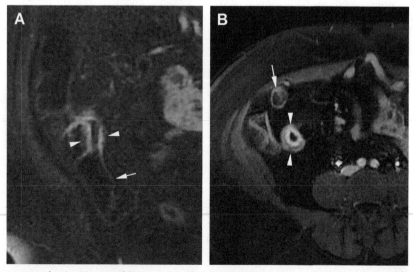

Fig. 8. MR enterography in 53-year-old woman with biopsy-proven Crohn disease. Coronal (*A*) and axial (*B*) three-dimensional T1-weighted fat-suppressed LAVA sequences demonstrate diseased ileum with mural stratification, characterized by mucosal hyperenhancement, surrounded by relatively poor submucosal enhancement (edema), in active disease. Compare normal (*arrows*) and abnormal bowel segments (*arrowheads*).

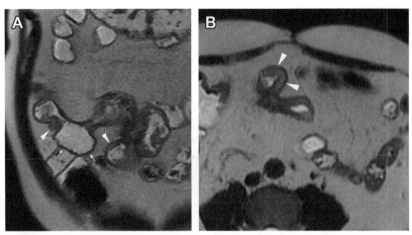

Fig. 9. MR enterography in a 48-year-old man with fistulating Crohn disease. Coronal (*A*) and axial (*B*) HASTE sequences show submucosal edema represented by mural high-signal intensity (*arrowheads*). This finding is associated with active inflammation. Enteric sacculation (*A, arrows*) is related to long-standing disease, both chronic and active.

hyperenhancement on MR enterography has demonstrated good correlation with the Crohn disease activity index and is the most sensitive finding in active disease, which significantly correlates with histologic findings.[7,45,46] Several studies have reported MR enterography sensitivities for

the detection of active inflammatory disease between 73% and 90%.[7,45,46]

Fistula-forming and perforating disease This subtype of disease is characterized by severe inflammation with progression to transmural

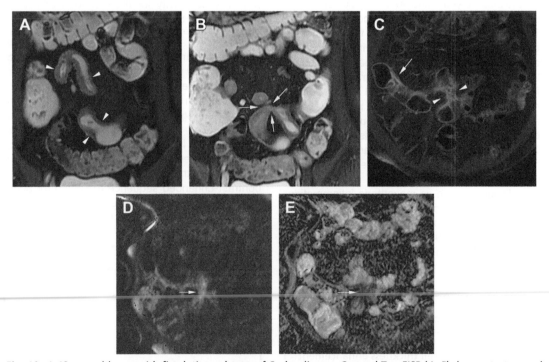

Fig. 10. A 48-year-old man with fistulating subtype of Crohn disease. Coronal TrueFISP (*A, B*) demonstrate mural thickening in skip lesions (*A, arrowhead*) associated with a complex ileoileal fistula (*B, arrows*). Coronal contrast-enhanced LAVA (*C*) showing mural hyperemia (*arrow*) and hyperenhancement of bowel wall loops adjacent to the fistula formation (*arrowheads*). There are skip lesions with mural hyperenhancement. Coronal DWI with b-value of 800 (*D*) and ADC map (*E*) demonstrating the water motion restriction in the active diseased area (*arrows*).

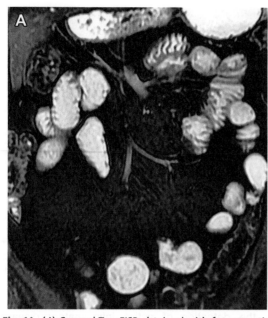
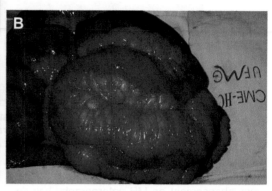

Fig. 11. (*A*) Coronal TrueFISP obtained with fat saturation showing mesenteric fibrofatty proliferation displacing small bowel loops. (*B*) A surgical specimen of a patient with Crohn disease demonstrates an extensive fibrofatty proliferation adjacent to the small bowel.

ulceration and fistulation. The cumulative risk of developing fistulas for patients with Crohn disease is 33% after 10 years and 50% after 20 years, with perianal fistulas being the most common type.[17] The imaging findings related to fistulae include bowel angulation associated with bowel wall contiguity and linear tracts between these bowel loops.[11] Multiplanar MR enterography is useful for a complete evaluation and avoidance of missed sinuses. Desmoplastic and/or fibrotic reactions in the mesentery around the fistula create a star appearance of the fistula (see **Figs. 7** and **10**). Inflamed fistulas can demonstrate intense contrast enhancement due to their higher vascular flow and hyperemia. Extraintestinal complications, such as mesenteric inflammation, abscesses, and involvement of adjacent viscera, can also be well depicted by MR enterography in patients with fistula-forming and perforating subtypes of Crohn disease. Rieber and colleagues[47] demonstrated that the sensitivity for

the detection of abscesses was 0% for conventional enteroclysis and 100% for MR enterography. The sensitivity for the diagnosis of fistulae was 17% and 83%, respectively.

Fibrostenotic disease This subtype of Crohn disease is characterized by the presence of strictures that may progress to bowel obstruction. The stricture can be classified as functionally significant if the upstream bowel dilatation is greater than 3 cm in diameter (**Fig. 12**). In the fibrostenotic subtype of the disease, low-level inhomogeneous mural enhancement is demonstrated, with no evidence of associated edema. In this setting, it is mandatory to evaluate the T2-weighted images and the contrast-enhanced sequence to search for acute wall edema and mural stratification and/or mucosal hyperenhancement, respectively. Differentiation

---

Box 3
Crohn disease, chronic phase: MR enterography findings

No or mild entire wall thickness enhancement

Fatty infiltration of the submucosal bowel wall layer

Mesentery fibrofatty infiltration

Box 4
Imaging-based classification of Crohn disease

Active inflammatory disease

Perforating and fistulating disease

Fibrostenotic disease

Reparative and regenerative disease

Data from Maglinte DD, Gourtsoyiannis N, Rex D, et al. Classification of small bowel Crohn's subtypes based on multimodality imaging. Radiol Clin North Am 2003;41(2):285–303.

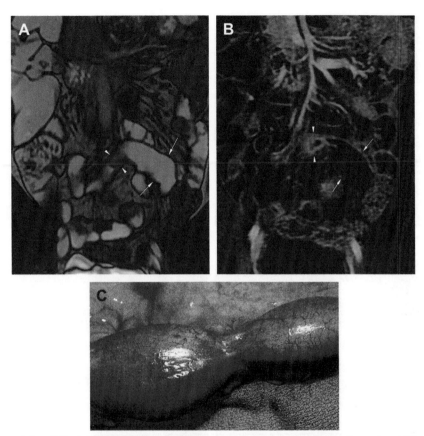

Fig. 12. Coronal TrueFISP obtained without fat saturation (*A*) and coronal three-dimensional T1-weighted fat saturated (LAVA) in a 43-year-old woman with fibrostenotic subtype of Crohn disease characterized by the presence of strictures (*arrowheads*) (*B*) associated with bowel obstruction and upstream bowel dilatation (*arrows*). (*C*) The surgical specimen demonstrating the fibrostenotic segment.

between fibrotic and edematous stenosis based on imaging findings is useful for selecting patients for medical (edematous stenosis) and surgical (fibrous stenosis) treatment.

Reparative or regenerative disease This subtype reflects inactive Crohn disease and may be associated with other forms of the disease located in different bowel loops. It is characterized by mucosal atrophy and presence of regenerative polyps. Minimal decrease in luminal diameter can be seen but there is no mural edema or evidence of active inflammation.

Evaluation of small bowel motility MR enterography allows assessment of bowel motility. The True-FISP dynamic cine sequences are becoming routine in MR enterography protocols and may add value to conventional anatomic findings by improving Crohn disease detection and determination of Crohn disease activity.[23–25] Evaluation of bowel motility can be used to distinguish between temporary collapsed and truly narrowed tracts, as

well as be a potential biomarker of activity (**Fig. 13**).[23,25,48] Froehlich and colleagues,[24] in a retrospective study evaluating the added value of acquiring coronal cine sequences with the standard MR enterography protocol, concluded that, in patients presenting with Crohn disease, lesions seem to be associated with motility changes, which can be useful in the diagnosis.

Beyond Crohn Disease: the Role of MR Imaging in the Evaluation of Other Small Bowel Diseases

MR enterography has an evolving, although less well documented role in the evaluation of other small-bowel diseases,[9,14] including various benign and malignant neoplasms arising in isolation or associated with polyposis syndromes (eg, Peutz-Jeghers), inflammatory conditions (eg, vasculitis and treatment-induced enteritis), infectious processes, celiac disease, diverticular disease, Meckel diverticulum, intussusception, systemic sclerosis,

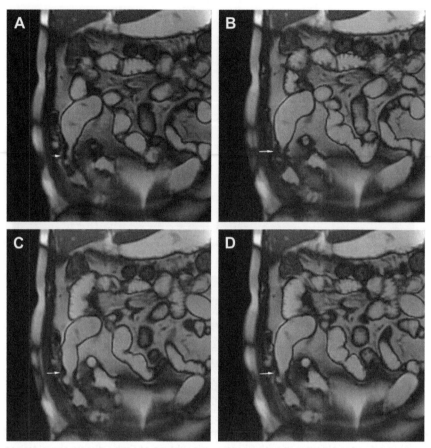

Fig. 13. MR enterography in the assessment of bowel motility. Coronal TrueFISP dynamic cine images in the same position (A–D). There are little peristaltic movements in the fibrostenotic segment (arrows) between the images, acquired at different times.

small-bowel obstructions, and bowel duplication (see **Box 1**). Although spatial resolution of MR imaging is lower than that of a CT scan, the main advantages of the former are the combination of good soft-tissue contrast, detection of extraenteric abnormalities, and lack of radiation exposure, which allows repeated data acquisition for functional bowel evaluation (see **Table 1**).

Distinction between inflammatory and neoplastic disorders may be difficult. T2-weighted imaging and gadolinium-enhanced fat-suppressed T1-weighted imaging (LAVA) play a pivotal role in characterizing wall thickening and identifying its cause: in a thickened bowel segment, a stratified enhancement pattern corresponding to the classic halo sign is useful for excluding malignant conditions.[9] This pattern is related to enhancing mucosa and edematous submucosa.

Another finding that may help differentiate benign from malignant disorders is the length of the thickened bowel segment: with few exceptions, thickening of a long segment of the small bowel indicates a benign condition.[9,49]

Small bowel tumors

Small bowel neoplasms are rare entities and often pose a diagnostic dilemma to radiologists, gastroenterologists, and oncologists.[44,50] Although rare, they are commonly included in the differential diagnosis of small bowel disease because of their nonspecific presenting symptoms. Patients may present with pain, obstruction, bleeding, anorexia, weight loss, perforation, or jaundice. The nonspecific nature of these symptoms and the lack of reliable clinical findings virtually assure significant delay in the diagnosis.[44,51] The most common small bowel tumors are adenocarcinoma, carcinoid tumor, lymphoma, and gastrointestinal stromal tumor. Nonmalignant small bowel tumors include hamartomatous polyps related to Peutz-Jeghers syndrome and hyperplastic polyps.

Identification and differentiation between benign and malignant small-bowel lesions with MR imaging can be difficult, particularly when they are small. Although any of these tumors may appear as focal intraluminal masses at MR enterography, small segments of focal bowel wall thickening or areas of increased mural enhancement may suggest neoplastic conditions. There is a paucity of data regarding the accuracy of MR enterography for the detection of small-bowel masses and its diagnostic performance has yet to be prospectively evaluated in a large series of subjects.[9] Suboptimal small-bowel distention can hide lesions and MR enteroclysis may be necessary in some cases. Masselli and colleagues[52] demonstrated a high accuracy of this method in a prospective study with 150 subjects who were clinically suspected of having small bowel neoplasm and the overall sensitivity, specificity, and accuracy in identifying subjects with small bowel lesions were 86%, 98%, and 97%, respectively.

To the authors' best knowledge, there is only one study that compared the accuracy of MR enterography in evaluating small bowel tumors to other methods. Gupta and colleagues[53] evaluated the utility of MR enterography compared with capsule endoscopy for the detection of small bowel polyps in 19 subjects with Peutz-Jeghers syndrome and found that there was no significant difference between these techniques for the detection of polyps larger than 10 mm. However, a larger number of polyps between 6 and 10 mm were detected with capsule endoscopy but not with MR enterography, compatible with the superior mucosal visualization achieved with the first modality.

Peutz-Jeghers syndrome is a genetic disorder with an autosomal dominant pattern of inheritance, characterized by multiple hamartomatous polyps throughout the gastrointestinal tract, mostly in the small bowel. The main problems in the management of patients with this syndrome are the long-term cancer risk and polyp-related complications.[9] In this setting, MR enterography may play a role in the surveillance of these patients, considering its accuracy in detecting polyps larger than 10 mm because these polyps have increased risk of malignant degeneration.[9,53]

MR enterographic features of adenocarcinomas include annular and constricting lesions, eccentric or circumferential wall-thickening with irregular borders, and moderate late-enhancement after administration of intravenous contrast media. Lymph node enlargement is not as marked in the presence of adenocarcinomas because it is in the setting of lymphomas.[9] MR enterography may also demonstrate metastases from bowel adenocarcinomas to lymph nodes, liver, and peritoneal surfaces.

MR enterographic appearances of carcinoid tumors of the small bowel vary, including a submucosal avidly enhancing nodule, uniform bowel wall-thickening, multifocal enhancing polypoid lesions in a segmental distribution, or numerous tiny enhancing lesions in a carpet-like configuration.[9,54] The tumor may also determine thickening, angulation, and fixation of ileal loops because of mesenteric fibrosis and desmoplasia, sometimes leading to obstruction and ischemia. An enlarged mesenteric lymph node is also a common finding.[54] Mesenteric carcinoid tumors have a maximum diameter of 2 to 4 cm and sometimes exhibit radiating spicule-like strands of tissue. The liver is the most common site for disease-spread and liver metastases are characteristically hypervascular.

A mildly enhancing exofitic mass or a long segment of circumferential bowel wall-thickening without proximal bowel obstruction, associated with adjacent lymphadenopathy or aneurysmal ulceration, is suggestive of lymphoma. The presence of splenic lesions or diffuse splenomegaly and retroperitoneal lymphadenopathy support the diagnosis. Sometimes lymphoma can mimic inflammatory bowel disease (**Fig. 14**). A homogeneous signal intensity on T2-weighted images combined with huge lymph node enlargement and splenomegaly may help distinguish lymphoma from Crohn disease.[10,55]

Celiac disease

Celiac disease, also known as gluten-sensitive enteropathy and nontropical sprue, is a chronic inflammatory intestinal disease with a multifactorial cause. It is an enteropathy induced by dietary gluten that affects the small intestine in genetically susceptible individuals. There are frequent associations with other autoimmune diseases such as type 1 diabetes mellitus, autoimmune thyroid disease, Addison disease, Sjögren syndrome, and systemic lupus erythematosis.[56]

The most common imaging finding is diffuse fluid-filled small bowel dilatation. MR enterography typically demonstrates an abnormal mucosal fold pattern of the small bowel, with villous atrophy in the proximal small bowel and compensatory hypertrophy of folds in the ileum, which results in reversal of the jejunoileal fold pattern (ileal jejunization).[9,44,56] Fewer than three folds per inch within the jejunum characterize villous atrophy. Other characteristic imaging findings include fold-thickening, bowel wall-thickening, mesenteric vascular engorgement, enlarged lymph nodes, and splenic atrophy. Imaging plays an important role in the identification of gastrointestinal complications of diseases such as intestinal lymphoma, intussusception, ulcerative jejunoileitis, cavitary mesenteric lymph node syndrome, and adenocarcinoma of the small bowel.[44]

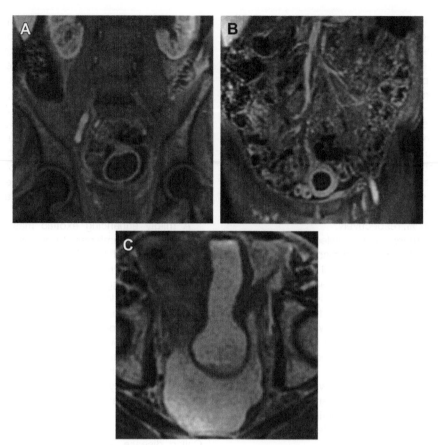

Fig. 14. MR enterography. Coronal postcontrast LAVA sequences (*A*) and (*B*) and axial HASTE (*C*) in a patient with biopsy-proven lymphoma. There is mural thickening of an ileal segment in the pelvis, simulating inflammatory disease.

EVALUATING PEDIATRIC PATIENTS WITH SUSPECTED OR CONFIRMED CROHN DISEASE

One important issue discussed in the literature is the evaluation of pediatric patients with suspected or confirmed Crohn disease with MR enterography, considering its lack of ionizing radiation.[57–60] It is well known that children are more vulnerable to the effects of ionizing radiation when compared with adults and are at a higher risk of suffering from the late effects of ionizing radiation because of their longer life expectancy.[61]

Most of the literature regarding the use of MR enterography in children demonstrates that this method successfully identifies small bowel and colon segments affected by Crohn disease, with sensitivities varying between 85.1% and 100%, taking CT enterography or histopathology as the reference standard.[57–59] Additionally, MR enterography provides an accurate noninvasive assessment of Crohn disease activity and mural fibrosis and can aid in establishing treatment strategies for symptomatic patients and in assessing therapeutic response.

In conclusion, MR enterography can be used as the first-line imaging modality in children with known or suspected Crohn disease. Some studies show that the severity of inflammation on MR enterography had a statistically significant positive correlation with the Pediatric Crohn Disease Activity Index (PCDAI).[60]

RADIATION DOSE CONSIDERATION

CT scans result in radiation doses that are very much at the high end of those produced in diagnostic radiology, because CT scans are effectively a large number of individual images that are electronically combined. The effective dose involved in a single CT scan is not large; however, it is typically two to six times larger than that from barium small-bowel follow-through. Results of a recent meta-analysis concluded that the use of a diagnostic modality, such as MR, that does not involve the use of ionizing radiation is preferable for the diagnosis of Crohn disease.[1] The carcinogenic effect of radiation can be particularly significant in patients with Crohn disease who already have an increased risk of developing gastrointestinal or hepatobiliary cancer and small bowel lymphoma. A recent study highlighted the high cumulative radiation doses given to subjects with Crohn disease, mainly due to the increased use of CT scanning.[62] In this study, CT scanning accounted for up to 84.7% of the cumulative dose given to Crohn disease patients and 15.5% of subjects had cumulative dose higher than 75 mSv.

SUMMARY

MR enterography plays a pivotal role in the evaluation of the small bowel. MR enterography is rapidly becoming the first-line imaging modality for the diagnosis of Crohn disease, especially in the pediatric population. Improvements in MR technology, such as fast scanning techniques and dynamic sequences, that allow evaluation of bowel motility, have permitted accurate diagnosis of complications of Crohn disease, including abscess, fistula, and stenosis.

CT enterography is preferred by some radiologist as the first imaging modality to evaluate small bowel diseases, regarding its higher resolution. At our department, we prefer using CT enterography as a baseline examination in most patients because of its consistent high quality; however, in the follow-up, MR enterography is the standard to help detect complications and to evaluate the response to therapy. However, MR enterography is gradually replacing CT enterography, mainly because it offers a number of advantages, including the absence of associated ionizing radiation exposure. It allows sequential imaging over prolonged periods of time, useful to assess small bowel peristalsis, multiplanar imaging capabilities, and superb contrast and temporal resolution.

Because MR enterography is more time-consuming than CT enterography and because the image quality is highly dependent on patients' cooperation, CT is the preferred imaging method in the elderly and in patients who have difficulty holding their breath. CT is also the preferred method in uncooperative patients and in the emergency setting.

There is a paucity of data regarding the accuracy of MR enterography for the detection of small-bowel disorders beyond Crohn disease; its diagnostic performance has yet to be prospectively evaluated in a large series of subjects with small bowel masses. The authors prefer using CT enterography as the first-line imaging modality because these patients usually do not present with chronic diseases, which would require multiple CT scans during their lifetime.

REFERENCES

1. Horsthuis K, Bipat S, Bennink RJ, et al. Inflammatory bowel disease diagnosed with US, MR, scintigraphy, and CT: meta-analysis of prospective studies. Radiology 2008;247(1):64–79.
2. Grand DJ, Harris A, Loftus EV Jr. Imaging for luminal disease and complications: CT enterography, MR enterography, small-bowel follow-through, and ultrasound. Gastroenterol Clin North Am 2012;41(2): 497–512.
3. Maglinte DD, Gourtsoyiannis N, Rex D, et al. Classification of small bowel Crohn's subtypes based on multimodality imaging. Radiol Clin North Am 2003; 41(2):285–303.
4. Hara AK, Alam S, Heigh RI, et al. Using CT enterography to monitor Crohn's disease activity: a preliminary study. AJR Am J Roentgenol 2008;190(6): 1512–6.
5. Ciaurriz-Munuce A, Fraile-Gonzalez M, Leon-Brito H, et al. Ionizing radiation in patients with Crohn's disease. Estimation and associated factors. Rev Esp Enferm Dig 2012;104(9):452–7.
6. Fidler JL, Guimaraes L, Einstein DM. MR imaging of the small bowel. Radiographics 2009;29(6): 1811–25.
7. Sinha R, Verma R, Verma S, et al. MR enterography of Crohn disease: part 2, imaging and pathologic findings. AJR Am J Roentgenol 2011;197(1):80–5.
8. Zappa M, Stefanescu C, Cazals-Hatem D, et al. Which magnetic resonance imaging findings accurately evaluate inflammation in small bowel Crohn's disease? A retrospective comparison with surgical pathologic analysis. Inflamm Bowel Dis 2011;17(4): 984–93.
9. Amzallag-Bellenger E, Oudjit A, Ruiz A, et al. Effectiveness of MR enterography for the assessment of small-bowel diseases beyond Crohn disease. Radiographics 2012;32(5):1423–44.
10. Masselli G, Gualdi G. MR imaging of the small bowel. Radiology 2012;264(2):333–48.
11. Masselli G, Gualdi G. CT and MR enterography in evaluating small bowel diseases: when to use which modality? Abdom Imaging 2012 [Epub ahead of print].
12. Masselli G, Casciani E, Polettini E, et al. Comparison of MR enteroclysis with MR enterography and conventional enteroclysis in patients with Crohn's disease. Eur Radiol 2008;18(3):438–47.
13. Cronin CG, Lohan DG, Mhuircheartaigh JN, et al. MRI small-bowel follow-through: prone versus supine patient positioning for best small-bowel distention and lesion detection. AJR Am J Roentgenol 2008;191(2):502–6.
14. Kavaliauskiene G, Ziech ML, Nio CY, et al. Small bowel MRI in adult patients: not just Crohn's disease-a tutorial. Insights Imaging 2011;2(5):501–13.

15. Sinha R, Verma R, Verma S, et al. MR enterography of Crohn disease: part 1, rationale, technique, and pitfalls. AJR Am J Roentgenol 2011;197(1):76–9.

16. Lee SS, Kim AY, Yang SK, et al. Crohn disease of the small bowel: comparison of CT enterography, MR enterography, and small-bowel follow-through as diagnostic techniques. Radiology 2009;251(3):751–61.

17. Tolan DJ, Greenhalgh R, Zealley IA, et al. MR enterographic manifestations of small bowel Crohn disease. Radiographics 2010;30(2):367–84.

18. Young BM, Fletcher JG, Booya F, et al. Head-to-head comparison of oral contrast agents for cross-sectional enterography: small bowel distention, timing, and side effects. J Comput Assist Tomogr 2008;32(1):32–8.

19. Oto A, Zhu F, Kulkarni K, et al. Evaluation of diffusion-weighted MR imaging for detection of bowel inflammation in patients with Crohn's disease. Acad Radiol 2009;16(5):597–603.

20. Ajaj W, Goyen M, Schneemann H, et al. Oral contrast agents for small bowel distension in MRI: influence of the osmolarity for small bowel distention. Eur Radiol 2005;15(7):1400–6.

21. McKenna DA, Roche CJ, Murphy JM, et al. Polyethylene glycol solution as an oral contrast agent for MRI of the small bowel in a patient population. Clin Radiol 2006;61(11):966–70.

22. Wiarda BM, Horsthuis K, Dobben AC, et al. Magnetic resonance imaging of the small bowel with the true FISP sequence: intra- and interobserver agreement of enteroclysis and imaging without contrast material. Clin Imaging 2009;33(4):267–73.

23. Menys A, Atkinson D, Odille F, et al. Quantified terminal ileal motility during MR enterography as a potential biomarker of Crohn's disease activity: a preliminary study. Eur Radiol 2012;22(11):2494–501.

24. Froehlich JM, Waldherr C, Stoupis C, et al. MR motility imaging in Crohn's disease improves lesion detection compared with standard MR imaging. Eur Radiol 2010;20(8):1945–51.

25. Girometti R, Zuiani C, Toso F, et al. MRI scoring system including dynamic motility evaluation in assessing the activity of Crohn's disease of the terminal ileum. Acad Radiol 2008;15(2):153–64.

26. Oto A, Kayhan A, Williams JT, et al. Active Crohn's disease in the small bowel: evaluation by diffusion weighted imaging and quantitative dynamic contrast enhanced MR imaging. J Magn Reson Imaging 2011;33(3):615–24.

27. Kiryu S, Dodanuki K, Takao H, et al. Free-breathing diffusion-weighted imaging for the assessment of inflammatory activity in Crohn's disease. J Magn Reson Imaging 2009;29(4):880–6.

28. Fleischer DE, Grimm IS, Friedman LS. Inflammatory bowel disease in older patients. Med Clin North Am 1994;78(6):1303–19.

29. Shanahan F. Crohn's disease. Lancet 2002;359(9300):62–9.

30. Horsthuis K, Stokkers PC, Stoker J. Detection of inflammatory bowel disease: diagnostic performance of cross-sectional imaging modalities. Abdom Imaging 2008;33(4):407–16.

31. Podolsky DK. Inflammatory bowel disease. N Engl J Med 2002;347(6):417–29.

32. Travis SP, Stange EF, Lemann M, et al. European evidence based consensus on the diagnosis and management of Crohn's disease: current management. Gut 2006;55(Suppl 1):i16–35.

33. Hara AK, Leighton JA, Heigh RI, et al. Crohn disease of the small bowel: preliminary comparison among CT enterography, capsule endoscopy, small-bowel follow-through, and ileoscopy. Radiology 2006;238(1):128–34.

34. Triester SL, Leighton JA, Leontiadis GI, et al. A meta-analysis of the yield of capsule endoscopy compared to other diagnostic modalities in patients with non-stricturing small bowel Crohn's disease. Am J Gastroenterol 2006;101(5):954–64.

35. Wold PB, Fletcher JG, Johnson CD, et al. Assessment of small bowel Crohn disease: noninvasive peroral CT enterography compared with other imaging methods and endoscopy–feasibility study. Radiology 2003;229(1):275–81.

36. Furukawa A, Saotome T, Yamasaki M, et al. Cross-sectional imaging in Crohn disease. Radiographics 2004;24(3):689–702.

37. Mazziotti S, Ascenti G, Scribano E, et al. Guide to magnetic resonance in Crohn's disease: from common findings to the more rare complicances. Inflamm Bowel Dis 2011;17(5):1209–22.

38. Sandborn WJ, Feagan BG, Lichtenstein GR. Medical management of mild to moderate Crohn's disease: evidence-based treatment algorithms for induction and maintenance of remission. Aliment Pharmacol Ther 2007;26(7):987–1003.

39. Florie J, Horsthuis K, Hommes DW, et al. Magnetic resonance imaging compared with ileocolonoscopy in evaluating disease severity in Crohn's disease. Clin Gastroenterol Hepatol 2005;3(12):1221–8.

40. Higgins PD, Caoili E, Zimmermann M, et al. Computed tomographic enterography adds information to clinical management in small bowel Crohn's disease. Inflamm Bowel Dis 2007;13(3):262–8.

41. Choi D, Jin Lee S, Ah Cho Y, et al. Bowel wall thickening in patients with Crohn's disease: CT patterns and correlation with inflammatory activity. Clin Radiol 2003;58(1):68–74.

42. Fletcher JG, Fidler JL, Bruining DH, et al. New concepts in intestinal imaging for inflammatory bowel diseases. Gastroenterology 2011;140(6):1795–806.

43. Desreumaux P, Ernst O, Geboes K, et al. Inflammatory alterations in mesenteric adipose tissue in Crohn's disease. Gastroenterology 1999;117(1):73–81.

44. Paulsen SR, Huprich JE, Fletcher JG, et al. CT enterography as a diagnostic tool in evaluating small bowel disorders: review of clinical experience with over 700 cases. Radiographics 2006;26(3):641–57 [discussion: 657–62].

45. Florie J, Wasser MN, Arts-Cieslik K, et al. Dynamic contrast-enhanced MRI of the bowel wall for assessment of disease activity in Crohn's disease. AJR Am J Roentgenol 2006;186(5):1384–92.

46. Low RN, Sebrechts CP, Politoske DA, et al. Crohn disease with endoscopic correlation: single-shot fast spin-echo and gadolinium-enhanced fat-suppressed spoiled gradient-echo MR imaging. Radiology 2002;222(3):652–60.

47. Rieber A, Aschoff A, Nussle K, et al. MRI in the diagnosis of small bowel disease: use of positive and negative oral contrast media in combination with enteroclysis. Eur Radiol 2000;10(9):1377–82.

48. Umschaden HW, Szolar D, Gasser J, et al. Small-bowel disease: comparison of MR enteroclysis images with conventional enteroclysis and surgical findings. Radiology 2000;215(3):717–25.

49. Hoeffel C, Crema MD, Belkacem A, et al. Multidetector row CT: spectrum of diseases involving the ileocecal area. Radiographics 2006;26(5):1373–90.

50. Van Weyenberg SJ, Meijerink MR, Jacobs MA, et al. MR enteroclysis in the diagnosis of small-bowel neoplasms. Radiology 2010;254(3):765–73.

51. Maglinte DD, O'Connor K, Bessette J, et al. The role of the physician in the late diagnosis of primary malignant tumors of the small intestine. Am J Gastroenterol 1991;86(3):304–8.

52. Masselli G, Polettini E, Casciani E, et al. Small-bowel neoplasms: prospective evaluation of MR enteroclysis. Radiology 2009;251(3):743–50.

53. Gupta A, Postgate AJ, Burling D, et al. A prospective study of MR enterography versus capsule endoscopy for the surveillance of adult patients with Peutz-Jeghers syndrome. AJR Am J Roentgenol 2010;195(1):108–16.

54. Kamaoui I, De-Luca V, Ficarelli S, et al. Value of CT enteroclysis in suspected small-bowel carcinoid tumors. AJR Am J Roentgenol 2010;194(3):629–33.

55. Umschaden HW, Gasser J. MR enteroclysis. Radiol Clin North Am 2003;41(2):231–48.

56. Shanbhogue AK, Prasad SR, Jagirdar J, et al. Comprehensive update on select immune-mediated gastroenterocolitis syndromes: implications for diagnosis and management. Radiographics 2010;30(6):1465–87.

57. Dillman JR, Ladino-Torres MF, Adler J, et al. Comparison of MR enterography and histopathology in the evaluation of pediatric Crohn disease. Pediatr Radiol 2011;41(12):1552–8.

58. Gee MS, Nimkin K, Hsu M, et al. Prospective evaluation of MR enterography as the primary imaging modality for pediatric Crohn disease assessment. AJR Am J Roentgenol 2011;197(1):224–31.

59. Chalian M, Ozturk A, Oliva-Hemker M, et al. MR enterography findings of inflammatory bowel disease in pediatric patients. AJR Am J Roentgenol 2011;196(6):W810–6.

60. Silverstein J, Grand D, Kawatu D, et al. Feasibility of using MR enterography for the assessment of terminal ileitis and inflammatory activity in children with Crohn disease. J Pediatr Gastroenterol Nutr 2012;55(2):173–7.

61. Palmer L, Herfarth H, Porter CQ, et al. Diagnostic ionizing radiation exposure in a population-based sample of children with inflammatory bowel diseases. Am J Gastroenterol 2009;104(11):2816–23.

62. Desmond AN, O'Regan K, Curran C, et al. Crohn's disease: factors associated with exposure to high levels of diagnostic radiation. Gut 2008;57(11):1524–9.

Magnetic Resonance Imaging of Rectal Cancer

Luciana Costa-Silva, MD, MSc[a],*,
Gina Brown, MBBS, MD, MRCP, FRCR[b]

KEYWORDS

- Magnetic resonance imaging • Neoplasm staging • Rectal neoplasms
- Diffusion magnetic resonance imaging • Image interpretation • Prognosis
- Neoplasm recurrence, Local • Treatment outcome

KEY POINTS

- High-resolution T2-weighted magnetic resonance imaging has emerged as the first-line imaging tool for multidisciplinary team decisions and is the most important sequence for evaluating rectal tumors.
- Rectal cancer staging is based on defining pertinent anatomy of the rectum and the surrounding structures, allowing for surgical planning and prognostic stage grouping.
- The primary goal of staging rectal cancer is to identify risk factors for distant or local recurrence to offer tailored treatments, based on individual prognosis.
- Some investigations are now focused on conservative management of rectal cancer, increasing the demand for radiologic evaluation of response to chemoradiation to distinguish responding from nonresponding tumors.
- Diffusion-weighted imaging may be a useful adjunctive tool for monitoring the response to chemoradiation therapy for rectal cancer.

INTRODUCTION AND BACKGROUND

Cancer is a major public health problem in the United States and many other parts of the world. A total of 1,660,290 new cancer cases and 580,350 deaths from cancer are projected to occur in the United States in 2013.[1] Among these cases, it is estimated that 102,480 will be new colorectal cases (39% from the rectum) and 50,830 will be cancer deaths. Worldwide, colorectal cancer is the third most common cancer in men (663,000 cases, 10.0% of the total) and the second in women (571,000 cases, 9.4% of the total).[2] Recent trends in the United States show a decreasing incidence of invasive colon and rectal cancers in both men and women, which can be attributed to adoption of colorectal screening programs with earlier detection and removal of precancerous polyps.[3]

Historically, prognosis of rectal cancer has been directly related to the extent of extramural spread into the mesorectum and the ability to achieve surgical clearance at the circumferential resection margins (CRMs),[4,5] and for patients not undergoing total mesorectal excision (TME) surgery, pelvic recurrence rates were strongly linked to nodal status. Quirke and colleagues[6] reported that microscopically positive resection margins occurred in up to 40% of patients treated by non-TME surgery, with local recurrence rates of 83%. Two advances in therapy have a substantial effect on reducing the frequency of local recurrence and improving survival: TME and preoperative neoadjuvant chemoradiation therapy (CRT). The adoption of preoperative radiation therapy for advanced tumors showed a substantial reduction in pelvic recurrence rates of clinically resectable rectal cancers from 20% to 10% in the first

[a] Department of Anatomy and Imaging, Federal University of Minas Gerais, Av. Prof. Alfredo Balena 190, Belo Horizonte 30130-100, Brazil; [b] Department of Radiology, Royal Marsden NHS Foundation Trust, Downs Road, Sutton, Surrey SM2 5PT, UK
* Corresponding author. Rua Antonio de Albuquerque 1021/901, Belo Horizonte 30112-011, Brazil.
E-mail address: costaluciana@ufmg.br

Magn Reson Imaging Clin N Am 21 (2013) 385–408
http://dx.doi.org/10.1016/j.mric.2013.01.006
1064-9689/13/$ – see front matter © 2013 Elsevier Inc. All rights reserved.

Stockholm trials, and this was associated with a survival benefit. More recently, the widespread adoption of TME techniques has reduced the rates of margin involvement in unselected rectal cancers undergoing TME surgery from up to 28% to less than 15% in the last decade.[6,7] Therefore, precise assessment of the distance of tumor to the mesorectal fascia by preoperative staging has become important for distinguishing between patients who will be cured by primary surgery and those who are at high risk for local disease recurrence because of the risk of circumferential margin involvement.[8]

High-resolution magnetic resonance (MR) imaging plays a pivotal role in the pretreatment assessment of the most important risk factors for local recurrence. However, another important role of MR imaging is in the evaluation of low rectal tumors, in which sphincter preservation is a challenge. Assessment of the safety of the TME plane is crucial, because sphincter function may be severely compromised by irradiation, but, on the other hand, perforation of a low rectal cancer during the TME dissection results in local recurrence that could be avoided by preoperative shrinkage of the tumor through radiotherapy. Because the mesorectum significantly tapers toward the top of the anal canal, tumors in this area can easily invade surrounding structures. Therefore careful assessment of the safety of the TME plane by MR imaging is essential. In a selected group of patients, CRT with delayed surgery increases the likelihood of preserving sphincter function, because of a downsizing and downstaging effect of induction therapy on the tumor, leading to improved resectability and local control.[9] Tumor shrinkage as a result of preoperative CRT is now a reality, and pathologically complete responses (CRs) are not uncommon.[10]

The success of this imaging technique depends on obtaining good-quality high-resolution T2-weighted images of the primary tumor, the mesorectal fascia, and mesorectal and pelvic sidewall lymph nodes. MR imaging can predict the CRM with high accuracy and consistency, allowing preoperative identification of patients at risk of recurrence that benefits from preoperative treatment, more extensive surgery, or both. The technique also enables the identification of patients whose disease is optimally treated with primary total mesorectal surgery alone, with preservation of the sphincter complex. Recent studies have shown that it is a reliable and reproducible technique with high specificity (92%) for predicting a negative CRM, the relationship of the tumor to the CRM, and the depth of tumor invasion outside the muscularis propria.[7,11] Furthermore, the MERCURY

(Magnetic Resonance Imaging and Rectal Cancer European Equivalence) trial centers[12] were able to select up to 33% of patients with good prognostic features who could undergo primary surgery without preoperative therapy and without developing local recurrence on long-term follow-up.

There are data indicating that pathologic response after preoperative chemoradiotherapy is a prognostic factor for disease-free survival (DFS) for advanced rectal cancer and magnetic resonance is a valuable tool to evaluate the tumor regression grade (TRG).[13,14] Moreover, there are some observational data that indicate that in patients with clinical CR, surgery may be avoided. Careful follow-up with a wait-and-see approach has produced impressive results, similar to those of radiation therapy for anal carcinoma.[15,16] These studies have used biopsy or excision of the scar to define CR. The potential role of MR imaging in not only identifying patients who are likely to have CR but also in monitoring those patients for tumor regrowth is under investigation in a prospective clinical trial (Deferral of Surgery trial, UKCRN ID 8565, National Cancer Research Institute, UK).

So, with the increasing availability of preoperative therapy and the proven ability of MR imaging to give accurate prognostic information, the radiologists' role in the preoperative multidisciplinary team decision-making process has become critical, because the information provided by the detailed imaging of the primary tumor guides the team to help achieve better outcomes for patients with rectal cancer.

NORMAL ANATOMY

Over the past years, the surgical anatomy of the pelvis has been reevaluated, because there is growing evidence of the benefits related to careful anatomic dissection in rectal cancer surgery. The complete removal of the tumor-containing rectum and its draining nodes as a distinct anatomic package is the essence of TME[5] and has resulted in reduced local recurrence rates.[17]

The rectum is that part of the gastrointestinal tract that extends from the upper end of the anal canal to the rectosigmoid junction and is approximately 15 cm in length. Anatomically, it can be divided into 3 segments: the low, mid, and high rectum. These segments correspond to the first 7 to 10 cm, the next 4 to 5 cm, and the last 4 to 5 cm (measuring from the anal verge), respectively.[18]

The proximal part of the anal canal is characterized by the insertion of the levator ani muscle onto the fibers that form the puborectalis sling. Recognition of the inferior limits of the rectum is important in determining the distance between the tumor and the puborectalis sling, which is crucial for sphincter preservation during surgery. There are some important structures that must be recognized on MR imaging scans: the rectal wall layers, the mesorectum, the mesorectal fascia, the retrorectal space, the rectosacral fascia, the peritoneal reflection, and the Denonvilliers fascia.

In cross section, the rectal wall consists of the mucosal layer, muscularis mucosae, submucosa, and muscularis propria (**Fig.** 1A). Most of the rectum lies below the peritoneal reflection, and so only the upper third is invested by the serosa or peritoneum. On MR imaging, the mucosal layer of the bowel wall is visible as a fine, low-signal-intensity line with the thicker, higher-signal-intensity submucosal layer beneath. The muscularis propria is shown on MR imaging as 2 distinct layers: the inner circular and the outer longitudinal layers. The outer layer has an irregular appearance and some surface interruptions caused by vessels entering the rectal wall, but readily distinguished from tumor by its lower signal intensity on high-resolution T2-weighted images.

The mesorectum is the fatty tissue shown on axial MR imaging as a high-signal-intensity structure that surrounds the rectum and contains lymph nodes, lymphatics, and vessels and is encircled by the mesorectal fascia, which represents the CRM when TME is used as the surgical technique. The mesorectal fascia is a layer encompassing the mesorectum, and it is best seen on axial and coronal MR images, appearing as a low-signal-intensity thin linear structure. It is optimally visualized on high-resolution thin-section MR imaging (see **Fig.** 1B). Benign lymph nodes within the mesorectum are shown as uniform-signal-intensity ovoid structures, with smooth-bordered margins and homogeneous texture. Benign or reactive nodes are predominantly high signal intensity on the T2 sequences, but can also be uniformly low or intermediate signal intensity and can be significantly enlarged despite being benign. Sometimes, a regular chemical shift artifact can be seen in 1 side of it.

The parietal fascia fuses with the sacral periosteum at the level of the sacral promontory and within the pelvis overlies the muscles of the pelvic wall. Anteriorly, this fascia is attached to the body of the pubis. On MR imaging, it appears isointense relative to the muscles and may not always be seen as a separate structure, but it can be clearly seen as a separate layer overlying the pelvic sidewall compartment and between the mesorectal fascia and presacral compartment (**Fig.** 2).

The retrorectal space is situated between the presacral parietal fascia and the mesorectal fascia. The presacral fascia is shown on sagittal MR imaging as a low-signal-intensity thin linear structure overlying the presacral vessels (**Fig.** 3). The mesorectal fascia is seen anterior to this structure, and the potential virtual space between these 2 fascial layers forms the retrorectal space and the plane of dissection in TME surgery.

The rectosacral fascia is a pelvic floor fascial structure of variable thickness, which is shown on sagittal MR imaging as an oblique low-signal-intensity band extending from the junction of the S3 and S4 vertebrae to the posterior wall of the rectum, adjacent to the anal sphincteric complex (**Fig.** 4).

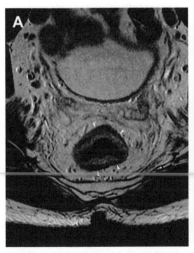 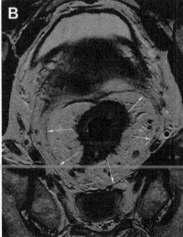

Fig. 1. Rectal wall and mesorectal fascia. Axial high-resolution T2-weighted fast spin-echo sequences showing the rectal wall layers (*A*) Muscularis propria (*white arrowheads*) has low signal intensity. (*B*) Low-signal-intensity mesorectal fascia surrounding the high-signal-intensity mesorectal fat (*white arrows*) and the peritoneal reflection (*red arrow*).

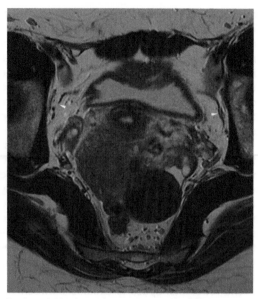

Fig. 2. Axial high-resolution T2-weighted fast spin-echo sequence. Parietal fascia is seen anterolaterally as a thin linear low-intensity layer at the lateral side of the pelvis.

The peritoneal reflection is easily seen on sagittal MR imaging as a low-signal-intensity thin linear structure that extends over the surface of the bladder posteriorly to its point of attachment

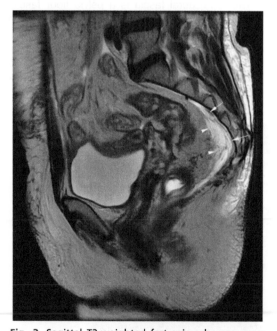

Fig. 3. Sagittal T2-weighted fast spin-echo sequence obtained in a 62-year-old man with a rectal carcinoma treated with chemoradiation shows the posterior fascial layers of the pelvis. Posterior mesorectal fascia (*white arrowheads*) is shown anteriorly and the presacral fascia is shown posteriorly (*white arrows*). There is fluid in the retrorectal space seen between these fascias.

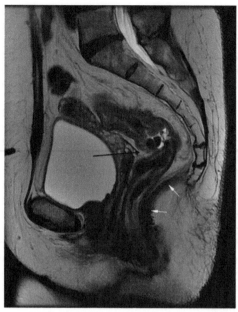

Fig. 4. Sagittal T2-weighted fast spin-echo sequence obtained in a 56-year-old man. Rectosacral fascia is seen as an oblique thick low-signal-intensity band extending posteriorly from the sacrum (S3–S4) to the rectum (*white arrows*). Notice the peritoneal reflection (*black arrow*).

onto the rectum. In men, the attachment site of the peritoneal reflection is the junction of the upper two-thirds and lower one-third of the rectum (see **Fig. 4**). In women, this site of attachment has more anatomic variations. The relationship between the rectal tumor and the peritoneal reflection is important in staging of the rectal cancer, because the tumors with invasion through the peritoneal reflection are categorized as stage T4a.

The Denonvilliers fascia is a well-developed fascia that derives from the urogenital septum during embryonal development. It forms a characteristic anterior surface of the mesorectum, on its lower part, and it is visible on axial MR imaging as a low-signal-intensity layer, adjacent to the prostate in men and as the rectovaginal septum behind the posterior vaginal wall in women (**Fig. 5**). Inferiorly, the septum extends to the perineal body.

IMAGING TECHNIQUE

Before the development of the modern phased-array pelvic surface coil, endorectal coils were the only method of obtaining high-resolution images of pelvic anatomic structures. The use of endorectal coils was limited in rectal cancer assessment, because of near-field artifact and luminal distortions created by the coils in direct

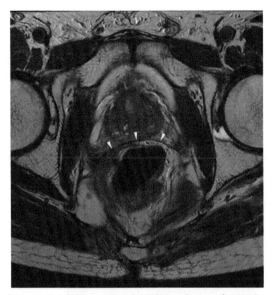

Fig. 5. Axial T2-weighted high-resolution fast spin-echo showing the Denonvilliers fascia (*arrowheads*) posteriorly relative to the prostate gland. TME comprises the rectum surrounded by complete mesorectum fat within an intact mesorectal fascial envelope including Denonvilliers fascia anteriorly. This fascia is seen below the point of attachment of the peritoneal reflection onto the anterior surface of rectum.

contact with the rectal wall. Further problems with endorectal coils, as with any endoluminal techniques such as endoanal ultrasonography, were the inability to evaluate stenosing tumors and to

fully evaluate the entire mesorectal lymph node drainage territory.

The introduction of phased-array coil systems improved staging of rectal cancer, which along with fast spin-echo T2-weighted sequences enabled high-resolution imaging oriented to the relevant surgical anatomic planes. These phased-array surface coils combined with a very high spatial resolution allowed detailed evaluation of the rectal wall and depiction of the surrounding important anatomy.

The technique for acquisition of the sequences has been previously described,[19] and the parameters are shown in **Table 1**.

A 1.5-T system is generally used with phased-array coils, which allow greater coverage of the anatomy when compared with the endorectal coils. The experience with a 3-T system in the high-resolution protocol is still limited, but it is likely that there are few or no benefits with this system for the staging of rectal cancer.[20]

Patients must be fully informed about the length of time required for MR imaging scanning (between 20 and 30 minutes) and must be positioned in the supine position in the scanner. There is no need to use purgative bowel preparation or enemas.[19,21] Antispasmodic agents are used to reduce pelvic small bowel motion. Gadolinium-enhanced T1-weighted imaging and fat saturation are not necessary, because these have not been shown to improve the diagnostic accuracy for staging of rectal cancer.[22]

Table 1
Recommended MR imaging parameters

	Sequence	FOV (mm)	Repetition Time/Echo Time	Slice (mm)	Matrix	NSA	Time (min:s)
Sagittal T2 From one pelvic sidewall to the other	TSE/23	250	3500/125	3 interleaved	304 × 512	4	6:36
Axial T2 Iliac crest to pelvic floor	TSE/22	420	3500/80	5 interleaved	352 × 512	1	1:38 SENSE 2
Axial T2 Perpendicular to the rectum	TSE/16	160	3500/120	3 interleaved	256 × 512	6	5:36
Oblique axial T2 To cover lymph node territory							
Coronal T2 Low tumors parallel to anal canal	TSE/16	160	3500/120	3 interleaved	256 × 512	6	5:36

Abbreviations: NSA, number of signal averages; SENSE, sensitivity encoding for fast MR imaging; TSE, turbo spin-echo.
Data from Brown G, Daniels IR, Richardson C, et al. Techniques and trouble-shooting in high spatial resolution thin slice MRI for rectal cancer. Br J Radiol 2005;78(927):245–51.

Initial localization images in the sagittal planes are needed to plan the high-resolution images (**Fig. 6**A–C). For this reason, the first series to be acquired is a sagittal, 25-cm field-of-view (FOV), 3-mm-thick T2-weighted sequence from 1 pelvic sidewall to the other, which enables identification of the primary tumor. It is essential that the referring surgeon has accurately indicated the tumor position (low, mid, or high rectal) to help proper planning of the sequences. The second series consists of large FOV axial sections (4–5 mm) of the whole pelvis. These first 2 sequences allow an overview of the pelvis and enable the primary tumor to be located with regard to the distance from the anal verge and puborectalis sling, but these are not adequate for T staging or nodal characterization, which are best undertaken using the high-resolution sequences described later.

The high-spatial-resolution sequence comprises a T2-weighted thin axial section (3 mm) through the rectal tumor and adjacent tissues.

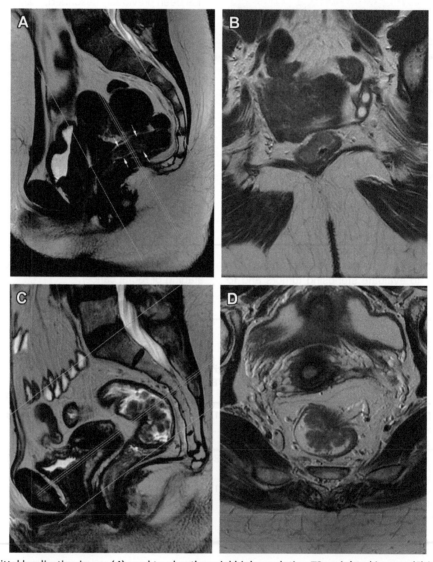

Fig. 6. Sagittal localization image (A) used to plan the axial high-resolution T2-weighted images (B) in a 54-year-old woman with a low-rectum adenocarcinoma (*white arrows in A*). (C, D) Sagittal initial localization image (C) and axial high-resolution T2-weighted images (D) in a 49-year-old woman with a pediculate midrectum mucinous adenocarcinoma. Note that the high-resolution T2-weighted thin-section axial sequence through the rectal tumor is obtained perpendicular to the long axis of the rectum at the level of the tumor (*orange and green lines in A and C*). Note also that the axial sequences must be extended 4 to 5 cm above the superior edge of tumor to make sure to cover the draining nodes and tumor deposits.

These sequences are angled perpendicular to the long axis of the rectum at the level of the tumor, using a 16-cm FOV (see **Fig. 6**B, D). The perpendicular plane is necessary; otherwise, the images may be misinterpreted because of partial volume effects. This sequence must be extended to at least 5 cm above the superior edge of the tumor to ensure coverage of draining nodes and tumor deposits (see **Fig. 6**A, C). Knowledge of the distribution pattern of mesorectal nodes may assist in preoperative radiotherapy planning if the tumor shows high-risk features.

The T2-weighted thin-section coronal sequence is optional for the upper-rectum and midrectum tumor, but mandatory for patients with low rectal cancers. This sequence consists of high-spatial-resolution thin sections (3 mm) parallel to the long axis of the rectum at the level of the tumor and it shows the levator muscles, including the puborectal, and the sphincter complex in relationship to the rectal wall (**Fig. 7**).

The routine use of diffusion-weighted imaging (DWI) is gradually increasing and preliminary data suggest that apparent diffusion coefficient (ADC) values may reflect tumor aggressiveness, but it is not clear whether this provides additional prognostic information compared with conventional T2-weighted high-resolution imaging and whether ADC values could influence treatment decisions.[23] The published data suggest that it is unlikely that the addition of DWI alters staging accuracy because of substantial overlap in ADC values between benign and malignant processes.[23–25]

Water diffusion is a physical process that results from the thermally driven, random motion of water molecules.[26,27] In a glass of water, molecules undergo free, thermally agitated diffusion (with a three-dimensional Gaussian distribution). The width of the Gaussian distribution expands with time, and the average square of this width per unit time gives the units of the ADC. In tissues, apparent diffusion is observed because the movement of water molecules is modified by their interactions with cell membranes and macromolecules in an environment. The restriction to flow of water molecules is determined by tissue cellularity and the integrity of the cell membrane. Tumors typically display restricted diffusion because of their hypercellularity.[28]

In our standard 1.5-T GE Signa HDxt system (General Electric Medical Systems, Milwaukee, WI), we use an 8-channel cardiac coil, with a spin-echo echo planar imaging sequence (repetition time [TR], 4500 milliseconds; echo time [TE], 80 milliseconds; flip angle, 90°; FOV, 280–360 mm; 16 number of averages; slice thickness, 4 mm; interslice gap, 0.4 mm; acquisition matrix, 128 × 100) with bandwidth of 1.953 Hz/pixel, with an imaging time of DWI of 3 minutes 36 seconds for 20 slices, b value (0, 500, 1000 s/mm²), and 3 directions. DWI is performed in the axial plane. The motion-probing gradient pulses are placed in the x-axis,

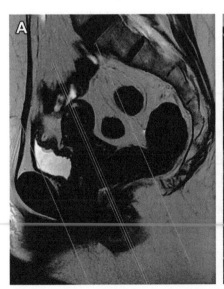
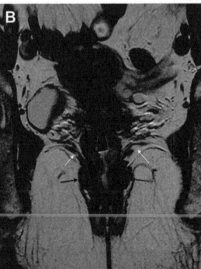

Fig. 7. Sagittal initial localization image (*A*) used to plan the coronal high-resolution thin-section T2-weighted sequences (*B*) in a 61-year-old woman with a low rectal adenocarcinoma extending to the anal canal (*red arrows*). The coronal sequence is parallel to the long axis of the rectum at the level of the tumor (*orange and green lines in A*) and shows the levator muscles (*white arrows*), including the puborectal (*black arrows*), and the sphincter complex in relationship to the rectal wall.

y-axis, and z-axis (all planes). The parameters are shown in **Table 2**.

IMAGING INTERPRETATION
Staging of the Primary Rectal Tumor

The American Joint Committee on Cancer guidelines, seventh edition, defines the criteria for the staging of primary rectal tumors. The process of T staging, T substaging, and N staging is shown in **Table 3**. The T staging is based on the invasion of the primary tumor through the rectal wall and its relationship to the submucosa and muscularis propria. Therefore, the best results for staging rectal cancer have been obtained through careful interpretation of thin-section, high-resolution, and small FOV T2-weighted images obtained perpendicular to the rectal wall.

T Staging

MR imaging should be analyzed by the radiologist assessing the primary rectal tumor in terms of stage; the degree of invasion outside the muscularis propria (extramural extension); and relationship to the mesorectal fascia, anal sphincter, and pelvic sidewall. The radiologist should first describe the height of the tumor, ideally from the anal verge, because this is a useful reference point for the referring surgeon, followed by the length of the tumor. The description of the morphologic appearances of the tumor must be categorized as polypoid, ulcerating, hemicircumferential, or circumferential (**Fig. 8**). On T2-weighted high-resolution images, a nonmucinous tumor is shown as a lesion of intermediate signal intensity with no areas of high signal intensity. Mucinous tumors appear as fluidlike high signal intensity on these T2-weighted images (**Fig. 9**). The following step

is the identification of the invasive portion of the tumor, which is the most worrisome area, corresponding to the most invasive portion of the tumor on the rectal wall and to the site of ulceration of the luminal component, at the same location.

T1 tumors are those in which there is invasion of the submucosa, represented by the identification of abnormal signal intensity replacing the normal submucosa (**Fig. 10**). The best way to distinguish T1 (submucosal invasion only) from T2 tumors (extension to the muscular layer) is to show partial preservation of the high signal intensity of the submucosa layer beneath the intermediate signal intensity of the tumor.

T2 tumors are those with extension into the muscularis propria, where abnormal intermediate signal intensity with partial-thickness or full-thickness involvement can be appreciated, but there is no extension of intermediate signal intensity to the mesorectal fat (**Fig. 11**). T3 tumors manifest as a broad bulge or nodular projection of abnormal intermediate signal intensity extending beyond muscularis propria in the mesorectal fat (**Fig. 12**). We do not recommend interpreting features such as desmoplastic reaction as tumor because this results in overstaging.[21,29] We advocate the use of T3 substaging as clinically more relevant than distinguishing T3 from T4 spread. The T substage takes into account the prognostic importance of depth of extramural spread from the outermost edge of the muscularis propria (extramural tumor extension) and enables recognition that a T3a tumor has an identical prognosis to a T2 tumor. The T3 stratification was originally developed by Hermanek as a modification of the TNM classification according to the following depths of extramural spread: T3a less than 1 mm spread, T3b 1 to 5 mm, T3c greater than 5–15 mm, and T3d greater than

Table 2
Diffusion-weighted imaging sequence parameters (Phillips, Best, The Netherlands; Siemens, Erlangen, Germany; and General Electric platforms, Milwaukee, Wisconsin.)

Parameter	Philips	Siemens	General Electric
FOV (cm)	280	220	280
Matrix size	112 × 256	138 × 256	128 × 100
TR	2500	3100	4500
TE	66	71	80
Parallel imaging factor	2	2	2
Number of signals average	4	8	16
Section thickness (mm)	5	5	4
Direction of motion-probing gradients	3 scan trace	3 scan trace	3 scan trace
Fat suppression	SPAIR	SPAIR	STIR
b factors (s/mm^2)	0,350,750	0,350,750	0,500, 1000

Abbreviations: SPAIR, spectral attenuated inversion recovery; STIR, short-tau inversion recovery.

Table 3
TNM staging of rectal tumors on MR imaging

TNM Stage	Description
Tx	Primary tumor cannot be evaluated
T0	No evidence of invasive primary tumor
T1	Invasion of submucosa by tumor; abnormal signal intensity has replaced part but not all of the submucosa
T2	Invasion but not penetration of muscularis propria; intermediate signal intensity in muscularis propria
T3	Invasion through muscularis propria; broad bulge or nodular projection of intermediate signal intensity extending beyond muscularis propria
a	<1 mm beyond the muscularis propria
b	1–5 mm beyond the muscularis propria
c	>5 and ≤15 mm beyond the muscularis propria
d	>15 mm beyond the muscularis propria
T4	Invasion of other organs
a	Abnormal signal intensity extends into adjacent organs through peritoneal reflection
b	Tumor invades visceral peritoneum
N0	No nodal metastasis
N1	1–3 perirectal or pericolic involved nodes
N2	≥4 perirectal or pericolic involved nodes
Mx	Cannot be assessed
M0	No metastasis
M1	Distant metastasis

15 mm. Both imaging and histopathologic assessment of T3 substage are performed by measuring the extramural tumor extension into the mesorectal fat in millimeters beyond the outermost edge of muscularis propria (see **Table 3**). T4 tumors are distinguished according to invasion of adjacent organs or structures (T4a) or have perforated the peritoneal reflection (T4b) (**Figs. 13** and **14**).

MR imaging is a well-established technique in the staging of advanced rectal cancers. Common sites of local infiltration of adjacent structures should be evaluated when examining advanced local tumors.[21] For mid and upper tumors, anterior invasion can involve the bladder, uterus, or seminal vesicles, as well as the peritoneum; lateral extension can involve the pelvic sidewall; and posterior extension can involve the sacrum. For low tumors, the common sites for stage T4 infiltration are the pelvic floor structures; the anal sphincter; the levator muscles; and the prostate, vagina, and coccyx.

Special attention should be given to lower rectal tumors, because they represent a greater challenge for the colorectal surgeon than the higher-level tumors. The conventional TNM staging systems for colorectal cancers are insufficient in these cases, because they do not account for

the anatomic considerations and the fact that the mesorectal envelope tapers at this level. We propose a special staging system that takes into account the relevant local anatomy, with the aim of providing more information to help the surgeon define the most appropriate plane (**Table 4**).[21,30,31] The margin positivity rate for abdominoperineal excision has been reported to be as much as 30%, compared with 10% for low anterior resections. The concept of the 2 planes for rectal cancer allows the surgeon and radiologist to plot a carefully defined route map for preoperative staging and to plan surgery.[30,32,33]

For the evaluation of the potential CRM involvement, measurements are taken from the outermost radial border of the tumor and its distance to the mesorectal fascia. The same distances must be measured for extramural venous invasion and tumor satellite/deposits (**Box 1**). A potentially positive margin is defined as tumor lying within 1 mm (<1 mm) of the mesorectal fascia.[7,8] Measurements are also taken when lymph nodes show definite features of malignant replacement (mixed signal intensity and extension through the nodal capsule by tumor), extramural vascular invasion, and tumor deposit or satellites may all result in a positive margin if lying within 1 mm of the mesorectal fascia.

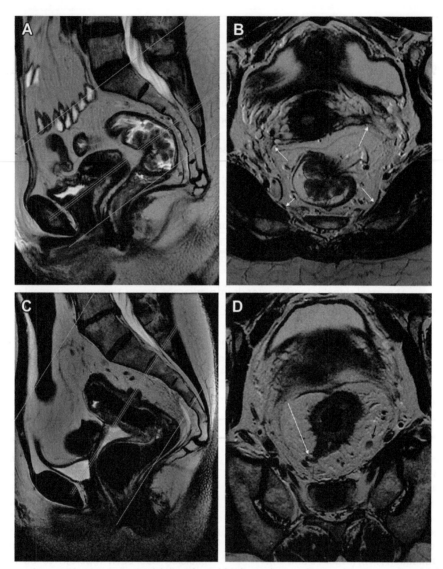

Fig. 8. Same patient as Fig. 6A, B. Sagittal (*A*) and axial high-resolution thin-section T2-weighted (*B*) sequences obtained in a 49-year-old woman with a midrectum adenocarcinoma. Note the stalk seen as a low-signal-intensity linear structure (*black arrowheads in A and B*) and the polypoid morphology appearance of this tumor that protrudes into the rectal lumen. (*C, D*) Sagittal (*C*) and axial T2-weighted (*D*) sequences in a 62-year-old woman with a circumferential rectal tumor. Notice the extramural venous invasion (*white arrow in D*) and a normal lymph node (*black arrow in D*). The red line corresponds to the CRM distance.

This measurement is important for the prevention of local recurrence after TME, because there is strong evidence that neoplastic involvement of the CRM is closely related to a high recurrence rate.[6,8,14,34] However, lymph nodes are a rare cause of circumferential margin involvement and a cause of margin involvement in only 1% to 2% of resected specimens, therefore defining a margin as involved must be based only on the clear evidence of a node with definite malignant features (mixed signal and irregularity of the nodal border).[35]

Extramural vascular invasion is an important and independent prognostic feature that can be readily identified on MR imaging.[36,37] It is defined by the presence of tumor itself beyond the muscularis propria, within the vessels, which are visualized as signal flow-void tubular structures on T2-weighted spin-echo sequences lying perpendicular to the rectal wall. Tumor invasion of the vessels is seen as irregular expansion of the extramural vessels by intermediate tumor signal intensity (**Fig. 15**).

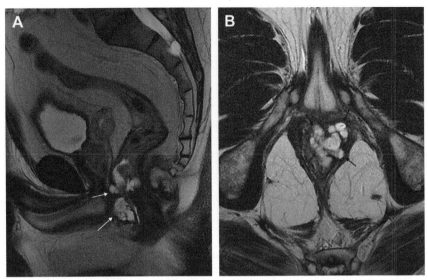

Fig. 9. Sagittal (*A*) and axial thin-section (*B*) T2-weighted fast spin-echo sequences obtained in a 47-year-old man with a mucinous low rectal adenocarcinoma that appears as high-signal-intensity fluidlike signal on these images. Notice that the tumor disrupts the inferior plane (*black arrows*) and that the anterior plane is not safe (*white arrows*).

For the prediction of T3 substage and high-risk features such as increasing depth of spread, venous invasion, and CRM infiltration, MR imaging is a highly accurate and reliable technique and represents a noninvasive tool for identifying those patients who are likely to benefit from neoadjuvant preoperative CRT as well as those who could safely undergo primary surgery TME without preoperative therapy.

N Staging

The next step is the evaluation of mesorectal and lateral pelvic sidewall lymph nodes. In TNM staging, 1 to 3 nodes are considered N1 and 4 or more are considered N2. In the past, radiologists have traditionally relied on measurements of nodal size for defining positive or negative nodes. However, when correlated to matched pathologic material, lymph node size criteria evaluation has

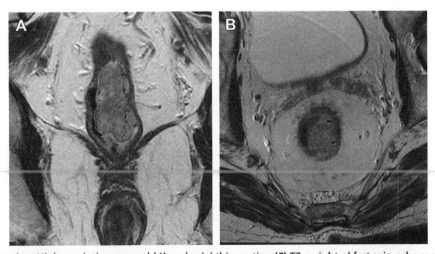

Fig. 10. T staging. High-resolution coronal (*A*) and axial thin-section (*B*) T2-weighted fast spin-echo sequences obtained in a 58-year-old man with rectal cancer show a T1 polypoid tumor (*white line drawing*) that has effaced submucosal layer, but the muscularis propria (*arrowhead in A and B*) beneath it is preserved. Black arrows show the stalk.

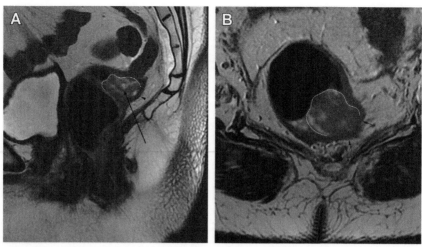

Fig. 11. T2 tumor. Sagittal (*A*) and axial high-resolution thin-section (*B*) T2-weighted fast spin-echo images in a 72-year-old woman with midrectal cancer show a polypoid lesion (*white line drawing in A and B*) that extends into the muscularis propria (*arrowhead in A and arrows in B*) with partial-thickness involvement, but there is no extension to the mesorectal fat. Notice that this tumor contains some mucin (*black arrow in A*).

been proved to be unreliable.[38,39] We therefore do not recommend evaluating lymph nodes by measuring size, because there is substantial overlap related to enlarged benign reactive nodes. Moreover, metastatic disease is frequently observed in nodes less than 5 mm in diameter. Brown and colleagues[38] mapped individual nodes harvested on pathology to the in vivo counterparts and reported that uniform smooth-bordered nodes with homogeneous signal intensity were nearly always benign. The presence of irregular borders or mixed signal intensity strongly correlated with node positivity, with an overall accuracy of 85% when tested prospectively using a high-resolution technique (**Fig. 16**).[39] Kim and colleagues[40] later confirmed these observations from a retrospective series and noted that the presence of a mottled heterogenic pattern was associated with 50% sensitivity and 95% specificity for malignant involvement. Their study also confirmed the relevance of spiculated or indistinct borders, with sensitivities of 45% and 36%, and specificities of 100% and 100%, respectively.

The clinical significance and management of involved pelvic sidewall lymph nodes in rectal cancer remains controversial. The MERCURY study group evaluated 325 patients and found that 38 had suspicious pelvic sidewall nodes

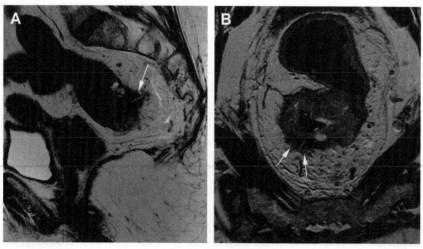

Fig. 12. T3 tumor. (*A, B*) T2-weighted sagittal (*A*) and oblique axial (*B*) images showing annular stage T3c tumor. Note 8 mm of extension (*red line*) beyond outer muscle coat (*white arrows in A and B*).

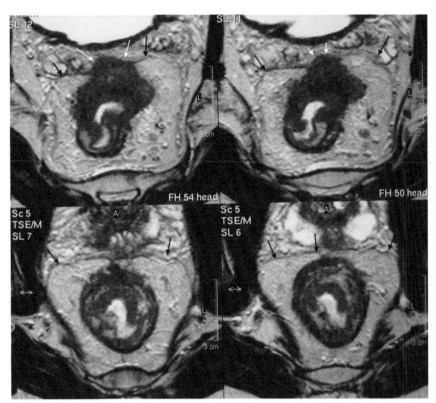

Fig. 13. T4 tumor. Axial high-resolution thin-section T2-weighted fast spin-echo images in an 82-year-old man with midrectal cancer show perforation and invasion through the peritoneal reflection (*white arrows*). The black arrows show the mesorectal fascia.

identified on baseline scans.[41] After a minimum of 5-year follow-up, these investigators found that MR imaging-suspected nodal pelvic involvement was associated with a worse 5-year overall survival (OS) and DFS for patients undergoing primary surgery, without preoperative therapy. However, among patients who received preoperative radiotherapy, the presence of MR imaging-suspected pelvic sidewall lymph nodes did not negatively affect survival. There were also strong associations between mesorectal nodal involvement detected by MR imaging and other adverse features such as extramural venous invasion, suggesting that suspicious pelvic sidewall nodes on MR imaging represented a more advanced disease state. MR imaging detection of nodal

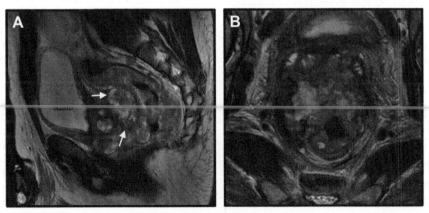

Fig. 14. T4b tumor. Sagittal (*A*) and axial (*B*) T2-weighted sequences showing a huge mucinous tumor invading the prostate gland (*white arrows in A*). In (*B*), black arrows show the mucin pools.

Table 4
Stages of low rectal tumors on MR imaging
Stage 1	Tumor confined to bowel wall but does not extend through full thickness; intact outer muscle coat
Stage 2	Tumor replaces muscle coat but does not extend into intersphincteric plane
Stage 3	Tumor invades intersphincteric plane or lies within 1 mm of levator muscle
Stage 4	Tumor invades external anal sphincter and is within 1 mm and beyond levators with or without invading adjacent organs signal intensity in muscularis propria

Data from Taylor FG, Swift RI, Blomqvist L, et al. A systematic approach to the interpretation of preoperative staging MRI for rectal cancer. AJR Am J Roentgenol 2008;191(6):1827–35.

disease in the pelvic sidewall compartment is therefore an adverse feature but does not seem to be independently prognostic for patient survival (**Fig. 17**).

Prognostic Factors Depicted by MR Imaging

The prospectively conducted MERCURY study of consecutive patients who have rectal cancer enabled validation of the MR imaging staging factors against the risks of local recurrence, distant failure, or both (**Box 2**). Based on these outcome data, the next generation of clinical trials is being designed to specifically address those risks, for example, the use of neoadjuvant therapy for patients who are at risk of distant metastases rather than local recurrence (**Fig. 18**).

POSTTREATMENT EVALUATION: HOW CAN MR IMAGING RESTAGE RECTAL CANCER AFTER CRT?

The standard treatment of advanced colorectal cancer includes performing neoadjuvant long-course CRT to downstage the tumor, followed by TME surgery, which have reduced local recurrence and improved rates of curative resection.[9,42] Assessment of treatment efficacy has principally relied on histopathologic evaluation of irradiated specimens after TME. These studies have shown that posttreatment pathologic T and N stage (ypT and ypN, respectively, where y represents postradiation therapy specimens and p pathologic

staging) can predict local recurrence, DFS, and OS, and several studies have shown that they are independent prognostic factors. Some retrospective studies have shown that complete pathologic response after preoperative CRT followed by definitive surgical resection for advanced rectal cancer resulted in decreased recurrence and improved DFS.[43] Tumor downstaging has been regarded as a marker for tumor radiosensitivity.

MR Imaging Technique

The MR imaging technique used for the posttreatment assessment must be the same as the one used in the pretreatment evaluation. T2 high-resolution images are recommended to distinguish tumor from fibrosis for accurate MR TRG staging. Comparison with pretreatment images is essential. Images should be acquired using the same angles as those used in the pretreatment scans to enable comparison, and pretreatment images are used to help locate the treated tumor, which may be difficult to visualize in patients who have had a good therapeutic response.

DWI on the Postneoadjuvant Treatment Evaluation

As described earlier, DWI is a functional MR imaging technique that uses differences in the extracellular movement of water protons to discriminate between tissues of varying cellularity. In tissues with normal cellularity, water protons can diffuse relatively freely, which results in a loss of signal on DWI. Conversely, in tissues with increased cellularity (tumor), diffusion of water is restricted, resulting in persistent high signal on DWI. DWI has been proposed as a means of predicting the response to treatment. Barbaro and colleagues,[44] in a prospective study of 62 consecutive patients, assessed the value of ADCs obtained from MR imaging before and after CRT for rectal cancer as treatment response predictors and found that low pretreatment ADCs of less than 1.0×10^{-3} mm^2/s correlated with poor TRG

Box 1
Distances to be obtained in relationship to mesorectal fascia (ie, potential MR imaging CRM, outer margin [mrCRM])
Main tumor to mrCRM
T3 substage suspicious lymph node to mrCRM
Extramural venous invasion to mrCRM
Tumor satellite/deposit to mrCRM

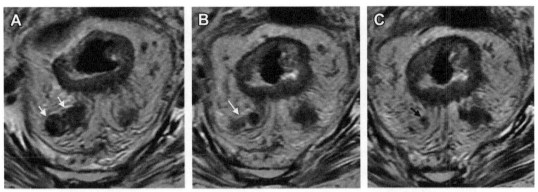

Fig. 15. Extramural venous invasion. 45-year-old woman with rectal cancer. Axial high-resolution T2-weighted images showing extramural venous invasion (*white arrows in A and B*) seen as irregular expansion of the extramural vessels with tissue with the same intermediate signal as the primary tumor. (*C*) The vessel returned to its normal diameter and the normal flow void is seen (*black arrow*).

scores. These investigators also observed that during treatment, the preoperative ADCs as well as the mean percentage of increase in tumor ADC was significantly greater in the responders than in the nonresponders. They showed that a preoperative ADC of 1.4×10^{-3} mm^2/s or greater had a positive and negative predictive value of 78.9% and 61.8%, respectively, to indicate therapeutic response.[44] On the other hand, Curvo-Semedo and colleagues[45] failed to show a relationship between pre-CRT ADC, post-CRT ADC, or ΔADC measurements that could be used to differentiate between patients with a CR and residual tumor. Radiation-induced proctitis and fibrosis were significant and independent predictors of diffusion restriction in patients achieving pathologic CR after treatment with neoadjuvant CRT for locally advanced rectal cancer, and pre-CRT tumor volume was observed to affect both variables.[24] Overall, many results regarding

DWI and ADC have been conflicting, and further work is necessary to validate the final impact of DWI on the management of patients undergoing chemoradiotherapy treatment.

MR Imaging Interpretation After CRT

On post-CRT T2-weighted MR imaging, areas of fibrosis appear as very low signal intensity, whereas areas of residual tumor have intermediate signal, similar to the baseline scans. Careful review of the high-resolution images enables identification of small foci of intermediate-signal-intensity viable tumor, within the fibrosis. Some tumors develop a colloid response with mucin production, which is shown on T2-weighted images as very-high-signal-intensity pools. The recommended evaluation of the MR imaging after CRT is described in **Box 3**. The use of a standardized approach for pathologic evaluation must be

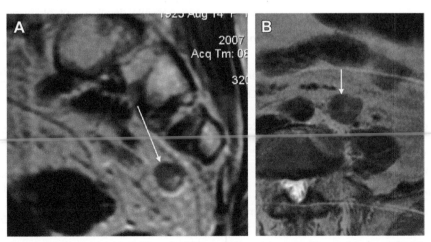

Fig. 16. Lymph node involvement. (*A, B*) 59-year-old man with rectal cancer. T2-weighted sagittal (*A*) and axial (*B*) images show obviously malignant nodes (*white arrows*) with irregular borders and mixed signal intensity.

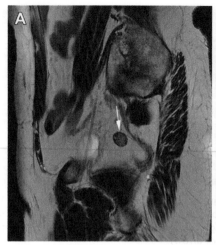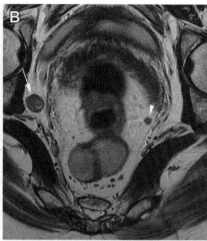

Fig. 17. Pelvic sidewall lymph node involvement. (*A, B*) 43-year-old patient, with T3d stage rectal cancer. Sagittal (*A*) and axial (*B*) images depicted irregular margins and a mottled heterogenic pattern (*white arrows in A and B*) in the right pelvic sidewall. (*B*) The arrowhead shows a small 4 mm malignant mesorectal node with irregular margins and mixed texture.

implemented to allow comparison between the results of various treatment approaches. As a consequence, reassessment of MR imaging scans after preoperative therapy has implications for surgical planning, timing of surgery, sphincter preservation, deferral of surgery for good responders, and development of further preoperative treatments for radiologically identified poor responders. Up to 24% of patients undergoing this treatment have pathologic CR in the final specimen. MR imaging is being investigated in a prospective trial not only as a means of identifying patients with a potential CR but also for monitoring continued tumor regression using serial MR follow-up imaging. In the clinical setting, the subgroup of patients with unfavorable post-treatment MR imaging parameters seem to be at

a higher risk of local or systemic recurrence after a standard TME resection. The surgeon may be warned of this risk preoperatively, and an extended dissection may need to be performed to avoid a potentially involved CRM. In future studies, this group could be considered for further therapy such as intensified or extended systemic chemotherapy, a radiotherapy boost, extension of the surgical resection, or more intensive postoperative follow-up.[46]

Histopathologic Tumor Grade Response

The use of preoperative CRT modifies the macro and microscopic aspects of the tumor appearance of rectal cancer. The features of treated tumors include marked fibrosis with or without replacement of neoplastic cells by inflammatory cells, and possible development of mucin production pools.

Histopathologists grade tumor response in 3 ways: first, assessment of the status of the CRM, followed by the evaluation of the depth of tumor spread and nodal status (ypT and ypN stage), and then, by evaluating TRG. TRG analysis may be considered a useful predictor of outcome in addition to T stage. T staging has limitations because it cannot always adequately show the extension of tumor regression (**Box 4**). For example, a tumor may regress so much that only a few viable tumor cells remain outside the rectal wall, so assigning pT3 status may not, on its own, fully reflect the true extent of tumor regression.

TRG as a measurement of response to neoadjuvant therapy was first described by Mandard and colleagues[47] in 1994, in esophageal carcinomas

---

Box 2

MR imaging validated prognostic factors for recurrence

MR imaging factors predicting local recurrence

Distance to the mesorectal fascia/potential CRM less than 1 mm

Low tumor extending into the intersphincteric plane or beyond (TME mesorectal plane of dissection is unsafe)

Peritoneal involvement

Factors predicting distant failure

Extramural tumor spread greater than 5 mm

Extramural venous invasion

Poor TRG

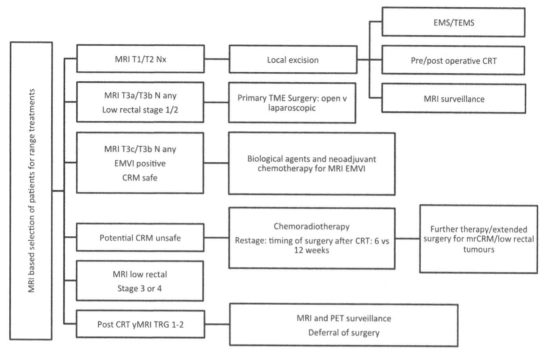

Fig. 18. An example of MR imaging evaluation being used to tailor treatment of patients in current international clinical trials of preoperative treatments. EMVI, extramural venous invasion; TEMS, transanal endoscopic microsurgery.

on a scale from 1 to 5 based on the presence of residual viable tumor cells and the extent of fibrosis. The Mandard modified grading, used for the evaluation of post-CRT rectal cancer, is defined as follows: grade 1 is the absence of residual tumor and fibrosis extending through the different layers of the rectal wall; grade 2 is defined by the presence of rare residual tumor cells scattered throughout the fibrosis; grade 3 is characterized by an increase in the number of residual viable tumor cells, but the fibrosis still predominates; grade 4 shows residual tumor outgrowing the fibrosis; and grade 5 is characterized by absence of any tumor regression.[13]

How to Assess Tumor Response Using MR Imaging

Imaging methods for assessing response after oncologic therapies continue to evolve. Although morphologic evaluation is the standard of reference, the added value of diffusion-weighted MR techniques is being evaluated. Histopathologic

---

Box 3
MR imaging evaluation after CRT

Description of the morphologic appearances of tumor, including any mucinous or necrotic components

Height of treated tumor from the anal verge compared with baseline pretreatment images

Length of treated tumor from the anal verge compared with baseline pretreatment images

MR imaging T stage and T substage, taking into account the depth of extramural spread

MR imaging TRG

Distance to the potential CRM and whether this appears potentially involved or clear

Presence of extramural venous invasion

Mesorectal and pelvic sidewall lymph node staging

Data from Patel UB, Taylor F, Blomqvist L, et al. Magnetic resonance imaging-detected tumor response for locally advanced rectal cancer predicts survival outcomes: MERCURY experience. J Clin Oncol 2011;29(28):3753–60.

Box 4
Histopathologic evaluation of tumor response

Assessment of the status of the CRM

Evaluation of the depth of tumor spread and nodal status (ypT and ypN stage)

Measurement of the extent of extramural spread beyond the muscularis propria

Evaluation of TRG

results and survival outcomes are always the standard of reference and validation, respectively. Various studies reported that MR imaging can be accurately used to evaluate CRT, and several different methods have been proposed for assessing response on MR imaging.[48,49]

These methods include posttreatment MR imaging T staging (ymrT [T stage on MR images obtained after CRT]), MR imaging-based tumor regression grading (mrTRG), volume reduction between baseline and after treatment, and modified Response Evaluation Criteria in Solid Tumors (mRECIST)[50] measurement (**Box 5**).

T Staging After CRT

ymrT (T stage on MR images obtained after CRT) is based on the interpretation of local extent of persistent tumor signal intensity relative to the layers of bowel wall on axial high-resolution T2-weighted images. Tumor response is represented by the replacement of tumor signal by low-signal-intensity fibrosis or the development of high-signal-intensity mucin pools; such areas are not considered to be tumor, and T stage is based on defining the extent of residual intermediate-signal-intensity tumor signal on high-resolution T2-weighted scans.

MR Imaging TRG Analysis

MR imaging TRG is based on principles similar to the pathologic TRG system originally described by Mandard and Dworak, and the degree of tumor replacement by fibrotic stroma is determined.[14,21,47,51,52] This is the most important method for evaluating tumor response. The MERCURY study group[14] has shown that it has been possible to develop an MR imaging-based tumor regression grading (mrTRG) system by applying the principles of histopathology TRG (**Table 5**). The tumor is assessed to determine if it is fibrous or if tumor signal intensity predominates. For this evaluation, a comparison between

the post-CRT and the baseline axial high-resolution images is necessary to determine the proportion of tumor that has become of low signal intensity, representing fibrosis, and the proportion that remains with intermediate signal intensity, representing viable tumor.

MR Imaging Volumetric Analysis

Maximal height is measured on a sagittal section, and transverse maximum diameters are assessed on axial slices. Tumor volume is obtained by multiplying tumor length, width, and height, and the percentage of volume reduction is calculated. Another way to calculate volume is to outline the tumors on a work station. The baseline scans are compared with the post-CRT scans.

MR Imaging mRECIST

Although RECIST criteria is considered a powerful method of evaluating response, inconsistencies arise in measuring geometrically irregular tumors, such as rectal cancers. Because measurement of multilobulated tumors cannot be reproduced, interobserver variability may be unacceptably high.[44] Maximum tumor length is best measured on sagittal images before and after treatment. CR is defined as complete disappearance of tumor. Partial response to treatment is defined as at least a 30% decrease in tumor length, taking as reference the baseline tumor length. Progression of the disease is defined as at least a 20% increase in tumor length, and stable disease is defined as neither sufficient shrinkage to qualify for partial response nor sufficient increase to qualify for progression of the disease.

This method has the major limitation of not taking into account extramural shrinkage or progression, which may be of greater prognostic or clinical relevance.

Patel and colleagues[49] compared the various methods of identifying good versus poor responders with the histopathologic standards of T stage (ypT) and tumor regression grading (TRG) and concluded that favorable and unfavorable histopathology were predicted by both ymrT and mrTRG, and therefore recommended these as optimal parameters for posttreatment assessment of rectal cancers treated with CRT.

WHAT DOES THE PHYSICIAN NEEDS TO KNOW?
The Surgeon's View

With the evolution of surgical techniques (TME) and the shift to neoadjuvant CRT in advanced rectal cancers, high-resolution MR plays a pivotal

---

> **Box 5**
> **Imaging methods for the assessment of chemoradiation or radiation therapies**
>
> Posttreatment MR imaging T staging
>
> MR imaging-based tumor regression grading (mrTRG)
>
> Volume reduction between baseline and after treatment
>
> Modified Response Evaluation Criteria in Solid Tumors (mRECIST) measurement

Table 5
TRG of rectal tumor on MR imaging

Grade	Response	
Grade 1	Complete radiologic response	No evidence of tumor signal intensity or fibrosis only
Grade 2	Good response	Dense hypointense fibrosis, minimal residual tumor
Grade 3	Moderate response	Mixed fibrosis/mucin and intermediate signal representing residual tumor, but fibrosis still predominates
Grade 4	Slight response	Minimal fibrosis/mucinous degeneration, tumor predominates
Grade 5	No response	Tumor has the same appearance as baseline

Data from Patel UB, Taylor F, Blomqvist L, et al. Magnetic resonance imaging-detected tumor response for locally advanced rectal cancer predicts survival outcomes: MERCURY experience. J Clin Oncol 2011;29(28):3753–60.

role for the surgeon. In the setting of primary rectal tumors, MR imaging is used to stage and identify patients at risk of recurrence who may benefit from preoperative CRT, more extensive surgery, or both.

A surgeon dealing with rectal cancers initially wants to differentiate between rectal tumors confined within the rectal wall and those that extend beyond the muscularis propria. The depth of invasion outside the muscularis propria must be assessed, because it has a prognostic value. Radiation therapy produces little survival benefit and results in significant morbidity when used to treat stage T1 to T2 or favorable-risk early-stage T3a/T3b tumors (<5 mm invasion outside the muscularis propria, MR extramural venous invasion [EMVI] negative, and mrCRM negative). However, radiation therapy has an important role in more advanced-stage T3c/T3d tumors (>5 mm invasion outside the muscularis propria), in which the risk of local and distant treatment failure increases.

The prognostic heterogeneity of stage T3 tumors is well known. The MERCURY study group reported that the mean difference between the MR-derived and histopathologically derived maximal extramural depth of the tumor was −0.05 mm ± 3.85 mm, so MR and histopathologic assessments of tumor spread were considered equivalent. Therefore, the ability of MR imaging to accurately separate patients according to prognostic risk by depth of spread is robust.[11]

Another important point is the relationship of the tumor to the potential CRM. Incomplete surgical removal of the circumferential tumor spread is believed to be the main cause of local recurrence after resection of rectal cancer. Several studies have shown that MR imaging is a consistent and reproducible technique, with high specificity (92%) for predicting a negative CRM.[7,8,53] High-resolution MR imaging with a phased-array coil

accurately predicted the distance from the tumor to the circumferential mesorectal plane of resection. A tumor-free margin measured on MR imaging of at least 1 mm can predict a histologic free margin with a high degree of certainty. The MR imaging prediction of the tumor-free margin is therefore reliable.

In relationship to the nodal staging, it is important to know which patients need to receive CRT and to map local nodal spread within and beyond the mesorectum. Although histopathologic nodal disease is an independent poor prognostic factor in patients with rectal cancer, and adversely affects survival, this does not hold true for MR imaging assessment.

Evaluation of local depth of spread, presence or absence of EMVI and CRM status using MR imaging have been shown to be more important and more easily reproducible than MR imaging assessment of nodal status. Furthermore, encapsulated lymph nodes are a rare cause of circumferential margin involvement occurring in only 1.3% of patients compared with direct tumor spread or tumor nodules as a cause of CRM involvement.

In surgical planning, the ability to consistently define a safe plane for both the radial and distal mesorectal dissection is desirable to ensure complete tumor and nodal clearance at surgery, thus reducing the risk of local pelvic recurrence. High-spatial-resolution MR imaging has proved useful in showing local tumor extent, particularly in relation to the mesorectal fascia.[7,11] Areas at risk of involvement after resection must be described in detail by the radiologist; important examples are the peritoneal reflection, rectosacral fascia, and presacral fascia.

Another important topic for the surgeon is low rectal cancer. The relation of the tumor to the sphincter complex and the ability to achieve clear radial and distal margins is key to the success of the operation. MR imaging can help the surgeon predetermine the planes of surgical excision, because the worst outcomes related to tumor perforation and margin positivity rates have been observed when the surgeon has committed to the mesorectal plane of surgery for the distal TME dissection instead of approaching the dissection in the extralevator plane at the outset. Preoperative MR imaging planning can prevent this situation. Various studies, including the MERCURY study, Dutch TME trial, the MRC CLASICC, and Leeds studies have shown that low rectal cancer treated with TME plane surgery with abdominoperineal excision resulted in surgical wasting and ensuing perforation of the tumors around the level of the puborectalis sling. These tumors were always more locally advanced than similar-height tumors undergoing anterior resection and had a worse outcome, as measured by margin involvement and perforation rates.[54–59] Therefore, accurate staging is required to determine the need for neoadjuvant therapy or an enhanced surgical procedure such as extralevator abdominoperineal excision or anteriorly enhanced abdominoperineal excision surgery (**Fig. 19**). It is therefore important to give a detailed description of the radial extent of the tumor to the mesorectal plane and intersphincteric plane by careful assessment of the sagittal, axial, and coronal images. The radiologist needs to give detailed information to the surgeon regarding the potential surgical planes available for resection that enable clear margins.

After CRT, the radiologist must evaluate tumor response to CRT, the T staging and substaging, N staging and CRM status, by measuring the distance between the CRM and the tumor. The extent of tumor regression carries prognostic significance and is related to OS and DFS.

The Radiation Oncologist's View

After the diagnosis of advanced rectal cancer, it is important to show the radiation oncologist the planning volumes for radiation therapy. A clear description of the tumor height and its relationship to the anal verge, puborectalis sling, and promontory is desirable, as is the distribution of nodal involvement.

Modern three-dimensional radiotherapy is based on CT. For rectal cancer, this therapy relies on target definition on CT, which is not the optimal imaging modality. The major limitation of CT is its low inherent contrast resolution. Targets defined by MR imaging could facilitate more accurate definition of tumor volumes than CT. O'Neill and colleagues[60] reported that tumor volumes defined on MR imaging were smaller, shorter, and further from the anal sphincter than CT-based volumes. This finding is relevant because sphincter/pelvic floor dysfunction is one of the predominant dose-limiting causes of toxicity for low-lying rectal tumors, and sphincter dysfunction is both dose and volume dependent. This situation remains a major challenge for patients and clinicians, but radiotherapy planning may result in smaller

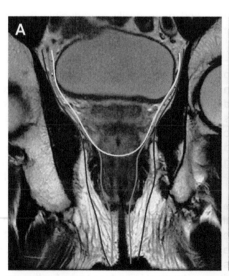
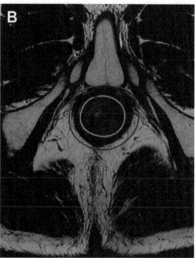

Fig. 19. T2-weighted axial (*A*) and coronal (*B*) high-resolution images of a 52-year-old man with a low rectal tumor. These images show the potential planes of surgical excision: TME anterior resection (*yellow line*), enhanced abdominoperineal excision (*yellow line*), intersphincteric abdominoperineal/ultralow anterior resection (*blue line*).

treatment volumes, which could lead to a reduction in dose to organs at risk and facilitate dose escalation.

It is increasingly becoming a common practice to use MR imaging in radiotherapy treatment planning for target volume delineation, because commercial radiotherapy treatment planning systems are capable of performing image registration or fusion between images acquired. The advantage of MR imaging compared with CT is its superior ability to discriminate soft tissues. This improved accuracy could lead to better tumor control as well as sparing of normal tissues. The target contours must include the rectal tumor itself and the MR imaging-based mesorectal and lateral sidewall lymph nodes with malignant involvement.

The Medical Oncologist's View

Preoperative identification of metastatic disease is of great value. Patients with synchronous metastatic disease may be submitted to different treatment pathways, which include different regimes of neoadjuvant chemotherapy, synchronous metastasectomy, and even metastasectomy before resection of the primary tumor.

For the medical oncologist, the prognostic factors are of significant importance.

The following are defined as MR imaging good prognosis:

- CRM clear on preoperative (tumor >1 mm to the mesorectal fascia)[7,11]
- No evidence of extramural venous invasion[36]
- Early MR imaging T stage (T2 or less, T3a, T3b) regardless of N stage[12,61]
- For low rectal tumors, good prognosis was defined as MR imaging stage 1 or 2 low rectal, namely tumor not encroaching into the intersphincteric plane or levators[56]

These prognostic factors are being reevaluated in many centers in terms of the best selection of patients who should receive preoperative CRT. There is a common use, in many centers, of routine neoadjuvant CRT for all T3 tumors; however, Taylor and colleagues,[12] in a multicenter study, reported that preoperative MR imaging could select patients with rectal cancer who have a good prognosis, which, with optimal preoperative selection and good-quality TME surgery, could achieve local recurrence rates of 1.7% in MR imaging-defined T3a/b regardless of nodal status.

MR imaging in identification of poor prognostic factors in rectal cancer is important.[11,36,40] However, the implications for preoperative staging and management have not been fully determined and are under evaluation in large multicenter phase 2 and phase 3 trials. Hunter and colleagues[62] studied 236 patients and, from the MR imaging identification of depth of spread, extramural venous invasion, and CRM status, hypothesized that these risk factors would be linked with a higher risk of developing synchronous metastatic disease. They found that when MR imaging identified high-risk patients (extramural venous invasion, >5 mm extramural invasion, involved CRM, or intersphincteric plane involved by tumor in low rectal tumors) a higher rate of synchronous metastatic disease was shown (20.7% in the high-risk group vs 4.2% in the low-risk group; odds ratio 6.0). It is hypothesized that more intensive preoperative investigation on initial staging, including fluorodeoxyglucose-positron emission tomography/computed tomography and liver MR imaging may improve outcomes, because of earlier selection of patients requiring chemotherapy and metastasectomy. More trials are needed to confirm the possibility of using induction neoadjuvant chemotherapy and the benefit of new regimes in MR imaging to identify high-risk patients.

SUMMARY

The introduction of MR imaging has helped in identifying prognostic staging information in patients diagnosed with rectal tumors. Rectal cancer staging is based on defining pertinent anatomy of the rectum and the surrounding structures. The primary goal of imaging methods is to accurately stage rectal cancer and to identify risk factors for local recurrence to offer a tailored treatment, based on individual prognosis. High-resolution T2-weighted imaging is the most important sequence in the MR imaging evaluation of rectal tumors, giving the opportunity to differentiate between tumors confined to the rectal wall and those that extend beyond the muscularis propria. The validated high-risk factors identifiable using MR imaging that are related to poor prognosis are: stage T3c or more, mesorectal fascia involvement, extramural venous invasion, and low rectal tumors. By definition, if a rectal tumor lies within 1 mm of the mesorectal fascia on high-resolution MR imaging scans, the surgical margin is deemed to be involved. No imaging modality is sufficiently reliable for determining the nodal status to plan treatments solely based on the presence or absence of nodes, and it is therefore advocated that more reliable measures such as extramural spread, venous invasion, and CRM status are used to guide treatment decisions.

Restaging locally advanced rectal cancer after neoadjuvant treatment is becoming relevant, and patients who achieve good response have a favorable prognosis. Some investigations are now focused on conservative management of rectal cancer, increasing the demand for radiologic evaluation of response to chemoradiation to distinguish responding from nonresponding tumors. DWI seems to be a promising tool for facilitating predictions and monitoring the response to CRT for rectal cancer.

MR imaging of the rectum has emerged as the first-line imaging tool for multidisciplinary team decisions.

REFERENCES

1. Siegel R, Naishadham D, Jemal A. Cancer statistics, 2013. CA Cancer J Clin 2013;63:11–30.
2. Ferlay J, Shin HR, Bray F, et al. Estimates of worldwide burden of cancer in 2008: GLOBOCAN 2008. Int J Cancer 2010;127(12):2893–917.
3. Center MM, Jemal A, Smith RA, et al. Worldwide variations in colorectal cancer. CA Cancer J Clin 2009;59(6):366–78.
4. Nagtegaal ID, Quirke P. What is the role for the circumferential margin in the modern treatment of rectal cancer? J Clin Oncol 2008;26(2):303–12.
5. Heald RJ, Ryall RD. Recurrence and survival after total mesorectal excision for rectal cancer. Lancet 1986;1(8496):1479–82.
6. Quirke P, Durdey P, Dixon MF, et al. Local recurrence of rectal adenocarcinoma due to inadequate surgical resection: histopathological study of lateral tumour spread and surgical excision. Lancet 1986;2(8514):996–9.
7. MERCURY Study Group. Diagnostic accuracy of preoperative magnetic resonance imaging in predicting curative resection of rectal cancer: prospective observational study. BMJ 2006;333(7572):779.
8. Taylor FG, Quirke P, Heald RJ, et al. One millimetre is the safe cut-off for magnetic resonance imaging prediction of surgical margin status in rectal cancer. Br J Surg 2011;98(6):872–9.
9. Sauer R, Becker H, Hohenberger W, et al. Preoperative versus postoperative chemoradiotherapy for rectal cancer. N Engl J Med 2004;351(17):1731–40.
10. Hiotis SP, Weber SM, Cohen AM, et al. Assessing the predictive value of clinical complete response to neoadjuvant therapy for rectal cancer: an analysis of 488 patients. J Am Coll Surg 2002;194(2):131–5 [discussion: 135–6].
11. MERCURY Study Group. Extramural depth of tumor invasion at thin-section MR in patients with rectal cancer: results of the MERCURY study. Radiology 2007;243(1):132–9.
12. Taylor FG, Quirke P, Heald RJ, et al. Preoperative high-resolution magnetic resonance imaging can identify good prognosis stage I, II, and III rectal cancer

best managed by surgery alone: a prospective, multi-center, European study that recruited consecutive patients with rectal cancer. Ann Surg 2011;253(4):711–9.
13. Bouzourene H, Bosman FT, Seelentag W, et al. Importance of tumor regression assessment in predicting the outcome in patients with locally advanced rectal carcinoma who are treated with preoperative radiotherapy. Cancer 2002;94(4):1121–30.
14. Patel UB, Taylor F, Blomqvist L, et al. Magnetic resonance imaging-detected tumor response for locally advanced rectal cancer predicts survival outcomes: MERCURY experience. J Clin Oncol 2011;29(28):3753–60.
15. Habr-Gama A, Perez RO, Nadalin W, et al. Operative versus nonoperative treatment for stage 0 distal rectal cancer following chemoradiation therapy: long-term results. Ann Surg 2004;240(4):711–7 [discussion: 717–8].
16. Maas M, Beets-Tan RG, Lambregts DM, et al. Wait-and-see policy for clinical complete responders after chemoradiation for rectal cancer. J Clin Oncol 2011;29(35):4633–40.
17. Havenga K, Enker WE, Norstein J, et al. Improved survival and local control after total mesorectal excision or D3 lymphadenectomy in the treatment of primary rectal cancer: an international analysis of 1411 patients. Eur J Surg Oncol 1999;25(4):368–74.
18. Iafrate F, Laghi A, Paolantonio P, et al. Preoperative staging of rectal cancer with MR imaging: correlation with surgical and histopathologic findings. Radiographics 2006;26(3):701–14.
19. Brown G, Daniels IR, Richardson C, et al. Techniques and trouble-shooting in high spatial resolution thin slice MRI for rectal cancer. Br J Radiol 2005;78(927):245–51.
20. Maas M, Lambregts DM, Lahaye MJ, et al. T-staging of rectal cancer: accuracy of 3.0 Tesla MRI compared with 1.5 Tesla. Abdom Imaging 2012;37(3):475–81.
21. Taylor FG, Swift RI, Blomqvist L, et al. A systematic approach to the interpretation of preoperative staging MRI for rectal cancer. AJR Am J Roentgenol 2008;191(6):1827–35.
22. Vliegen RF, Beets GL, von Meyenfeldt MF, et al. Rectal cancer: MR imaging in local staging–is gadolinium-based contrast material helpful? Radiology 2005;234(1):179–88.
23. Curvo-Semedo L, Lambregts DM, Maas M, et al. Diffusion-weighted MRI in rectal cancer: apparent diffusion coefficient as a potential noninvasive marker of tumor aggressiveness. J Magn Reson Imaging 2012;35(6):1365–71.
24. Jang KM, Kim SH, Choi D, et al. Pathological correlation with diffusion restriction on diffusion-weighted imaging in patients with pathological complete response after neoadjuvant chemoradiation therapy

for locally advanced rectal cancer: preliminary results. Br J Radiol 2012;85(1017):e566–72.

25. Lambregts DM, Maas M, Riedl RG, et al. Value of ADC measurements for nodal staging after chemoradiation in locally advanced rectal cancer–a per lesion validation study. Eur Radiol 2011;21(2):265–73.

26. Le Bihan D. Molecular diffusion nuclear magnetic resonance imaging. Magn Reson Q 1991;7(1):1–30.

27. Bammer R. Basic principles of diffusion-weighted imaging. Eur J Radiol 2003;45(3):169–84.

28. Qayyum A. Diffusion-weighted imaging in the abdomen and pelvis: concepts and applications. Radiographics 2009;29(6):1797–810.

29. Brown G, Richards CJ, Newcombe RG, et al. Rectal carcinoma: thin-section MR imaging for staging in 28 patients. Radiology 1999;211(1):215–22.

30. Shihab OC, Moran BJ, Heald RJ, et al. MRI staging of low rectal cancer. Eur Radiol 2009;19(3):643–50.

31. Shihab OC, Heald RJ, Rullier E, et al. Defining the surgical planes on MRI improves surgery for cancer of the low rectum. Lancet Oncol 2009;10(12):1207–11.

32. Shihab OC, How P, West N, et al. Can a novel MRI staging system for low rectal cancer aid surgical planning? Dis Colon Rectum 2011;54(10):1260–4.

33. Shihab OC, Taylor F, Salerno G, et al. MRI predictive factors for long-term outcomes of low rectal tumours. Ann Surg Oncol 2011;18(12):3278–84.

34. Hall NR, Finan PJ, al-Jaberi T, et al. Circumferential margin involvement after mesorectal excision of rectal cancer with curative intent. Predictor of survival but not local recurrence? Dis Colon Rectum 1998;41(8):979–83.

35. Shihab OC, Quirke P, Heald RJ, et al. Magnetic resonance imaging-detected lymph nodes close to the mesorectal fascia are rarely a cause of margin involvement after total mesorectal excision. Br J Surg 2010;97(9):1431–6.

36. Smith NJ, Barbachano Y, Norman AR, et al. Prognostic significance of magnetic resonance imaging-detected extramural vascular invasion in rectal cancer. Br J Surg 2008;95(2):229–36.

37. Smith NJ, Shihab O, Arnaout A, et al. MRI for detection of extramural vascular invasion in rectal cancer. AJR Am J Roentgenol 2008;191(5):1517–22.

38. Brown G, Richards CJ, Bourne MW, et al. Morphologic predictors of lymph node status in rectal cancer with use of high-spatial-resolution MR imaging with histopathologic comparison. Radiology 2003; 227(2):371–7.

39. Brown G, Radcliffe AG, Newcombe RG, et al. Preoperative assessment of prognostic factors in rectal cancer using high-resolution magnetic resonance imaging. Br J Surg 2003;90(3):355–64.

40. Kim JH, Beets GL, Kim MJ, et al. High-resolution MR imaging for nodal staging in rectal cancer: are there any criteria in addition to the size? Eur J Radiol 2004; 52(1):78–83.

41. MERCURY Study Group. Relevance of magnetic resonance imaging-detected pelvic sidewall lymph node involvement in rectal cancer. Br J Surg 2011; 98(12):1798–804.

42. Kapiteijn E, Marijnen CA, Nagtegaal ID, et al. Preoperative radiotherapy combined with total mesorectal excision for resectable rectal cancer. N Engl J Med 2001;345:638–46.

43. Theodoropoulos G, Wise WE, Padmanabhan A, et al. T-level downstaging and complete pathologic response after preoperative chemoradiation for advanced rectal cancer result in decreased recurrence and improved disease-free survival. Dis Colon Rectum 2002;45(7):895–903.

44. Barbaro B, Fiorucci C, Tebala C, et al. Locally advanced rectal cancer: MR imaging in prediction of response after preoperative chemotherapy and radiation therapy. Radiology 2009;250(3):730–9.

45. Curvo-Semedo L, Lambregts DM, Maas M, et al. Rectal cancer: assessment of complete response to preoperative combined radiation therapy with chemotherapy–conventional MR volumetry versus diffusion-weighted MR imaging. Radiology 2011; 260(3):734–43.

46. O'Neill BDP, Brown G, Heald RJ, et al. Non-operative treatment after neoadjuvant chemoradiotherapy for rectal cancer. Lancet Oncol 2007;8(7):625–33.

47. Mandard AM, Dalibard F, Mandard JC, et al. Pathologic assessment of tumor regression after preoperative chemoradiotherapy of esophageal carcinoma. Clinicopathologic correlations. Cancer 1994;73(11): 2680–6.

48. Yeo SG, Kim DY, Kim TH, et al. Tumor volume reduction rate measured by magnetic resonance volumetry correlated with pathologic tumor response of preoperative chemoradiotherapy for rectal cancer. Int J Radiat Oncol Biol Phys 2010;78(1):164–71.

49. Patel UB, Brown G, Rutten H, et al. Comparison of magnetic resonance imaging and histopathological response to chemoradiotherapy in locally advanced rectal cancer. Ann Surg Oncol 2012; 19(9):2842–52.

50. Eisenhauer EA, Therasse P, Bogaerts J, et al. New response evaluation criteria in solid tumours: revised RECIST guideline (version 1.1). Eur J Cancer 2009; 45(2):228–47.

51. Patel UB, Blomqvist LK, Taylor F, et al. MRI after treatment of locally advanced rectal cancer: how to report tumor response–the MERCURY experience. AJR Am J Roentgenol 2012;199(4):W486–95.

52. Dworak O, Keilholz L, Hoffmann A. Pathological features of rectal cancer after preoperative radiochemotherapy. Int J Colorectal Dis 1997;12(1):19–23.

53. Beets-Tan RG, Beets GL, Vliegen RF, et al. Accuracy of magnetic resonance imaging in prediction of tumour-free resection margin in rectal cancer surgery. Lancet 2001;357(9255):497–504.

54. Shihab OC, Brown G, Daniels IR, et al. Patients with low rectal cancer treated by abdominoperineal excision have worse tumors and higher involved margin rates compared with patients treated by anterior resection. Dis Colon Rectum 2010;53(1):53–6.

55. Salerno G, Chandler I, Wotherspoon A, et al. Sites of surgical wasting in the abdominoperineal specimen. Br J Surg 2008;95(9):1147–54.

56. Salerno GV, Daniels IR, Moran BJ, et al. Magnetic resonance imaging prediction of an involved surgical resection margin in low rectal cancer. Dis Colon Rectum 2009;52(4):632–9.

57. Nagtegaal ID, van de Velde CJ, Marijnen CA, et al. Low rectal cancer: a call for a change of approach in abdominoperineal resection. J Clin Oncol 2005; 23(36):9257–64.

58. Guillou PJ, Quirke P, Thorpe H, et al. Short-term endpoints of conventional versus laparoscopic-assisted surgery in patients with colorectal cancer (MRC CLASICC trial): multicentre, randomised controlled trial. Lancet 2005;365(9472):1718–26.

59. Marr R, Birbeck K, Garvican J, et al. The modern abdominoperineal excision: the next challenge after total mesorectal excision. Ann Surg 2005;242(1): 74–82.

60. O'Neill BD, Salerno G, Thomas K, et al. MR vs CT imaging: low rectal cancer tumour delineation for three-dimensional conformal radiotherapy. Br J Radiol 2009;82(978):509–13.

61. Merkel S, Mansmann U, Siassi M, et al. The prognostic inhomogeneity in pT3 rectal carcinomas. Int J Colorectal Dis 2001;16(5):298–304.

62. Hunter CJ, Garant A, Vuong T, et al. Adverse features on rectal MRI identify a high-risk group that may benefit from more intensive preoperative staging and treatment. Ann Surg Oncol 2012;19(4):1199–205.

Multiparametric Magnetic Resonance Imaging of the Prostate

Jaime Araujo Oliveira Neto, MD[a],*,
Daniella Braz Parente, MD, PhD[b]

KEYWORDS

- Prostate cancer • MRI • Multiparametric • Diffusion weighted • Dynamic contrast enhanced
- Magnetic resonance spectroscopy • Diagnostic • Staging

KEY POINTS

- There is plenty of room for improvement in the current standard of care for prostate cancer.
- The combined use of anatomic and functional information provided by the multiparametric approach increases the accuracy of MR imaging in detecting and staging prostate cancer.
- Some MR imaging findings in prostate cancer correlate with tumor aggressiveness.
- Multiparametric MR imaging–guided biopsies have a higher tumor detection rate and better correlate with final Gleason grade than random systematic ones.
- Multiparametric MR imaging improves the risk assessment of patients with prostate cancer and can aid in the selection of patients for radical treatment or active surveillance.

INTRODUCTION

Prostate cancer (PCa) is the second most frequently diagnosed cancer worldwide and the sixth leading cause of cancer death in men.[1] According to Globocan, PCa accounts for 13.6% of the total new cases of cancer and is responsible for 6% of the total cancer deaths per year.[2]

The 2 most commonly used tests for the diagnosis of PCa are serum prostate specific antigen (PSA) level measurement and digital rectal examination (DRE).[3] However, DRE has a low positive predictive value[4] and a low interobserver agreement among urologists.[5] PSA levels correlate with PCa risk but no threshold level provides an acceptable combination of sensitivity and specificity. Up to 32% of men with positive biopsies have PSA levels lower than 4.0 ng/mL and up to 79% of men with PSA serum levels higher than 4.1 ng/mL do not have PCa.[6] When PCa is suspected on the basis of elevated serum PSA levels or abnormal DRE, the diagnosis must be confirmed with systematic transrectal ultrasound (TRUS)-guided biopsies.[3] Systematic random TRUS-guided biopsies sample only a small fraction of the prostate and are known to give false-negative results in a significant number of patients, often requiring repeated biopsy procedures, which are associated with discomfort and potential morbidity.[7] Magnetic resonance (MR) imaging offers an alternative assessment technique that has been shown to be highly accurate for the detection of clinically significant PCa and can be used to identify areas of greater likelihood of cancer to be sampled during TRUS-guided biopsies.[8]

PCa mortality has been declining since the middle 1990s and part of the decline is probably because of early diagnosis and improvements in treatments with curative intent.[1] On the other

[a] D'Or Institute for Research and Education, Labs D'Or – Grupo Fleury and Quinta D'Or Hospital, Rua Mario Pederneiras 25/501, Rio de Janeiro 22261–020, Brazil; [b] D'Or Institute for Research and Education, Labs D'Or – Grupo Fleury, Rua General Garzon 100/1002, Rio de Janeiro 22470-010, Brazil
* Corresponding author.
E-mail address: jaimeaoneto@gmail.com

Magn Reson Imaging Clin N Am 21 (2013) 409–426
http://dx.doi.org/10.1016/j.mric.2013.01.004

hand, it is known that many patients die *with* PCa but not *from* PCa and between 23% and 42% of screen-detected PCa would not have been diagnosed in the absence of screening.[9] The differentiation of patients who will benefit from treatment from those who will not is a key step in the management of PCa and the Gleason score has proven to be the most important clinical parameter in measuring the risk of mortality from PCa.[10] Because PCa is often heterogeneous, and areas with different grades of differentiation are commonly present in one patient, systematic TRUS-guided biopsies of the prostate are known to yield a misleading Gleason score in a significant number of patients.[11] Gleason scores obtained from MRI-guided prostate biopsies correlate better with the final Gleason score than systematic random biopsies.[12]

Depending on local staging and risk assessment, treatment options for patients with PCa include prostatectomy, radiotherapy, hormone ablation, and active surveillance.[3] DRE alone is not accurate enough for local staging, so clinical nomograms that combine clinical stage (determined by means of DRE), serum PSA levels, and the Gleason grade in the biopsy specimen were developed.[13] MR imaging can detect significant extracapsular extension (ECE) of PCa[14] and the addition of MR imaging information to clinical nomograms increases the accuracy for local staging.[15]

Contemporary MR imaging of the prostate combines anatomic images from high-resolution T2-weighted (T2W) sequences and functional information obtained from diffusion-weighted imaging (DWI), dynamic contrast-enhanced imaging (DCEI), and MR spectroscopy (MRS), in a multiparametric approach (mpMR imaging). This article describes some aspects of each of these techniques and the clinical impact of mpMR imaging in the detection, characterization, and staging of PCa.

MR IMAGING TECHNIQUES
High-Resolution T2W Sequences

In T2W images, the peripheral zone of the prostrate has hyperintense signal, whereas the central and transition zones have low signal, allowing the zonal anatomy of the prostate to be clearly delineated. The prostate capsule is also demonstrated as a thin line of low signal intensity surrounding the gland.[16]

High-resolution T2W images are used for PCa detection, localization, and staging and should be obtained in the sagittal, axial, and coronal planes, the last 2 planes perpendicular and parallel to the line between the rectum and the prostate, respectively. A consensus meeting by European uroradiologists on MR imaging for the detection, localization, and characterization of PCa has outlined minimum and optimum slice thickness and spatial resolution parameters for MR imaging sequences (Table 1).[17]

Peripheral zone PCa is typically a lesion of low signal intensity in T2W images (Fig. 1A), but the growth pattern and the aggressiveness of the tumor can alter its appearance. Tumors composed of densely packed malignant glands (dense tumors) can be diagnosed using T2W images, but sparse malignant glands intermixed with normal tissue (sparse tumors) are not significantly different from the surrounding normal tissue and are not readily detected on MR imaging. Sparse tumors tend to be less aggressive than dense tumors,[18] which indicates a correlation between tumor detectability and aggressiveness.

Certain benign conditions of the prostate, including chronic prostatitis, scars, and postbiopsy hemorrhage can result in low signal intensity areas on the T2W images, and can be misdiagnosed as cancer.[19] Although postbiopsy hemorrhage may be a source of confusion, sometimes the hemorrhage can support detection of a suspect lesion

---

Table 1
Minimum requirements for acquisition protocols

Technique	Slice Thickness 1.5 T	Slice Thickness 3.0 T	In-Plane Resolution 1.5 T	In-Plane Resolution 3.0 T	Other
T2W	4 mm	3 mm	0.7 × 0.7 mm	0.5 × 0.5 mm	
DWI	5 mm	4 mm	2.0 × 2.0 mm	1.5 × 1.5 mm	b values of 0, 100, and 800 s/mm² for ADC map calculation and 1400 s/mm² for trace images only.
DCE	4 mm	4 mm	1.0 × 1.0 mm	0.7 × 0.7 mm	Temporal resolution of at least 15 s.

Abbreviations: ADC, apparent diffusion coefficient; DCE, dynamic contrast enhanced; DWI, diffusion-weighted image; T2W, T2-weighted.

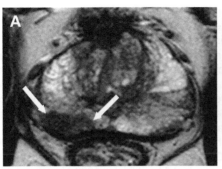
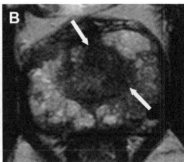

Fig. 1. High-resolution axial T2W MR images (3 mm) of PCa at 3 T (phased-array coil). (*A*) There is a low–signal intensity lesion on the right peripheral zone (*white arrows*) at the mid-third of the prostate, with no signs of capsular invasion. At prostatectomy, the lesion was classified as Gleason grade 7 (4 + 3) prostate adenocarcinoma. (*B*) An ill-defined homogeneous low–signal intensity area in the left transition zone (*white arrows*) at mid-third of the prostate in another patient. TRUS-guided biopsy (MR imaging oriented) showed a Gleason grade 8 (4 + 4) prostate adenocarcinoma on the corresponding position.

because of what is called the "hemorrhage exclusion sign," when the tumor presents as an isointense area on the T1W images, surrounded by hyperintense hemorrhage.[20] For lesions presenting as low signal intensity on the T2W images, wedge shape and diffuse extension without mass effect are the best predictors of benignity, whereas diffuse extension with mass effect and irregular shape and size are associated with malignancy.[21]

The detection of tumors located in the transition zone is more challenging. Because the signal intensities of benign prostatic hyperplasia (BPH) and PCa usually overlap on the T2W images, other imaging features have to be used to make the diagnosis, namely homogeneous low T2W signal intensity, ill-defined margins, lack of capsule, lenticular shape, and extension into the fibromuscular stroma (see **Fig. 1**B).[22]

The acquisition of high-resolution T2W images of the prostate is the first and most important step in the mpMR imaging protocol. These sequences are the basis of PCa MR imaging evaluation and play an important role in both location and staging of PCa (**Box 1**).

DWI

Recently, the technological developments of echo-planar imaging (EPI), high-amplitude gradients, multichannel coils, and the introduction of parallel imaging have extended the applications of DWI to the abdomen and pelvis.[23] DWI measures the microscopic random motion of molecules in a fluid, termed Brownian motion. In a simple solution, the diffusion depends on the temperature and the viscosity of the fluid. Biologic components, mainly cell membranes, form barriers to the free motion of water, thus restricting

diffusion.[24] Diffusion tends to be more restricted in tissues with a high cellular density and a narrow extracellular space, such as neoplastic tissue, so DWI is currently an important imaging technique in oncology.[23]

The sensitivity of the DWI sequence to molecular motion can be adjusted by modifying the "b value" parameter (the b value depends on the amplitude, duration, and time interval between the paired gradients used to generate the DWI sequence). Two separate image sets are generated in DWI acquisition: the trace image and an apparent diffusion coefficient (ADC) map. Signal intensity on the

---

Box 1
T2W hypointense lesions

Peripheral zone

Predictors of malignancy

- Mass effect

- Round or oval

- Irregular contours

Predictors of benignity

- No mass effect

- Linear or wedge shaped

Transition zone

Predictors of malignancy

- Homogeneous low T2W signal intensity

- Ill-defined margins,

- Lack of capsule

- Lenticular shape

- Extension into the fibromuscular stroma

DWI trace images reflects the amount of restriction to diffusion but also the T2W characteristics of the tissue ("T2 shine through" effect). The ADC map is obtained by using data from DWI trace images with at least 2 different b values and does not reflect T2W characteristics.

ADC levels are significantly lower in PCa tissue than in noncancerous prostate, allowing the detection of PCa.[25] PCa demonstrates high signal intensity on the DWI trace images obtained at high b values and has low signal intensity on the ADC maps (**Fig. 2**). Both the trace images and the ADC map should be assessed when detecting PCa using DWI because some tumors are diagnosed only on the ADC maps and others are visible only on the trace images.[26] Recent studies have shown a correlation between the ADC and the Gleason score, with lower ADCs corresponding to increasing Gleason scores.[27,28] Because ADC values are lower in BPH than in the peripheral zone, the accuracy for detection of PCa in the transition zone is significantly lower and even lower in the prostate base.[29]

Factors including imaging hardware and choice of imaging parameters, including b values, can have a significant impact on the calculated ADC, precluding the recommendation of a universal numeric ADC threshold for the diagnosis of PCa.[30] An optimal b value for PCa detection has not yet been established. Although some studies report better results with b values higher than 1000 s/mm^2,[31,32] others do not.[33] Increasing b values to this "ultra-high" level (ie, b >1000 s/mm^2) can increase tumor visibility, especially in the transition zone (**Fig. 3**), but also leads to an increase in the minimum allowed echo time and more pronounced image distortion artifacts that might compromise overall image quality. The recent Prostate MR Guidelines 2012 proposed by the European Society of Urogenital Radiology (ESUR) suggests the use of 3 b values of 0, 100, and 800–1000 s/mm^2 (see **Table 1**).[34]

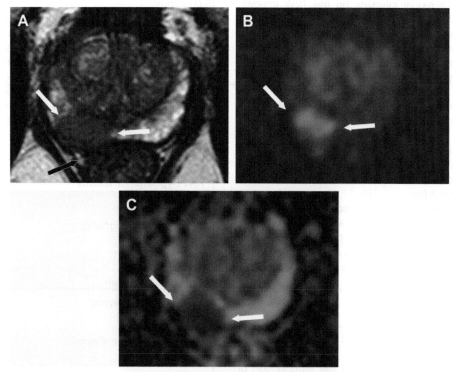

Fig. 2. High-resolution 3-mm axial T2W, trace DWIs (b value = 1000 s/mm^2) and ADC map of PCa at 3 T (phased-array coil) at level of prostate mid-third to apex. (*A*) T2W image shows a hypointense lesion on the right peripheral zone (*white arrows*); note the extension of the hypointense tissue beyond the capsule and the obliteration of the recto-prostatic angle (*black arrow*), which indicates extracapsular extension. The lesion is hyperintense on the trace DWI (*B*), and hypointense on the ADC map (*C*) with a very low mean ADC (0.74 × 10^{-3} mm^2/s). The identification of a lesion on both the ADC map and trace DWI is a more specific finding than is the identification of the lesion on either image alone. The very low mean ADC suggests a more aggressive tumor. TRUS-guided biopsy (MR imaging oriented) showed a Gleason grade 9 (4 + 5) prostate adenocarcinoma on the corresponding position.

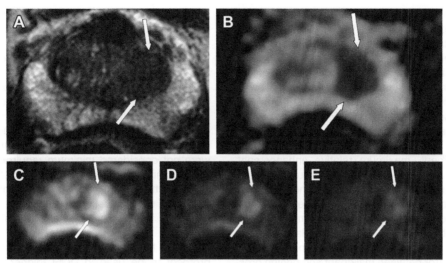

Fig. 3. High-resolution 3-mm axial T2W, trace DWIs (b values of 1000, 1500, and 2000 s/mm²) and ADC map of PCa at 3 T (phased-array coil) at level of prostate mid-third to base. (*A*) T2W image shows an ill-defined homogeneous low–signal intensity area in the left transition zone (*white arrows*), with low signal intensity on the ADC map (*B*). Note that the lesion is slightly hyperintense on the trace DWI with b = 1000 s/mm² (*C*) and becomes progressively more conspicuous as the b value increases to 1500 s/mm² (*D*) and 2000 s/mm² (*E*). The imaging noise also increases with the higher b values. TRUS-guided biopsy (MR imaging oriented) showed a Gleason grade 7 (3 + 4) prostate adenocarcinoma on the corresponding position.

In conclusion, DWI is a fast and simple technique that not only increases accuracy in detection but also provides additional quantitative information that correlates with PCa aggressiveness.

DCEI

Solid tumors, including PCa, cannot grow to a significant size without neoangiogenesis. Compared with the vasculature in normal organs, these newly formed vessel networks have an increased flow and blood volume, the capillaries are more permeable, and the fractional volume of the extracellular extravascular space (EES) is proportionally larger.[35] A simple comparison of pregadolinium and postgadolinium images is not enough to demonstrate those differences[36] and so DCEI was developed.

When a low-molecular-weight contrast agent reaches the capillaries, initially it leaks into the EES and later, when the intravascular concentration diminishes because of renal excretion, the contrast agent diffuses back out of the EES into the intravascular space and is filtered out.[37] DCEI uses sequential fast T1W images acquired before, during, and after intravenous injection of a gadolinium chelate to evaluate the kinetics of the uptake and clearance of the contrast agent and differentiate tumors from normal tissue. The most frequently used sequences to implement DCEI are fast 3-dimensional (3D) T1W gradient-echo sequences with or without fat suppression. Because there has to be a trade-off between temporal and spatial resolution, the ideal imaging protocol to implement DCEI is yet to be defined. To accurately assess the enhancement kinetics of PCa, a high temporal resolution is necessary, at the cost of limited spatial resolution. A higher spatial resolution can be obtained at the cost of lower temporal resolution and consequently less accurate description of the enhancement kinetics.[37] A consensus meeting by European uroradiologists on MR imaging for the detection, localization, and characterization of PCa has outlined the minimum and optimum parameters for DCEI of the prostate (see **Table 1**).[17]

There are several different approaches to DCEI: quantitative, semiquantitative, qualitative, and simple visual analysis.

The quantitative approach uses high temporal resolution images and pharmacokinetic modeling to derive the kinetic parameters including the transfer constant (K^{trans}, volume transfer constant between blood plasma and EES), rate constant (K_{ep}, rate constant between EES and blood plasma), and v_e (volume of extravascular extracellular space per unit volume of tissue), all of which are increased in PCa compared with the normal peripheral zone of the prostate tissue.[38] The signal intensity of the images must be converted into contrast agent concentration (by means of a T1 mapping) and the arterial input function must be measured to calculate the kinetic parameters from DCEI data.[37] Because the values obtained reflect the underlying physiologic phenomena, they are reproducible and relatively independent of MR equipment and imaging parameters, allowing comparison of data from different institutions.

The semiquantitative DCEI approach uses simple descriptors derived from the signal intensity–time curve, such as the time to peak contrast enhancement, maximum relative enhancement, wash-in rate (speed of contrast uptake), and washout rate (rate of contrast clearance). Prostate cancer lesions tend to show earlier and more intense contrast enhancement compared with normal tissue and washout in later phases (**Fig. 4**).[37] Wash-in seems to be the most accurate discriminator between malignant and benign prostatic tissue and, on multivariate analysis, a combination of wash-in and washout provides better discriminatory capability than either parameter alone.[39] This approach has the advantage of being simple to implement and is not subject to the assumptions of the model-based quantitative technique that may not be valid for every tissue or tumor type.[37] On the other hand, semiquantitative descriptors are subject to variations in temporal resolution, pulse sequence parameters, rate of contrast administration, and scaling factors. These variations limit the comparison of data from different institutions and hamper the definition of universal diagnostic thresholds.[40]

The qualitative DCEI approach is implemented by assessing the shape of the signal intensity–time curve. Signal intensity–time curves are classified as steady (type I), plateau (type II), or washout (type III) (see **Fig. 4**).[41] Type III curves are the most indicative of PCa, especially for a focal asymmetric enhancing lesion; however, this finding is not totally specific, and types I and II curves can be seen in patients presenting with PCa as well.[41] The assessment of the shape of the signal intensity–time curve is very simple to implement and because it does not require a very high temporal resolution, longer acquisition times can be used with higher spatial resolution. Bloch and colleagues[14,42] reported a substantial increase in the accuracy of MRI in predicting ECE with the addition of high spatial resolution (low temporal resolution) DCEI and color-coded parametric maps that combined wash-in rate and the shape of the signal intensity–time curve using 1.5-T and 3.0-T magnets.

Simple visual inspection exploits the fact that PCa lesions tend to show early enhancement and can be detected as hyperintense lesions in the "arterial" phases of DCEI (see **Fig. 4**). Girouin

and colleagues[43] described a better sensitivity in the localization of malignant lesions using DCEI with simple visual inspection of images compared with the T2W images alone, although they also reported a lower specificity.

The European Consensus Meeting on MRI for the Detection, Localization, and Characterization of Prostate Cancer could not reach a consensus on the best approach to analyzing DCEI data. Quantitative or semiquantitative DCE-MR imaging were not considered minimum requirements but are recommended as optimal practice.[17] The recent Prostate MR Guidelines 2012 proposed by the ESUR suggest using the qualitative approach based on the shape of the signal intensity–time curves.[17]

Despite the ongoing debate on the best imaging protocol to be used in DCEI (higher spatial vs higher temporal resolution) and the best approach to analyze the data (quantitative, semiquantitative, qualitative, or simple visual analysis), DCEI adds accuracy to the detection and staging of PCa and should be used as an optimal practice.

MRS

In MRS, the position of each metabolite peak in the output graph reflects the resonant frequencies or chemical shifts of its hydrogen protons, and the area of each peak reflects the relative concentration of that metabolite. The dominant peaks observed in prostate MRS are from protons in citrate (2.60 ppm), creatine (3.04 ppm), and choline compounds (3.20 ppm). A range of smaller peaks related to polyamine protons may be observed at approximately 3.15 ppm.[44]

Citrate is a normal constituent of prostatic tissue and its production is dramatically reduced or lost in PCa because of changes in cellular function.[45] Increased concentrations of choline-containing metabolites are related to an increased cell turnover and have also been associated with the presence and progression of PCa.[45] Because it is not possible to differentiate choline peaks from creatine peaks on the spectra obtained at common clinical field strengths, the ratio of choline plus creatine to citrate is used as a metabolic biomarker for PCa.[44]

MRS improves the detection and risk assessment of PCa, and measured peak ratios have also been shown to correlate with tumor aggressiveness (**Fig. 5**).[45] The ESUR Prostate MR Guidelines 2012 suggest using either a qualitative or a quantitative approach for interpreting prostate MRS. The qualitative approach is based on visual analysis of the citrate and choline/creatine peaks and a lesion is deemed suspect of significant cancer if the choline/creatine peak is higher than

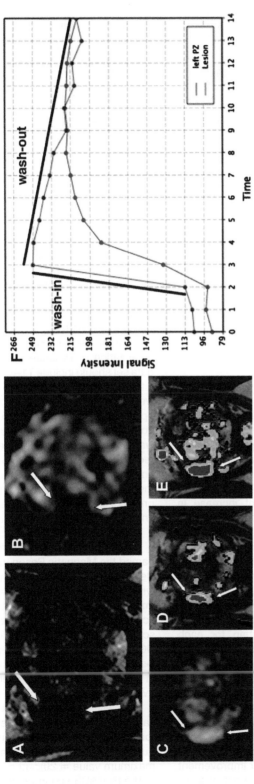

Fig. 4. mpMR image consisting of high-resolution 3-mm axial T2W, ADC map and DCE imaging of PCa at 3 T (phased-array coil) at level of the prostate apex. (A) T2W image shows a subtle ill-defined low-signal intensity area in the right lateral peripheral zone (white arrows). The lesion has low signal intensity on the ADC map (B). In early-phase DCE image (C), the lesion shows strong enhancement. Semiquantitative parametric maps superimposed on T2W images show that the lesion has intense contrast wash-in (D) and washout (E). (F) Signal intensity–time curve of the lesion shows a type III curve (blue) and the normal left peripheral zone shows a type II curve (red). The black lines indicate the concept of wash-in and washout. The lesion is indeterminate on the T2W image and the diagnostic confidence significantly increases with the analysis of the functional images. Random systematic biopsies showed a Gleason grade 7 (3 + 4) prostate adenocarcinoma on the right apex.

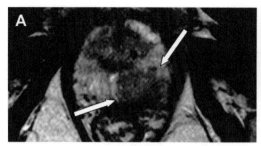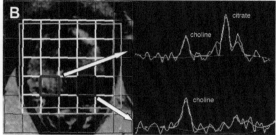

Fig. 5. MRS of PCa at 3 T (phased-array coil). (A) Axial 3-mm T2W images at level of the prostate mid-third to apex, shows a large hypointense lesion on the left peripheral zone. (B) A 3D MRS shows a normal spectrum on the right peripheral zone (red box) with normal choline plus creatine-to-citrate ratio of 0.48. In the voxel placed over the lesion on the left peripheral zone (blue box), the curve shows an increased choline peak and the citrate peak is markedly reduced. Random systematic biopsy showed Gleason grade 9 (4 + 5) prostate adeno-carcinoma on the left apex.

the citrate peak in at least 3 adjacent voxels. In the quantitative approach, the areas of the peaks are measured and choline plus creatine-to-citrate ratios higher than 0.72 in at least 2 adjacent voxels are considered to indicate malignant tissue, whereas ratios between 0.58 and 0.72 are considered ambiguous.[34]

MPMR IMAGING

One of the greatest advances in prostate MR imaging grew from the recognition that no single technique is able to adequately detect and characterize PCa. The combination of anatomic T2W images and the functional techniques described previously has been shown to increase the predictive power of MR imaging for detection and staging of PCa (see Fig. 4). Tanimoto and colleagues[46] reported a significant increase in the area under the receiver operating curve (AUC) for the detection of PCa as they transitioned from a protocol with T2W images only (AUC = 0.711), to a protocol combining T2W imaging and DWI (AUC = 0.905), and finally to a more complete protocol including T2W imaging, DWI, and DCEI (AUC = 0.966). Turkbey and colleagues[47] also reported a higher sensitivity for the combination of T2W images, MRS, and DCEI than for each sequence alone. In that study, each of the 3 MR imaging modalities provided an independent (ie, additive) predictive value for the detection of cancer. Interestingly, Riches and colleagues[48] found that the ability to identify cancer increased significantly with the use of a combination of any 2 functional parameters over the use of individual parameters, but the addition of a third functional parameter did not cause any further improvement in sensitivity or specificity. The ideal set of techniques to be used in prostate mpMR imaging has

not yet been defined but the combination of T2W images with 2 functional techniques seems to provide a reasonable compromise between accuracy and examination duration.

Accordingly, the ESUR Prostate MR Guidelines suggest the use of T2W images plus 2 functional techniques.[34] In the European Consensus Meeting on MRI for the Detection, Localization, and Characterization of Prostate Cancer, the phrase "the data set should include T1-weighted, T2-weighted, diffusion-weighted, and contrast-enhanced MRI" was considered appropriated as a minimum and optimum imaging requirement. MRS was not considered a minimum requirement and there was not a consensus as to whether it is an optimum requirement.[17] Because MRS is the most complex and time consuming of the functional techniques, the choice to include it in a multiparametric protocol should be based on personal experience and skill levels.

The ESUR Prostate MR Guidelines suggest a unified scoring system for mpMR imaging, named the Magnetic Resonance Prostate Imaging Reporting and Data System (MR PI-RADS),[34] which follows the steps of the BI-RADS (Breast Imaging Reporting and Data System).[49] In this scoring system, each lesion is scored on a 5-point scale for each sequence (T2W imaging, DWI, DCEI, MRS); the criteria for assigning scores to lesions identified by each technique are described in Table 2. Additionally, each lesion is given an overall score that indicates its chance of being a clinically significant cancer.[34] The maximum value depends on the number of sequences performed (2 sequences: maximum value = 10; 3 sequences: maximum value = 15; 4 sequences: maximum value = 20).

The PI-RADS scoring system was recently validated in a cohort of patients having repeat biopsy

Table 2
Prostate Imaging Reporting and Data System scoring system

Likert Scale

Score 1	Clinically significant disease highly unlikely to be present
Score 2	Clinically significant cancer unlikely to be present
Score 3	The presence of clinically significant cancer is equivocal
Score 4	Clinically significant cancer likely to be present
Score 5	Clinically significant disease highly likely to be present

T2-weighted Imaging for the Peripheral Zone

Score	Description
1	Uniform high signal intensity
2	Linear, wedge-shaped, or geographic areas of lower signal intensity, usually not well demarcated
3	Intermediate appearances not in categories 1/2 or 4/5
4	Discrete, homogeneous low-signal focus/mass confined to the prostate
5	Discrete, homogeneous low–signal intensity focus with extracapsular extension/invasive behavior or mass effect on the capsule (bulging), or broad (>1.5-cm) contact with the surface

T2-weighted Imaging for the Transition Zone

Score	Description
1	Heterogeneous transition zone adenoma with well-defined margins: "organized chaos"
2	Areas of more homogeneous low signal intensity; however, well marginated, originating from the transition zone/benign prostatic hyperplasia
3	Intermediate appearances not in categories 1/2 or 4/5
4	Areas of more homogeneous low signal intensity; however, well marginated, originating from the transition zone/benign prostatic hyperplasia
5	Same as 4, but involving the anterior fibromuscular stroma or the anterior horn of the peripheral zone, usually lenticular or water-drop shaped

Diffusion-weighted Imaging

Score	Description
1	No reduction in ADC compared with normal glandular tissue; no increase in signal intensity on any high–b value image ($\geq$b800)
2	Diffuse, hyper signal intensity on $\geq$b800 image with low ADC; no focal features; however, linear, triangular, or geographic features are allowed
3	Intermediate appearances not in categories 1/2 or 4/5
4	Focal area(s) of reduced ADC but isointense signal intensity on high–b value images ($\geq$b800)
5	Focal area/mass of hyper signal intensity on the high–b value images ($\geq$b800) with reduced ADC

Dynamic Contrast Enhanced Imaging

Score	Description
1	Type 1 enhancement curve
2	Type 2 enhancement curve
3	Type 3 enhancement curve
+1	For focal enhancing lesion with curve type 2–3
+1	For asymmetric lesion or lesion at an unusual place with curve type 2–3

(continued on next page)

Table 2
(continued)

Quantitative Magnetic Resonance Spectroscopy	
Score	**Description**
1	(Col + Cr)/Citrate ≤0.44 peripheral zone and ≤0.52 transition zone
2	(Col + Cr)/Citrate 0.44–0.58 peripheral zone and 0.52–0.66 transition zone
3	(Col + Cr)/Citrate 0.58–0.72 peripheral zone and 0.66–0.80 transition zone
4	(Col + Cr)/Citrate 0.72–0.86 peripheral zone and 0.80–0.94 transition zone
5	(Col + Cr)/Citrate >0.86 peripheral zone and > 0.94 transition zone

Qualitative Magnetic Resonance Spectroscopy	
Score	**Description**
1	Citrate peak height exceeds choline peak height >2 times
2	Citrate peak height exceeds choline peak height times >1, <2 times
3	Choline peak height equals citrate peak height
4	Choline peak height exceeds citrate peak height >1, <2 times
5	Choline peak height exceeds citrate peak height 2 times

Abbreviation: ADC, apparent diffusion coefficient.

using an mpMR imaging protocol that included T2W imaging, DWI, and DCEI and a TRUS fusion-guided system to superimpose mpMR imaging-determined suspicious areas on 3D TRUS images. Both random systematic and targeted cores were biopsied, followed by core-by-core analysis of pathology and mpMR imaging characteristics of the core locations. Higher PI-RADS scores were observed in segments with positive cores and the rate of positive cores increased proportionally to PI-RADS scores for each sequence and for the overall sum of the scores. The area of the receiver operating characteristic curve was estimated at 0.855 and using a threshold of 9 for the sum of the scores yielded a sensitivity of 67% and a specificity of 92%. Only 5% of the positive cores corresponded to areas where the sum of the scores was less than 9.[50]

mpMR imaging can overcome some of the limitations of each isolated technique to increase overall detection and diagnosis accuracy. The recently proposed MR PI-RADS is a step toward a more uniform interpretation of mpMR imaging.

HARDWARE

There is not currently a consensus on the choice of hardware to be used in prostate MR imaging. In 1994, Hricak and colleagues[51] demonstrated better staging performance using an endorectal coil than using only an external phased array coil, a finding later confirmed in a meta-analysis

report in 2002.[52] Since then, there have been several improvements in coil and pulse sequence design, and more recent studies present accuracies ranging from 86% to 96% in detection[46,50] and ranging from 68% to 89% in staging[53] of PCa performed at 1.5 T using only external phased array coils. However, the American College of Radiology Appropriateness Criteria on Pretreatment Staging Prostate Cancer still suggests endorectal MR imaging as the modality of choice for the local staging of high-risk PCa,[54] whereas the European Consensus on MRI for the Detection, Localization, and Characterization of Prostate Cancer decided that imaging could be adequately performed at 1.5 T with an external phased array coil only,[17] and the ESUR Prostate MR Guidelines 2012 suggest a protocol without an endorectal coil for the detection of PCa and a protocol with an endorectal coil for the local staging of PCa.[34]

MRI at 3.0 T provides images with higher signal-to-noise ratios and, theoretically, this increase in signal-to-noise ratio could remove the need for the endorectal coil, leading to better patient acceptance and lower costs. However, some studies have demonstrated better image quality at 1.5 T with endorectal coils than at 3.0 T with external phased array coils, although with equivalent staging performance.[55,56] The European Consensus on MRI for the Detection, Localization, and Characterization of Prostate Cancer decided that imaging should be performed at 3.0 T to reach an optimum level of detection but there was no consensus as to whether an endorectal coil should be part of the requirements for optimum imaging.[17] Currently, the best signal-to-noise ratio and spatial resolution for the evaluation of the prostate can be obtained with a combination of 3.0 T and an endorectal coil.[57–59]

Current practices for prostate MR imaging differ between Europe and the United States; endorectal coils are used more frequently in the United States.[17] It is not yet clear if the better image quality obtained with an endorectal coil results in better patient management or if the more simple approach using external phased array coils provides equivalent quality of care while allowing more widespread use of the method.

CLINICAL INDICATIONS FOR PROSTATE MR IMAGING
MR Imaging and Tumor Aggressiveness

As stated previously, the Gleason grade is the single most important clinical parameter in measuring the risk of mortality from PCa[10] and various studies report an inverse correlation between median ADC and the Gleason grade (see **Fig. 2**).[27,28,60,61] In a study of 56 patients, using prostatectomy specimens as the reference standard, Hambrock and colleagues[27] demonstrated that ADC can discern low-grade from combined intermediate-grade and high-grade lesions with an AUC of 0.90.

A correlation between imaging and Gleason grade has been shown for the other techniques described previously as well. In a study of 54 patients, using prostatectomy specimens as the reference standard, Kobus and colleagues[61] found that to differentiate low-grade from higher-grade tumors, the MRS choline plus creatine-to-citrate ratio had an AUC of 0.71 in the peripheral zone and 0.90 in the transition zone (see **Fig. 5**). Anatomic high-resolution T2W imaging also correlates with tumor aggressiveness. Wang and colleagues[62] showed that the tumor-to-muscle signal intensity ratio on the T2W images in the peripheral zone has an inverse correlation with the Gleason score. Thus, lower signal intensity on the T2W images means a more undifferentiated tumor.

The correlation between DCEI and tumor aggressiveness is not so clear. A good correlation was recently demonstrated between washout gradient and the Gleason grade.[63] On the other hand, so far no correlation has been found between tumor aggressiveness and DCEI quantitative kinetic parameters.[63,64]

There is a clear correlation between imaging and tumor aggressiveness but, at present, the lack of standardization for MR imaging magnets and acquisition protocols and the significant overlap in the values obtained at ADC maps and MRS among the different levels of tumor aggressiveness prevent the establishment of universal threshold values to be used in clinical practice.

MR Imaging–Directed Biopsies: Detecting Prostate Cancer

According to the 2012 version of the National Comprehensive Cancer Network (NCCN) Clinical Practice Guidelines on the Early Detection of Prostate Cancer, the diagnostic tests used in the screening of PCa are serum PSA level measurement and DRE, followed by random systematic TRUS-guided biopsies in patients with positive findings. Furthermore, patients with a negative biopsy but continued clinical suspicion should undergo a repeat biopsy.[65] This is a common clinical occurrence and in some cases the patient may be submitted to 4 or even more biopsies before reaching a final diagnosis (**Fig. 6**).[7]

If a repeat biopsy is required, MR imaging can be used to detect suspicious areas to be targeted during TRUS-guided biopsies. There are 3 different manners in which an MR imaging–detected lesion can be targeted at biopsy: (1) direct targeting within the magnet using MR-compatible devices; (2) use of fusion software to allow an MR imaging–defined lesion to be identified on ultrasound during a TRUS-guided biopsy procedure; or (3) cognitive targeting, in which the physician reviews the MR imaging data before the procedure and attempts to target the suspected area during the TRUS-guided biopsy using anatomic landmarks as reference.[8]

A systematic review of the literature on image-guided biopsies of the prostate using MR imaging–derived targets indicates that most studies reported superior performance for MR imaging–guided biopsies over random systematic ones. The pooled efficiency (number of clinically significant PCas/number of men biopsied) of the targeted sampling was 70% compared with 40% for the standard approach and the standard approach resulted in a diagnosis of insignificant PCa (ie, small low Gleason-grade lesions) in 10% of biopsied men.[8] In a prospective study of 555 patients who were biopsy-naive, Haffner and colleagues[66] reported a higher diagnostic accuracy for detection of significant cancer for cognitively targeted biopsies than for random systematic biopsies (0.98 vs 0.88, respectively). In that study, however, 12 significant tumors were detected only by the targeted approach and 13 significant tumors were detected only by the systematic approach, potentially demonstrating the importance of implementing both

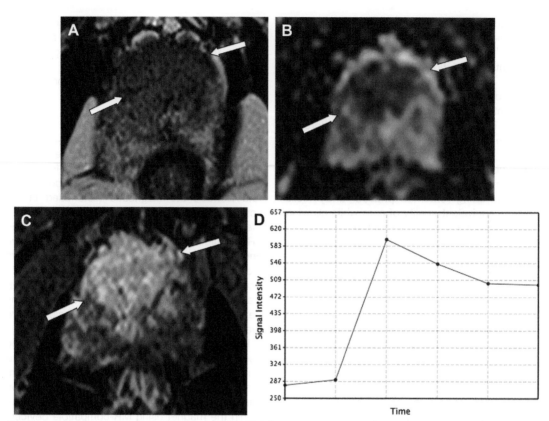

Fig. 6. mpMR image consisting of high-resolution T2W images, ADC map, and DCE imaging at 1.5 T (phased-array coil) in a 62-year-old patient with PSA level of 11.1 ng/mL and previously negative TRUS-guided biopsy. (*A*) Axial 3-mm T2W image at the prostate apex shows a large ill-defined and homogeneous hypointense area in the ventral transition zone (*white arrows*), with signs of extension into the anterior fibromuscular stroma. (*B*) ADC map (b values of 0, 400, and 800 s/mm²) shows restricted diffusion in the lesion with very low mean ADC (0.61 × 10⁻³ mm²/s). DCE imaging shows intense enhancement on early-phase (*C*) and a type III time–signal intensity curve (*D*). Random systematic biopsies showed a Gleason 6 (3 + 3) prostate adenocarcinoma. Patient was submitted to a radical prostatectomy and the histopathologic analysis of the specimen revealed a Gleason 7 (4 + 3) prostate adenocarcinoma.

biopsy approaches. Another prospective study of 101 patients reported higher positivity rate of targeted biopsies than systematic biopsies, and the difference increased with the degree of suspicion based on MRI. For low, moderate, and high suspicion based on MRI, the positivity rates on targeted and systematic biopsies were 4.8% versus 3.8%, 20.7% versus 12.3%, and 53.8% versus 29.9%, respectively.[67] Regardless of the guiding method, MR imaging–targeted biopsies detect more tumors than systematic biopsies and the degree of suspiciousness has a direct correlation with the positivity rate.

Low apical and anterior tumors are particularly difficult to detect in systematic biopsies. Anterior prostate tumors account for 21% of all PCas and are more often missed on systematic biopsies.[68] A study that evaluated the accuracy of prostate

biopsy on anterior tumors reported 98% correctly detected tumors in targeted biopsies using mpMR imaging compared with 46% in random systematic biopsies.[69]

Although controversial, some advocate the use of MR imaging even before the first prostate biopsy because prebiopsy imaging can avoid the problems associated with interpreting images containing postbiopsy hemorrhaging and also increase the detection of significant PCa while avoiding biopsy in those with insignificant disease.[70,71]

In conclusion, mpMR imaging–guided prostate biopsies detect more tumors than systematic biopsies. In the clinical setting of rising PSA levels and a negative biopsy, the choice to perform the second biopsy under direct or indirect MR imaging guidance should be strongly considered.

MR Imaging–Directed Biopsies: Characterizing Prostate Cancer

Random systematic biopsies of the prostate not only often miss the diagnosis of PCa but also yield incorrectly low Gleason grade in 34% to 38% of patients (see **Fig. 6**).[11] A recent study compared the performance of systematic and mpMR imaging/TRUS fusion-targeted biopsies in 195 patients with a previous negative transrectal biopsy and reported that none of the high-grade tumors were missed by targeted biopsies whereas approximately half were not detected by systematic biopsies.[72] Hambrock and colleagues[12] compared the performance rate of systematic biopsies and MR imaging–guided biopsies when aiming at the lowest signal areas on the ADC maps and using prostatectomy specimens as the reference standard. The positive predictive value for true low-grade tumors was 92% for MR imaging–guided biopsies and 45% for systematic biopsies. Undergrading of tumors with Gleason grades 4 or 5 was only 5% for MR imaging–guided biopsies and 46% for systematic biopsies. Undergrading of more than one level was observed in 57% of systematic biopsies and in none of the MR imaging–guided biopsies.

In summary, the Gleason grade from MR imaging–guided biopsies better correlates with the true Gleason grade of prostatectomy specimens and aggressive diseases can be missed if the clinician relies only on random systematic biopsies. The use of MR imaging–guided biopsies provides a better risk assessment and the individualization of therapeutic strategies.

Active Surveillance

Active surveillance involves actively monitoring the course of the disease with plans to intervene with curative intent if the cancer progresses. According to the NCCN Clinical Practice Guidelines in Oncology–Prostate Cancer, active surveillance is the appropriate course of action for men with very low-risk PCa (Gleason score ≤6, PSA <10 ng/mL, and fewer than 3 positive biopsies, none with more than 50% cancer involvement) when life expectancy is fewer than 20 years, or for men with low-risk PCa (Gleason score ≤6, PSA <10 ng/mL) when life expectancy is fewer than 10 years.[65] A large cohort showed a good outcome with this treatment paradigm over a mean follow-up of almost 7 years.[73]

The fear of underestimating the cancer burden with systematic TRUS-guided prostate biopsies and missing the opportunity to perform a radical curative treatment is one of the greatest barriers to the more widespread acceptance of active surveillance. This fear is in part justified by the fact that most of the reclassification of cancers in active surveillance protocols is actually attributable to underestimation of the amount of disease at the initial diagnosis and not true progression. Tumors in the anterior region of the transition zone are particularly prone to underestimation of both volume and Gleason grade.[74]

mpMR imaging cancer assessment has been shown to correlate with findings in follow-up biopsies and could help reduce the probability of underestimating cancer burden.[75–77] ADC is the most significant predictor of adverse findings on repeat biopsy and subsequent progression to radical treatment,[75,76] but the same may not hold true for MRS, as one study did not find a correlation between metabolite ratios and predicted outcome.[77] A recent study prospectively evaluated the impact of mpMR imaging (T2W imaging, DWI, and DCEI images) on disease reclassification in 60 patients on active surveillance, followed by a targeted biopsy for confirmation. Seventy-seven percent of patients with suspicious findings in mpMR imaging were reclassified at confirmation biopsy, as compared with 9% reclassification of patients with normal mpMR imaging. Most missed large tumors were located in the anterior or the transitional zone.[78]

mpMR imaging appears to have the potential to noninvasively identify candidates for active surveillance who harbor occult adverse disease and it should be offered to patients before confirmation biopsies. One possible future application of mpMR imaging is to monitor patients under active surveillance protocols and perform biopsies only if a suspected finding is demonstrated.

Staging

Local staging defines treatment recommendations[65] and may influence the surgical strategy in radical prostatectomy.[79] Staging is mostly based on T2W sequences and the imaging criteria used to define ECE are irregular bulging of the prostatic contour, loss of capsule, obliteration of the rectoprostatic angle, asymmetry of the neurovascular bundle, low signal intensity indicative of cancer in the periprostatic fat (**Fig. 7**), and low signal intensity in the seminal vesicles.[34] Using a 3D T2W sequence, Cornud and colleagues[80] compared the staging performance of direct versus indirect signs of ECE. Using only direct signs (presence of a hypointensity in any periprostatic area) provided a high specificity (96%), but at the expense of a low sensitivity (55%). The addition of indirect signs (tumor contact with the capsule and a capsular signal defect with or without

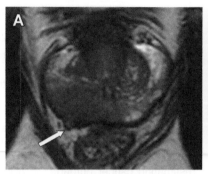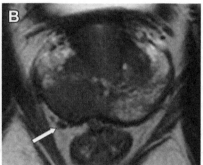

Fig. 7. Staging. High-resolution T2W imaging at 3.0 T with phased-array coil shows a large hypointense area in the right peripheral zone at the level of the mid-prostate to apex in (A) and in a slightly higher level in (B), highly suspicious for prostate carcinoma. Note the irregularity of the prostate capsule (*white arrow* in A) and asymmetric thickening of the right neurovascular bundle (*white arrow* in B), direct signs of extracapsular extension. At radical prostatectomy, the histopathologic analysis showed a pT3a Gleason grade 9 (4 + 5) prostate adenocarcinoma.

capsular bulging) resulted in a significant increase in sensitivity to 84%, at the expense of a modest (but significant, $P = .004$) reduction in specificity to 89% (**Box 2**).

mpMRI may offer improvements in traditional MR imaging–based local staging. DCEI data can help identifying ECE, demonstrating early enhancement of extracapsular tumor or asymmetric enhancement of neurovascular bundles (**Fig. 8**).[14,42,53] DWI may facilitate the detection of PCa lesions and indirectly increase the performance of T2W images; however, because of its intrinsic low spatial resolution, DWI does not have a direct role in the local staging. The addition of MRS to T2W imaging has been shown to increase the accuracy of local staging[81] and staging nomograms.[15] The contribution of MRS is also indirect, as it can demonstrate the extent of the tumor, which is associated with a risk of ECE, but it cannot directly detect tumor tissue outside of the prostate gland.

There is great heterogeneity in the performance of MR imaging in the staging of PCa, with sensitivities for ECE extension varying from 30% to 91%.[44] Endorectal MR imaging at 1.5 T[82] and 3.0 T[59] provides better information than nonendorectal imaging for ECE extension. Differences in staging performance between experienced and less experienced radiologists also have been consistently demonstrated.[53,83,84] Futterer and colleagues[84] reported that the addition of DCEI significantly increased the accuracy for less experienced readers, but not for the experienced reader.

Microscopic foci of ECE might be missed in MR imaging analysis because of insufficient tissue contrast or spatial resolution, resulting in limited correlation to histopathology.[85] Such a limitation may not be critical for patient management, however, because it has been shown that patients with focal capsular penetration and patients with organ-confined disease might have the same rate of postoperative disease recurrences.[86] Recent studies have shown that when focal (less than 1 mm) ECE is excluded, the accuracy for the detection of overall T3 stage is improved.[14,80] Manzone and colleagues[87] found a postoperative recurrence rate of PCa of 24% in patients with no ECE, which was similar to the recurrence rate of patients with equivocal ECE at MR imaging (27%) and significantly lower than the recurrence rate of patients with definite ECE at MR imaging (61.5%). They suggested that small foci of extracapsular disease that are not definitely identified using endorectal MR imaging might not be a determinant of patient outcome.

Local staging of PCa not only influences the choice of treatment modality but may also be used for surgical planning. Hricak and colleagues[79] showed that MR imaging information on the status of the neurovascular bundle could improve the surgeon's decision on whether a

---

Box 2
Imaging criteria for extracapsular extension

- Irregular bulging of the prostatic contour
- Loss of capsule
- Obliteration of the rectoprostatic angle
- Asymmetry of the neurovascular bundle
- Low signal intensity indicative of cancer in the periprostatic fat
- Low signal intensity in the seminal vesicles
- Extensive tumor contact with the capsule (indirect sign)

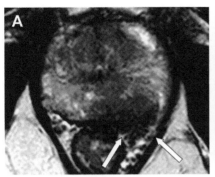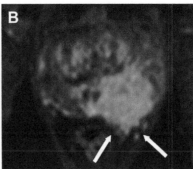

Fig. 8. Staging. High-resolution T2W imaging and DCE imaging at 3.0 T with phased-array coil (same patient as in Fig. 5). Axial T2W image (*A*) shows a large hypointense area in the left peripheral zone at the level of the mid-prostate to apex. There is extensive irregularity of the prostate capsule (*white arrows* in *A*) with obliteration of the recto-prostatic angle and extension of the T2W hypointense tissue to the neurovascular bundle. (*B*) On early-phase DCE image, the lesion shows intense enhancement and the features of extracapsular extension are also shown.

nerve-sparing surgery could be performed or if a more aggressive approach was necessary. After analyzing the MR images, the initial surgical plan was changed in 106 of 270 patients; in 36 patients to a more conservative approach, and in 67 patients to a more aggressive approach. The change in surgical plan was considered appropriate in respectively 90% and 67% of cases.

In conclusion, mpMR imaging information on local staging can improve the risk assessment and serve as a road map for surgical planning.

SUMMARY

The development of prostate MR imaging is an ongoing process that includes both technical and clinical aspects. From the technical point of view, the main advance in the past few years was the development of imaging protocols that combine the described MR imaging techniques in a multiparametric approach. The combination of functional and anatomic information has an additive effect that increases overall accuracy. Lack of standardization of imaging protocols and diagnostic criteria is still a problem that hampers the comparison of results among different institutions and precludes the realization of large multicenter trials. To that effect, the recently proposed ESUR Prostate MR Guidelines and the PI-RADS scoring system represent an initial step toward universal standards in PCa detection and evaluation.

From the clinical point of view, the most important recent development was the conclusion that even though MR imaging cannot reliably demonstrate small low-grade tumors, it provides good accuracy in the detection of significant cancer and there is a correlation between imaged parameters and tumor aggressiveness. This information

can be used to direct biopsies to achieve a higher tumor-detection rate and biopsy results that better reflect the true Gleason grade, resulting in better risk assessment and improved therapeutic decisions, particularly in the selection of patients for active surveillance. mpMR imaging also offers improved clinical staging of PCa but so far has not been incorporated into preoperative guidelines.

So far, imaging has had a secondary role in PCa. The improved accuracy provided by mpMR imaging and a better understanding of the clinical significance of the imaging findings can pave the way to a more direct role of MR imaging in patient management.

REFERENCES

1. Jemal A, Bray F, Center MM, et al. Global cancer statistics. CA Cancer J Clin 2011;61(2):69–90.
2. Ferlay J, Shin HR, Bray F, et al. Globocan 2008. Prostate cancer incidence, mortality and prevalence worldwide in 2008. 2008. Available at: http://globocan.iarc.fr. Accessed August 18, 2012.
3. Thompson I, Thrasher JB, Aus G, et al. Guideline for the management of clinically localized prostate cancer: 2007 update. J Urol 2007;177(6):2106–31.
4. Crawford ED, DeAntoni EP, Etzioni R, et al. Serum prostate-specific antigen and digital rectal examination for early detection of prostate cancer in a national community-based program. The Prostate Cancer Education Council. Urology 1996;47(6): 863–9.
5. Smith DS, Catalona WJ. Interexaminer variability of digital rectal examination in detecting prostate cancer. Urology 1995;45(1):70–4.
6. Arcangeli CG, Ornstein DK, Keetch DW, et al. Prostate-specific antigen as a screening test for prostate cancer. The United States experience. Urol Clin North Am 1997;24(2):299–306.

7. Djavan B, Ravery V, Zlotta A, et al. Prospective evaluation of prostate cancer detected on biopsies 1, 2, 3 and 4: when should we stop? J Urol 2001;166(5): 1679–83.

8. Moore CM, Robertson NL, Arsanious N, et al. Image-guided prostate biopsy using magnetic resonance imaging–derived targets: a systematic review. Eur Urol 2013;63(1):125–40.

9. Wolf AM, Wender RC, Etzioni RB, et al. American Cancer Society guideline for the early detection of prostate cancer: update 2010. CA Cancer J Clin 2010;60(2):70–98.

10. Egevad L, Granfors T, Karlberg L, et al. Prognostic value of the Gleason score in prostate cancer. BJU Int 2002;89(6):538–42.

11. Divrik RT, Eroglu A, Sahin A, et al. Increasing the number of biopsies increases the concordance of Gleason scores of needle biopsies and prostatectomy specimens. Urol Oncol 2007;25(5):376–82.

12. Hambrock T, Hoeks C, Hulsbergen-van de Kaa C, et al. Prospective assessment of prostate cancer aggressiveness using 3-T diffusion-weighted magnetic resonance imaging—guided biopsies versus a systematic 10-core transrectal ultrasound prostate biopsy cohort. Eur Urol 2012;61(1):177–84.

13. Kundra V, Silverman PM, Matin SF, et al. Imaging in oncology from the University of Texas M. D. Anderson Cancer Center: diagnosis, staging, and surveillance of prostate cancer. Am J Roentgenol 2007; 189(4):830–44.

14. Bloch BN, Genega EM, Costa DN, et al. Prediction of prostate cancer extracapsular extension with high spatial resolution dynamic contrast-enhanced 3-T MRI. Eur Radiol 2012;22(10):2201–10.

15. Wang L, Hricak H, Kattan MW, et al. Prediction of organ-confined prostate cancer: incremental value of MR imaging and MR spectroscopic imaging to staging nomograms. Radiology 2006;238(2):597–603.

16. Hricak H, Dooms GC, McNeal JE, et al. MR imaging of the prostate gland: normal anatomy. AJR Am J Roentgenol 1987;148(1):51–8.

17. Dickinson L, Ahmed HU, Allen C, et al. Magnetic resonance imaging for the detection, localisation, and characterisation of prostate cancer: recommendations from a European consensus meeting. Eur Urol 2011;59(4):477–94.

18. Langer DL, van der Kwast TH, Evans AJ, et al. Intermixed normal tissue within prostate cancer: effect on MR imaging measurements of apparent diffusion coefficient and T2—sparse versus dense cancers. Radiology 2008;249(3):900–8.

19. Ikonen S, Kivisaari L, Tervahartiala P, et al. Prostatic MR imaging. Accuracy in differentiating cancer from other prostatic disorders. Acta Radiol 2001;42(4): 348–54.

20. Purysko AS, Herts BR. Prostate MRI: the hemorrhage exclusion sign. J Urol 2012;188(5):1946–7.

21. Cruz M, Tsuda K, Narumi Y, et al. Characterization of low-intensity lesions in the peripheral zone of prostate on pre-biopsy endorectal coil MR imaging. Eur Radiol 2002;12(2):357–65.

22. Akin O, Sala E, Moskowitz CS, et al. Transition zone prostate cancers: features, detection, localization, and staging at endorectal MR imaging. Radiology 2006;239(3):784–92.

23. Koh DM, Collins DJ. Diffusion-weighted MRI in the body: applications and challenges in oncology. AJR Am J Roentgenol 2007;188(6):1622–35.

24. Le Bihan D, Breton E, Lallemand D, et al. MR imaging of intravoxel incoherent motions: application to diffusion and perfusion in neurologic disorders. Radiology 1986;161(2):401–7.

25. Issa B. In vivo measurement of the apparent diffusion coefficient in normal and malignant prostatic tissues using echo-planar imaging. J Magn Reson Imaging 2002;16(2):196–200.

26. Rosenkrantz AB, Kong X, Niver BE, et al. Prostate cancer: comparison of tumor visibility on trace diffusion-weighted images and the apparent diffusion coefficient map. AJR Am J Roentgenol 2011; 196(1):123–9.

27. Hambrock T, Somford DM, Huisman HJ, et al. Relationship between apparent diffusion coefficients at 3.0-T MR imaging and Gleason grade in peripheral zone prostate cancer. Radiology 2011;259(2):453–61.

28. Vargas HA, Akin O, Franiel T, et al. Diffusion-weighted endorectal MR imaging at 3 T for prostate cancer: tumor detection and assessment of aggressiveness. Radiology 2011;259(3):775–84.

29. Kim JH, Kim JK, Park BW, et al. Apparent diffusion coefficient: prostate cancer versus noncancerous tissue according to anatomical region. J Magn Reson Imaging 2008;28(5):1173–9.

30. Thormer G, Otto J, Reiss-Zimmermann M, et al. Diagnostic value of ADC in patients with prostate cancer: influence of the choice of b values. Eur Radiol 2012; 22(8):1820–8.

31. Metens T, Miranda D, Absil J, et al. What is the optimal b value in diffusion-weighted MR imaging to depict prostate cancer at 3T? Eur Radiol 2012; 22(3):703–9.

32. Ohgiya Y, Suyama J, Seino N, et al. Diagnostic accuracy of ultra-high-b-value 3.0-T diffusion-weighted MR imaging for detection of prostate cancer. Clin Imaging 2012;36(5):526–31.

33. Kim CK, Park BK, Kim B. High-b-value diffusion-weighted imaging at 3 T to detect prostate cancer: comparisons between b values of 1,000 and 2,000 s/mm2. AJR Am J Roentgenol 2010;194(1):W33–7.

34. Barentsz JO, Richenberg J, Clements R, et al. ESUR prostate MR guidelines 2012. Eur Radiol 2012;22(4): 746–57.

35. Folkman J, Beckner K. Angiogenesis imaging. Acad Radiol 2000;7(10):783–5.

36. Mirowitz SA, Brown JJ, Heiken JP. Evaluation of the prostate and prostatic carcinoma with gadolinium-enhanced endorectal coil MR imaging. Radiology 1993;186(1):153–7.

37. McMahon CJ, Bloch BN, Lenkinski RE, et al. Dynamic contrast-enhanced MR imaging in the evaluation of patients with prostate cancer. Magn Reson Imaging Clin N Am 2009;17(2):363–83.

38. Tofts PS, Brix G, Buckley DL, et al. Estimating kinetic parameters from dynamic contrast-enhanced T(1)-weighted MRI of a diffusable tracer: standardized quantities and symbols. J Magn Reson Imaging 1999;10(3):223–32.

39. Isebaert S, De Keyzer F, Haustermans K, et al. Evaluation of semi-quantitative dynamic contrast-enhanced MRI parameters for prostate cancer in correlation to whole-mount histopathology. Eur J Radiol 2012;81(3):e217–22.

40. Verma S, Turkbey B, Muradyan N, et al. Overview of dynamic contrast-enhanced MRI in prostate cancer diagnosis and management. Am J Roentgenol 2012; 198(6):1277–88.

41. Ito H, Kamoi K, Yokoyama K, et al. Visualization of prostate cancer using dynamic contrast-enhanced MRI: comparison with transrectal power Doppler ultrasound. Br J Radiol 2003;76(909):617–24.

42. Bloch BN, Furman-Haran E, Helbich TH, et al. Prostate cancer: accurate determination of extracapsular extension with high-spatial-resolution dynamic contrast-enhanced and T2-weighted MR imaging—initial results. Radiology 2007;245(1): 176–85.

43. Girouin N, Mège-Lechevallier F, Tonina Senes A, et al. Prostate dynamic contrast-enhanced MRI with simple visual diagnostic criteria: is it reasonable? Eur Radiol 2006;17(6):1498–509.

44. Hoeks CM, Barentsz JO, Hambrock T, et al. Prostate cancer: multiparametric MR imaging for detection, localization, and staging. Radiology 2011;261(1): 46–66.

45. Kurhanewicz J, Vigneron DB. Advances in MR spectroscopy of the prostate. Magn Reson Imaging Clin N Am 2008;16(4):697–710, ix–x.

46. Tanimoto A, Nakashima J, Kohno H, et al. Prostate cancer screening: the clinical value of diffusion-weighted imaging and dynamic MR imaging in combination with T2-weighted imaging. J Magn Reson Imaging 2007;25(1):146–52.

47. Turkbey B, Pinto PA, Mani H, et al. Prostate cancer: value of multiparametric MR imaging at 3 T for detection—histopathologic correlation. Radiology 2010;255(1):89–99.

48. Riches SF, Payne GS, Morgan VA, et al. MRI in the detection of prostate cancer: combined apparent diffusion coefficient, metabolite ratio, and vascular parameters. AJR Am J Roentgenol 2009;193(6): 1583–91.

49. Molleran V, Mahoney MC. The BI-RADS breast magnetic resonance imaging lexicon. Magn Reson Imaging Clin N Am 2010;18(2):171–85, vii.

50. Portalez D, Mozer P, Cornud F, et al. Validation of the European Society of Urogenital Radiology scoring system for prostate cancer diagnosis on multiparametric magnetic resonance imaging in a cohort of repeat biopsy patients. Eur Urol 2012; 62(6):986–96.

51. Hricak H, White S, Vigneron D, et al. Carcinoma of the prostate gland: MR imaging with pelvic phased-array coils versus integrated endorectal–pelvic phased-array coils. Radiology 1994;193(3): 703–9.

52. Engelbrecht NE, Aaberg TM Jr, Sung J, et al. Neovascular membranes associated with idiopathic juxtafoveolar telangiectasis. Arch Ophthalmol 2002; 120(3):320–4.

53. Renard-Penna R, Roupret M, Comperat E, et al. Accuracy of high resolution (1.5 tesla) pelvic phased array magnetic resonance imaging (MRI) in staging prostate cancer in candidates for radical prostatectomy: results from a prospective study. Urol Oncol 2011. [Epub ahead of print].

54. Israel GM, Francis IR, Roach M III, et al. American College of Radiology appropriateness criteria—pretreatment staging prostate cancer. 2005. Available at: http://www.acr.org/~/media/A939E3544ACA4B5B881342 F34B3804A4.pdf. Accessed October 31, 2012.

55. Sosna J, Pedrosa I, Dewolf WC, et al. MR imaging of the prostate at 3 tesla. Acad Radiol 2004;11(8): 857–62.

56. Beyersdorff D. MRI of prostate cancer at 1.5 and 3.0 T: comparison of image quality in tumor detection and staging. Am J Roentgenol 2005;185(5): 1214–20.

57. Bloch BN, Rofsky NM, Baroni RH, et al. 3 Tesla magnetic resonance imaging of the prostate with combined pelvic phased-array and endorectal coils; initial experience(1). Acad Radiol 2004;11(8):863–7.

58. Cornfeld DM, Weinreb JC. MR imaging of the prostate: 1.5T versus 3T. Magn Reson Imaging Clin N Am 2007;15(3):433–48.

59. Heijmink SW, Futterer JJ, Hambrock T, et al. Prostate cancer: body-array versus endorectal coil MR imaging at 3 T–comparison of image quality, localization, and staging performance. Radiology 2007; 244(1):184–95.

60. Bittencourt LK, Barentsz JO, Miranda LC, et al. Prostate MRI: diffusion-weighted imaging at 1.5T correlates better with prostatectomy Gleason grades than TRUS-guided biopsies in peripheral zone tumours. Eur Radiol 2011;22(2):468–75.

61. Kobus T, Vos PC, Hambrock T, et al. Prostate cancer aggressiveness: in vivo assessment of MR spectroscopy and diffusion-weighted imaging at 3 T. Radiology 2012;265(2):457–67.

62. Wang L, Mazaheri Y, Zhang J, et al. Assessment of bio-logic aggressiveness of prostate cancer: correlation of MR signal intensity with Gleason grade after radical prostatectomy. Radiology 2008;246(1):168–76.

63. Chen YJ, Chu WC, Pu YS, et al. Washout gradient in dynamic contrast-enhanced MRI is associated with tumor aggressiveness of prostate cancer. J Magn Reson Imaging 2012;36(4):912–9.

64. Oto A, Yang C, Kayhan A, et al. Diffusion-weighted and dynamic contrast-enhanced MRI of prostate cancer: correlation of quantitative MR parameters with Gleason score and tumor angiogenesis. AJR Am J Roentgenol 2011;197(6):1382–90.

65. Mohler JL, Armstrong AJ, Bahnson RR, et al. Prostate cancer, version 3.2012 featured updates to the NCCN guidelines. J Natl Compr Canc Netw 2012; 10(9):1081–7.

66. Haffner J, Lemaitre L, Puech P, et al. Role of magnetic resonance imaging before initial biopsy: comparison of magnetic resonance imaging—targeted and systematic biopsy for significant prostate cancer detection. BJU Int 2011;108(8 Pt 2):E171–8.

67. Pinto PA, Chung PH, Rastinehad AR, et al. Magnetic resonance imaging/ultrasound fusion guided prostate biopsy improves cancer detection following transrectal ultrasound biopsy and correlates with multiparametric magnetic resonance imaging. J Urol 2011;186(4):1281–5.

68. Bott SR, Young MP, Kellett MJ, et al. Anterior prostate cancer: is it more difficult to diagnose? BJU Int 2002;89(9):886–9.

69. Ouzzane A, Puech P, Lemaitre L, et al. Combined multiparametric MRI and targeted biopsies improve anterior prostate cancer detection, staging, and grading. Urology 2011;78(6):1356–62.

70. Ahmed HU, Kirkham A, Arya M, et al. Is it time to consider a role for MRI before prostate biopsy? Nat Rev Clin Oncol 2009;6(4):197–206.

71. Villers A, Marliere F, Ouzzane A, et al. MRI in addition to or as a substitute for prostate biopsy: the clinician's point of view. Diagn Interv Imaging 2012; 93(4):262–7.

72. Vourganti S, Rastinehad A, Yerram NK, et al. Multi-parametric magnetic resonance imaging and ultra-sound fusion biopsy detect prostate cancer in patients with prior negative transrectal ultrasound biopsies. J Urol 2012;188(6):2152–7.

73. Klotz L, Zhang L, Lam A, et al. Clinical results of long-term follow-up of a large, active surveillance cohort with localized prostate cancer. J Clin Oncol 2010;28(1):126–31.

74. Ouzzane A, Puech P, Villers A. MRI and surveillance. Curr Opin Urol 2012;22(3):231–6.

75. van As NJ, de Souza NM, Riches SF, et al. A study of diffusion-weighted magnetic resonance imaging in men with untreated localised prostate cancer on active surveillance. Eur Urol 2009;56(6):981–7.

76. Giles SL, Morgan VA, Riches SF, et al. Apparent diffusion coefficient as a predictive biomarker of prostate cancer progression: value of fast and slow diffusion components. Am J Roentgenol 2011; 196(3):586–91.

77. Fradet V, Kurhanewicz J, Cowan JE, et al. Prostate cancer managed with active surveillance: role of anatomic MR imaging and MR spectroscopic imaging. Radiology 2010;256(1):176–83.

78. Margel D, Yap SA, Lawrentschuk N, et al. Impact of multiparametric endorectal coil prostate magnetic resonance imaging on disease reclassification among active surveillance candidates: a prospective cohort study. J Urol 2012;187(4):1247–52.

79. Hricak H, Wang L, Wei DC, et al. The role of preoperative endorectal magnetic resonance imaging in the decision regarding whether to preserve or resect neurovascular bundles during radical retropubic prostatectomy. Cancer 2004;100(12):2655–63.

80. Cornud F, Rouanne M, Beuvon F, et al. Endorectal 3D T2-weighted 1mm-slice thickness MRI for prostate cancer staging at 1.5Tesla: should we reconsider the indirect signs of extracapsular extension according to the D'Amico tumor risk criteria? Eur J Radiol 2012;81(4):e591–7.

81. Yu KK, Scheidler J, Hricak H, et al. Prostate cancer: prediction of extracapsular extension with endorectal MR imaging and three-dimensional proton MR spectroscopic imaging. Radiology 1999;213(2): 481–8.

82. Futterer JJ, Engelbrecht MR, Jager GJ, et al. Prostate cancer: comparison of local staging accuracy of pelvic phased-array coil alone versus integrated endorectal-pelvic phased-array coils. Local staging accuracy of prostate cancer using endorectal coil MR imaging. Eur Radiol 2007;17(4):1055–65.

83. Mullerad M, Hricak H, Wang L, et al. Prostate cancer: detection of extracapsular extension by genitourinary and general body radiologists at MR imaging. Radiology 2004;232(1):140–6.

84. Futterer JJ, Engelbrecht MR, Huisman HJ, et al. Staging prostate cancer with dynamic contrast-enhanced endorectal MR imaging prior to radical prostatectomy: experienced versus less experienced readers. Radiology 2005;237(2):541–9.

85. Jager GJ, Ruijter ET, van de Kaa CA, et al. Local staging of prostate cancer with endorectal MR imaging: correlation with histopathology. AJR Am J Roentgenol 1996;166(4):845–52.

86. Epstein JI, Carmichael MJ, Pizov G, et al. Influence of capsular penetration on progression following radical prostatectomy: a study of 196 cases with long-term followup. J Urol 1993;150(1):135–41.

87. Manzone TA, Malkowicz SB, Tomaszewski JE, et al. Use of endorectal MR imaging to predict prostate carcinoma recurrence after radical prostatectomy. Radiology 1998;209(2):537–42.

MR Imaging of the Pelvic Floor
Defecography

Alice C. Brandão, MD*, Paula Ianez, MD

KEYWORDS

- Pelvic imaging MR • Defecography MR • Anatomy pelvic floor • Pelvic floor dynamics
- Anatomic and functional abnormalities

KEY POINTS

- Magnetic resonance (MR) imaging defecography makes it possible to evaluate the pelvic floor in its entirety with high-resolution images at rest and dynamic sequences.
- Defecography by MR imaging provides an accurate evaluation of the morphology and function of the anorectal and pelvic muscles and organs involved in pelvic floor dynamics.
- MR defecography identifies the diseases affecting the evacuation mechanism, providing information essential for surgical planning and choice of treatment approach.

INTRODUCTION

Functional disorders of the pelvic floor, such as pelvic organ prolapse, defecatory dysfunction, and urinary and fecal incontinence, represent a common health problem, especially in women. The integrity of the pelvic floor can be compromised by childbirth, pelvic surgery, obesity, constipation, age, genetic factors, and heavy physical exertion.[1] It is estimated that pelvic floor disorder affects more than 15% of multiparous women and that 10% to 20% of patients seek medical care in gastrointestinal clinics for evacuation dysfunction.[2] These conditions often significantly affect the quality of life and result in a variety of symptoms.

Clinical evaluation of patients with pelvic floor dysfunction is difficult. Symptoms, such as constipation, incontinence, and pain, are nonspecific and physical examination is frequently inaccurate. As a consequence, imaging is becoming popular as an adjunct tool for the assessment of pelvic floor abnormalities.[1]

Magnetic resonance (MR) imaging is certainly an invaluable tool in the management of those patients because it provides detailed anatomic information. MR imaging makes it possible to view the pelvic floor in its entirety and multiple compartments, both at rest and dynamically.

In this article, the authors discuss the following:

- The MR imaging details of pelvic floor anatomy
- The MR imaging technique
- The most commonly observed anatomic and functional abnormalities

ANATOMY

A basic knowledge of the pelvic floor anatomy is fundamental to imaging interpretation and understanding of dysfunction. The pelvic floor is divided into 3 compartments: anterior, middle, and posterior. The anterior compartment contains the bladder and urethra; the middle contains the uterus, cervix and vagina; and the posterior contains the rectum and anal canal. The support of the structures arises from the attachment of the muscles, endopelvic fascia, and ligaments to the pelvic bones. In this article, the authors emphasize

Disclosures: None.
Funding Sources: None.
Clínica Felippe Mattoso, 700 Americas Avenue, 319, Barra da Tijuca, Rio de Janeiro 30112011, Brazil
* Corresponding author.
E-mail address: brandaosalomao@gmail.com

Magn Reson Imaging Clin N Am 21 (2013) 427–445
http://dx.doi.org/10.1016/j.mric.2013.01.007
1064-9689/13/$ – see front matter © 2013 Elsevier Inc. All rights reserved.

the female pelvic floor anatomy because functional disorders occur especially in women.

Pelvic Floor

The pelvic floor is a complex, integrated, multilayer system that provides active and passive support. The involved structures are the fascia and ligaments, the pelvic fascia, the pelvic diaphragm, and the urogenital diaphragm (**Box 1**).[3]

Fascia and ligaments provide passive support, whereas the muscles of the pelvic floor, mainly the levator ani, provide active support. The fascia is attached to the bone ring of the pelvis, with the ligament formed from fascia condensations (**Fig. 1**).[3]

The pelvic floor has 3 layers from superior to inferior, the pelvic fascia, pelvic diaphragm, and urogenital diaphragm, with their associated supportive structures, which are intimately to urogenital region, urethra, anal sphincter, and vaginal in women.[3]

The components of the pelvic organ support system are integrated, and they interact and compensate each other.

Pelvic Fascia

Pelvic fascia is a delicate and special structure that envelops the pelvic viscera and maintains the support of the bladder, urethra, uterus, vagina, and rectum in their respective anatomic relationships (**Box 2**).

It is not a true fascia on histology and may be better described as endopelvic connective tissue. However, the structure of this fascia differs greatly from connective tissue that forms the tendon sand ligaments in other parts of the body. The endopelvic fascia comprises a meshwork of collagen, smooth muscle cells, fibroblasts, elastin, and neurovascular and fibrovascular bundles.[4] It is a continuous sheet that goes from the pelvic viscera under the peritoneum to the pelvic diaphragm and laterally attaches to the pelvic bony (**Fig. 2**).

The endopelvic fascia forms transverse and vertical layers of fascia. It is referred to by different names: (1) *pubocervical* between the bladder and the vagina; (2) *rectovaginal* between the vagina

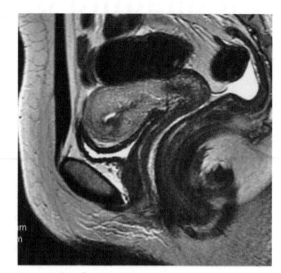

Fig. 1. Pelvic floor. Sagittal plane. Levator ani muscle.

and rectum; (3) *parametrium* at the uterine level, extending from the cervix to the pelvic sidewall; (4) *paracolpium* at the vaginal level, extending from the vagina to the pelvic sidewall; and (5) *tendineus* arcus, which is a lateral condensation of the fascia.[4]

The pubocervical fascia is a transverse anterior layer that extends from the pubis anteriorly to the cervix posteriorly, between the bladder, the urethra, and the vagina, from the pericervical ring to the perineal membrane of the urogenital triangle, which subsequently fuses to the pubic bone, and laterally inserts at the arcus tendineus fascia. The pubocervical fascia originates ligaments of the supporting system of the urethra and the bladder neck, which connect the urethra with the vagina, pubis, and levator ani. The ligaments are (1) the periurethral ligament, originating from the pubococcygeus muscle (levator ani muscle) coursing ventrally to the urethra; (2) the paraurethral ligament, connecting the lateral wall of the urethra to the periurethral ligament; and (3) the pubourethral ligament, connecting the urethra to the arcus tendineus fasciae (see **Fig. 2**).[5] Lesions in the pubocervical fascia will result in an anterior vaginal wall prolapse, including cystocele and urethral hypermobility (**Fig. 3**).

Box 1
Pelvic floor layers
Pelvic fascia
Pelvic diaphragm
Urogenital diaphragm
Urogenital region

Box 2
Pelvic fascia components
Pubocervical fascia
Rectovaginal fascia
Parametrium and paracolpium
Tendineus arcus fascia

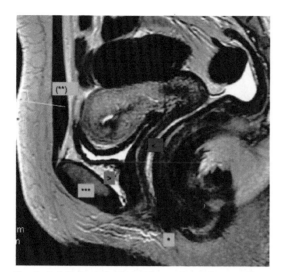

Fig. 2. Pelvic fascia is a continuous sheet that envelops the pelvic viscera (bladder, urethra, uterus, vagina, and rectum) under the peritoneum (*double asterisk*) to the pelvic diaphragm, attached to the perineal body (*asterisk*), arcus tendineus fascia and pelvic bony (*triple asterisk*). Pubocervical fascia (>) extends from the pubis anteriorly to the cervix posteriorly, between the bladder, the urethra, and the vagina; rectovaginal fascia (<) is a layer of connective tissue fused to the undersurface of the posterior vaginal wall and anteriorly to the rectum, suspended superiorly by the cervix attachment of the cardinal-uterosacral ligaments, distally attached to the perineal body.

The rectovaginal fascia is a layer of connective tissue fused to the undersurface of the posterior vaginal wall and anteriorly to the rectum, suspended superiorly by the cervix attachment of the cardinal-uterosacral ligaments, distally attached to the perineal body, and laterally to the arcus tendineus. It is an important structure that supports

the posterior compartment analogous to the pubocervical fascia in the anterior compartment. Between this fascia and the rectum lie the rectovaginal space and the pararectal fascia, which is an important plane for dissection and contains blood vessels, nerves, and lymph nodes, which supply the rectum. Lesions in the rectovaginal fascia will result in a posterior wall prolapse, including rectocele and enterocele (see **Fig. 3**).

The parametrium and paracolpium are part of the pelvic fascia at the uterus and vaginal level, respectively, extending from the cervix and the vagina to the pelvic sidewall. They are very close to the cardinal and uterosacral ligaments.

The uterosacral ligament forms the pericervical ring with fibers involving the cervix and upper vagina. The uterosacral and the cardinal ligaments together form an important, complex support system to the uterus and upper one-third of the vagina. The bilateral cardinal ligaments blend laterally with the parietal fascia of the pelvic sidewall muscles and the uterosacral ligaments with the presacral fascia (**Fig. 4**). Lesions in the pericervical rings promote uterus and vaginal prolapse.

The arcus tendineus fascia has 2 dense aggregations of the fascia, the arcus tendineus fascia pelvis and the arcus tendineus levator ani, which provide important passive lateral support. The arcus tendineus fascia pelvis provides lateral anchoring for the anterior vaginal wall where it supports the urethra, whereas the arcus tendineus levator ani provides anchoring for the levator ani muscles.[3]

Although the arcus tendineus fascia is too small to be visualized, its position can be inferred from the angle formed between the levator ani and the surface of the internal obturator muscles.[6]

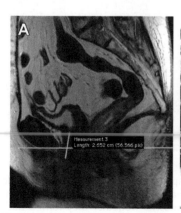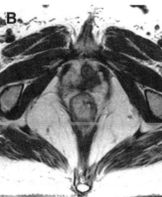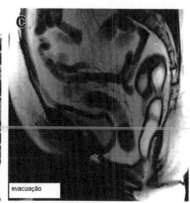

Fig. 3. (*A*) Cystocele and urethral hypermobility. Sagittal T2-weighted image. Note inferior translation of the urethra under the pubic bone. (*B*) Axial T2-weighted image. A defect of the right urethral support ligaments and paravaginal fascia can be noted. (*C*) MR defecography. Sagittal plane. FIESTA sequence. Cystocele. Posterior bladder wall descended below the pubococcygeal line. Note peritoneocele and enterocele.

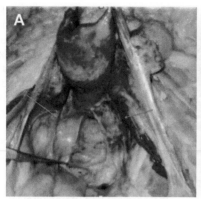
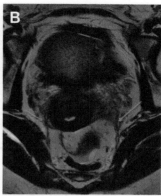

Fig. 4. The uterosacral and cardinal ligaments. Ligament complex support of the uterus and vagina. The utero-sacral forms the pericervical ring (*arrows*) and the cardinal ligaments blend laterally with the parietal fascia. (*A*) Dissection of the uterosacral ligament (*arrows*). (*B*) Axial T-yweighted image. The pericervical ring. The uterosac-ral ligament (*arrow*) blending with presacral fascia and cardinal ligaments laterally with the parietal fascia of the pelvic sidewall muscles. ([*A*] *Courtesy of* Roberto Carvalhosa, MD, Rio de Janeiro; with permission.)

Pelvic Diaphragm

The pelvic diaphragm comprises the levator ani and coccygeus muscles (**Box 3**).

The levator ani is the major muscle of the pelvic diaphragm, which maintains a constant basal tone and closes the urogenital hiatus, preventing incontinence and prolapse (see **Fig. 1**).

It is attached to the pubis and laterally to the arcus tendineus levator ani. This muscle is formed by inseparable parts of a single unit. However, several segments of the levator ani have been described in terms of their visceral insertions, such as the paired iliococcygeus and pubococcygeus muscles.

The ventromedial part of the levator ani, called the pubovisceralis or pubococcygeus muscle, is a thick, slinglike bundle of fibers arising from the inner aspect of the pubis, passing beside the urethra, vagina, and anorectum, and attaching to the vagina and anorectum (**Fig. 5**).

The slinglike configuration of the ventromedial part of the pubococcygeal muscle makes this muscle an important component of the pelvic floor involved in the genesis of prolapse and urinary incontinence. Tonic contraction of the two parts of this muscle closes the urogenital and anorectal

hiatus, which provides a supportive platform during normal activity and standing as well as a contraction reflex to increased intra-abdominal pressures.[6]

The pubovaginal, puborectal, and pubococcygeal muscles compose this muscle. The pubovaginal muscle has a horseshoe shape, inserts in the lateral and posterior vagina wall, and helps to support the vagina. The puborectal muscle suspends the rectum at the anorectal junction, with a slinglike configuration around the anal canal and rectum. It controls the descent of the feces and is considered part of the external anal

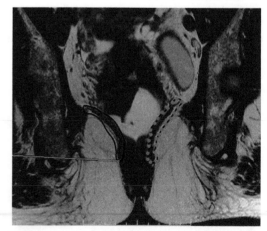

Fig. 5. Pelvic diaphragm diagram. Levator ani muscle, composed by paired iliococcygeus (*blue line*) and pubococcygeus muscles. Together they form a thick, slinglike bundle of fibers arising from the inner aspect of the pubis, passing beside the urethra, vagina, and anorectum, and attaching to the vagina and anorectum.

Box 3
Pelvic diaphragm
Levator ani muscle
Pubococcygeus muscle   Pubovaginal, puborectal, and pubococcygeal muscles
Iliococcygeus muscle
Coccygeus muscle

sphincter. The pubococcygeal part is the larger portion; is Y shaped, inserting on the coccyx (the levator plate); and also helps control the passage of stool (see **Fig. 5**; **Fig. 6**). Between their lateral components there is a space (the levator hiatus) that contains the urethra, vagina, and rectum.

The iliococcygeus muscle is the less dynamic levator ani muscle. It is located above the pubococcygeal muscle, originates from the arcus tendineus levator ani along the lateral pelvic sidewalls and extends posterior to the rectum, working as a musculofascial layer (see **Figs. 5** and **6**).

The coccygeus muscle is a less active muscle that is posterior to the levator ani and extends from the ischial spines to the lateral margins of the coccyx.[6] These muscles are readily visible on MR imaging (see **Fig. 6**).

The sacral nerve roots, S2 through S4, innervate the levator ani via the pudendal nerve. These roots cross the pelvic floor and are stretched and compressed during labor, increasing the chance for injury.[7]

Urogenital Diaphragm

The urogenital diaphragm, also called the *deep perineal space* or *perineal membrane*, has a horizontal configuration, situated caudal to the pelvic diaphragm, superior to the superficial perineal pouch, and anterior to the perineal body and external anal sphincter.[3] It has a triangular configuration from the anterior and lateral pubic bone attachments (pubic simphysis and ischiopubic rami) to the posterior perineal body.[8]

It is comprised of several muscles. The primary muscle of the urogenital diaphragm is the deep transverse muscle of the perineum, which originates at the inner surface of the ischial ramus, extends across the perineal membrane, and is readily visible at MR imaging. The other muscles compose the urethral and urethrovaginal sphincter (**Fig. 7**).

The urogenital diaphragm has attachments to surrounding structures, including the vagina, perineal body, external anal sphincter, and bulbocavernous muscle.[3]

Urethra

The female urethra is approximately 4.5 cm long and exhibits a ventral concavity behind the pubic bone. Two-thirds of the urethra is above the levator ani (pelvic diaphragm). In continent patients, the normal position of the urethra should be entirely retropubic, above or at the inferior pubic level.[5]

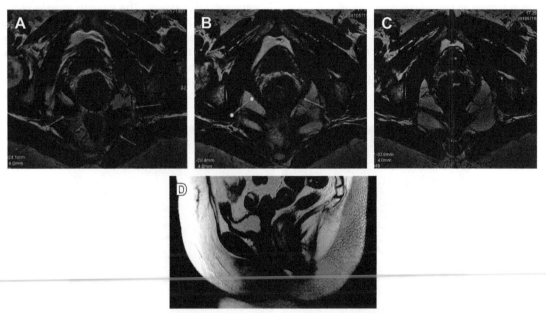

Fig. 6. Levator ani muscle. (*A*) Axial T2-weighted image. Iliococcygeus (*arrows*) muscle located above the pubococcygeal muscle, originates along the lateral pelvic sidewalls, and extends posterior to the rectum. (*B*) Axial T2-weighted image. Pubococcygeus muscles (*arrows*) compose the ventromedial part of the levator ani, composed of the pubovaginal, puborectal, and pubococcygeal muscles. (*C*) Axial T2-weighted image. The pubovaginal and puborectal muscles. The levator hiatus is formed between their lateral components, which contains the urethra, vagina, and rectum. (*D*) Axial T2-weighted image. The pubococcygeal muscle. Y-shaped part of this muscle, inserting on the coccyx (the levator plate muscles).

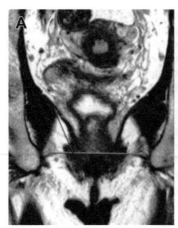
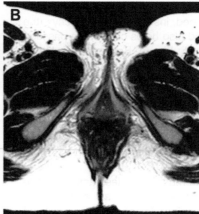

Fig. 7. Urogenital diaphragm. (*A*) Coronal T-yweighted image. This diaphragm (*blue line*) has a horizontal configuration and is situated caudal to the pelvic diaphragm (*red line*), superior to the superficial perineal pouch and anterior to the perineal body and external anal sphincter. (*B*) Axial T2-weighted image. This diaphragm has a triangular shape and is situated anterior to the perineal body and external anal sphincter. It contains the transverse muscle of the perineum and urethral and urethrovaginal sphincter.

In patients presenting with stress incontinence, a short urethra as well as an inferior translation of the urethra, with the lower segment of the urethra lying below the pubis, may be demonstrated (see **Fig. 3**; **Fig. 8**).[5]

The mucosa and submucosa and the internal and external sphincter compose the urethra and can be readily visible at high-resolution MR imaging in almost all individuals (see **Fig. 8**).

The proximal one-third of the urethra is lined with pseudostratified columnar epithelium. The folds of urothelial tissue, with rich submucosal vascular plexuses, mucosal secretions, and urethral smooth muscle, all contribute to passive urethral closure.

The urethral sphincter is comprised of involuntary inner smooth muscle that is continuous with the bladder as well as the voluntary external sphincter (rhabdosphincter), which is comprised of striated muscle. The inner smooth muscle sphincter extends throughout the proximal two-thirds of the urethra, and its tension is distributed relatively uniformly and contributes to about one-third of the intraurethral pressure. The smooth muscle of the urethra has high signal intensity on T2-weighed MR images and demonstrates enhancement after intravenous administration of contrast medium. This finding is probably caused by the specific histologic characteristics of smooth muscles (see **Fig. 8**). Lesions in the proximal sphincter muscle

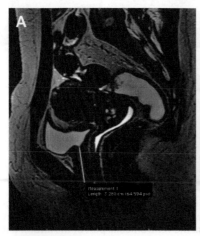
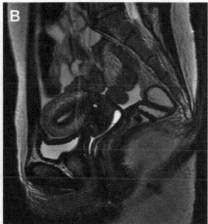

Fig. 8. (*A*) Usual female urethra configuration. It is approximately 4.5 cm long, situated behind the pubic bone, with two-thirds of the urethra retropubic above or at the inferior pubic level. The *green line* represents the urethral length. (*B*) Usual female urethra signal intensity. Sagittal T2-weighted image. Urethral sphincter. The smooth muscle of the urethra shows high signal intensity on T2-weighed image.

promote widening of the proximal urethra at the vesicle neck, called funneling (**Fig. 9**).[5]

Urethral and Bladder Neck Supporting Structures

Fascia and ligament support of the urethra and the bladder neck is vital to preserve urinary continence (**Box 4**).[3]

Vesicopelvic, urethropelvic, and pubourethral ligaments and fascia give anterior and lateral support to the bladder neck and urethra by means of attachment to the pubic bone and arcus tendineus fasciae pelvis.[3]

The pubocervical fascia originates ligaments of the supporting system of the urethra and the bladder neck, which connect the urethra with the vagina, pubis, and levator ani and can be easily identified with high-resolution MR imaging in almost all individuals. There is no consensus about these structures. However, the pubocervical fascia originates the periurethral ligament, which inserts directly into the levator ani muscle; the paraurethral ligament, connecting the lateral wall of the urethra to the periurethral ligament; and the pubourethral ligament, connecting the urethra to the arcus tendineus fasciae (**Fig. 10**).

The pubovesical ligament or muscle, an extension of detrusor smooth muscle coursing through the retropubic space to the arcus tendineus

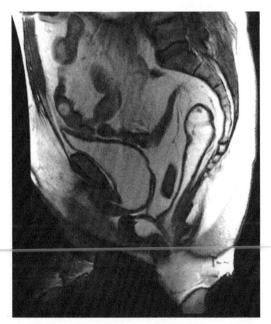

Fig. 9. Sagittal FIESTA defecography. Proximal sphincter lesion. Note widening of the proximal urethra at the vesicle neck, named funneling. Note cystocele, peritoneocele, and intussusception.

> **Box 4**
> **Ligaments of the supporting system of the urethra**
>
> Periurethral ligament
> Paraurethral ligament
> Pubourethral ligament

fasciae pelvis, has been identified at high-resolution MR imaging in a cadaver and may assist in opening the bladder neck during voiding. The bladder neck position is influenced by connections between the puborectalis muscle, vagina, and proximal urethra.[3] Lesions in the periurethral ligaments can be partial or incomplete and may cause urethral hypermobility with stress incontinence (see **Fig. 3**).[5]

Urogenital Region

The urogenital region forms the superficial part of the anterior pelvic floor. The external genital muscles of the perineum, the bulbocavernous (bulbospongiosus) muscle, and the ischiocavernous muscle lie within this region, as does the urethrovaginal sphincter in women.[3]

In women, the bulbocavernous muscle inserts into the pubic arch and the root and dorsum of the clitoris and has attachments to the vagina and urogenital diaphragm. The external genital muscles are visible with high-resolution MR imaging in all individuals.[3]

Vagina

The vaginal wall comprises smooth muscle and connective tissue (collagen and elastin) (**Box 5**).[3]

The vaginal support is composed of the pericervical ring, pelvic fascia, urogenital diaphragm, and arcus tendineus levator ani. DeLancey[9] describes 3 levels of vaginal support: (1) level I is the uterosacral-cardinal complex; (2) level II is the arcus tendineus fascia pelvis; and (3) level III is the perineal membrane and arcus tendineus levator ani (**Fig. 11**).

The uterosacral-cardinal complex supports the uterus and upper one-third of the vagina, with fibers involving the cervix and blending with the upper vagina (see **Fig. 4**).

The midvagina, level II support, is provided by the attachment of the vaginal muscularis to the arcus tendineus fascia pelvis and the intact vaginal muscularis. The anterior wall is bridged bilaterally between the arcus tendineus fascia pelvis. This hammock of vaginal tissue lies beneath the urethra and may be a vital component of urinary

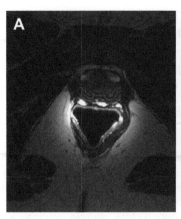
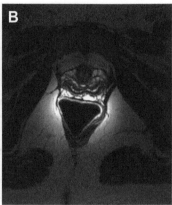
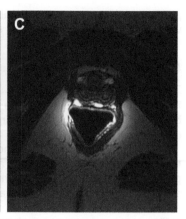

Fig. 10. Periurethral ligaments. (*A*) Axial T2-weighted image with endorectal coil. This ligament inserts directly into the levator ani muscle. (*B*) Axial T2-weighted image with endorectal coil. This ligament connects the lateral wall of the urethra to the periurethral ligament. (*C*) Axial T2-weighted image with endorectal coil. This ligament connects the urethra to the arcus tendineus fasciae.

continence. The urethra is compressed against this tissue when abdominal pressure is increased, as during coughing (**Fig. 12**).

The rectovaginal fascia and the perineal membrane maintain the third level of vagina support. Also, the vagina is attached to the levator ani at the level of the urogenital diaphragm. Its wall is surrounded by adipose tissue containing an extensive venous plexus.

When the support is intact, the vagina has an H-shaped configuration on the MR axial images. When there is a tear in the rectovaginal fascia or pubococcygeal muscle, the vagina loses this configuration, is asymmetric, and retracts toward the lesion (see **Fig. 12**).[5]

Perineal Body

Directly anterior to the anal sphincter is the perineal body (central tendon of the perineum). In men, it is posterior to the spongious and cavernous bodies and their related muscles, whereas in women it lies within the anovaginal septum. Many structures insert fibers into the perineal body, including the external anal sphincter, the deep and superficial transverse muscles of the perineum (urogenital diaphragm), and the bulbocavernous and puborectalis (pubococcygeus) muscles. The superficial transverse muscle of the perineum spans the dorsal edge of the urogenital diaphragm and elevates the perineal body (see **Fig. 2**).

Anal Sphincter

The anal canal sphincter contains muscular and neurovascular components and is surrounded by the fat-containing ischioanal space. The epithelial

Box 5	
Pelvic floor lesion related to a specific pelvic floor component	
Pelvic Floor Component	**Lesion**
Pubocervical fascia	Anterior vaginal wall prolapse, including cystocele and urethral hypermobility
Rectovaginal fascia	Rectocele and peritoneocele
Perivaginal ring	Uterus and vaginal prolapse
Urethral sphincter	Funneling
Lesion in the periurethral ligaments	Urethral hypermobility with stress incontinence

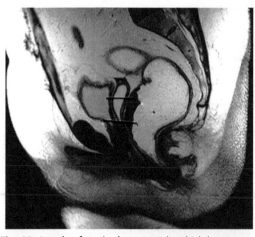

Fig. 11. Levels of vaginal support: level I (*above superior blue line*), uterosacral-cardinal complex; level II (*between blue lines*), arcus tendineus fascia pelvis; and level III (*below inferior blue line*), perineal membrane and arcus tendineus levator ani.

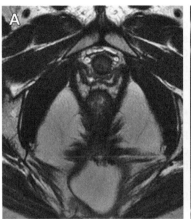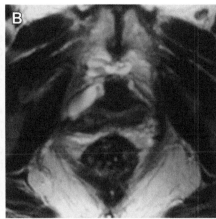

Fig. 12. (*A*) Vagina with an intact support has an H-shaped configuration on the axial T2-weighted image. The vaginal tissue supports the urethra and, together with the pubovaginal muscle, compresses the urethra when abdominal pressure is increased. (*B*) Paravaginal support tear. Tear in the pubococcygeal muscle, with an asymmetric vagina, retracted toward the lesion on the right side.

lining of the distal part of the anal canal is stratified squamous epithelium, richly supplied by sensory receptors that are concentrated mostly at the dentate line. This line demarcates the junction with the proximal columnar epithelium, which is devoid of sensory receptors. The mechanism of anal continence is similar to that of urinary control, with the anal lining and its underlying vascular spaces, the anal cushions, playing a major role in sealing the anal canal.[3]

The anal sphincters form cylindrical layers between which lies the longitudinal muscle and internal and external sphincter. The internal sphincter forms the innermost muscular layer and is the terminal condensation of the circular rectal smooth muscle. The internal sphincter extends from the anorectal junction to approximately 1.0 to 1.5 cm below the dentate line. It comprises smooth muscle fibers with autonomous innervations from sympathetic presacral nerves.[3]

The longitudinal muscle is the continuation of longitudinal muscle of the rectal wall. The longitudinal muscle is closely related to the subcutaneous external sphincter, whereas others have stated that this muscle passes through the subcutaneous external sphincter to terminate in the perianal skin.

The external sphincter is the outermost muscle of the distal anal canal and comprises several parallel bundles. It is a circular structure and is shorter anteriorly in women. The external sphincter extends approximately 1 cm beyond the internal sphincter. The superior part of the external sphincter is fused with or intimately related to the puborectalis muscle. Anteriorly, it is closely related to the superficial transverse muscle of the perineum and the perineal body. Posteriorly, the muscle is continuous with the

anococcygeal ligament. All sphincter muscles are readily seen on MR imaging, but the internal sphincter is best seen at the endoanal MR imaging. The muscle is under voluntary control and innervated by the pudendal nerves.[3]

MR IMAGING TECHNIQUE

MR imaging can add important information to the diagnosis of urethral and anal incontinence and to the diagnosis of pelvic prolapse. MR images acquired with phased-array coil have an increased spatial resolution and signal-to-noise ratio.

Detailed demonstration of the urethra, sphincter, supporting ligaments, and levator ani became possible with this superior soft tissue contrast, and the images provide valuable information about the anatomy discussed earlier and lesion assessment.

The MR protocol should include axial, sagittal, and coronal T2-weighted high-resolution images.

For the dynamic pelvic floor imaging, fast T2-weighted imaging (single-shot fast spin echo, half-Fourier acquisition turbo spin echo, and FIESTA [fast imaging employing steady-state acquisition]) should be performed during rest and strain.

MR imaging should be performed in a 1.5T or 3T unit, with a phased-array coil, to improve signal-to-noise ratio, such as the cardiac phased-array coil.

Dynamic MR Defecography Technique

A variety of approaches to perform dynamic MR imaging of the pelvic floor have been advocated. Generally, most centers perform a 3-phase examination consisting of (1) Valsalva imaging, (2) a squeeze maneuver to assess puborectalis contraction, and (3) simulated defecation using rectal contrast to examine for rectal abnormalities and pelvic organ prolapse.

The authors' standard MR protocol includes patient preparation, instruction, and positioning and MR technique.

Patient Preparation

The patient preparation consists of 2 parts: preparation at home and at the radiology department. At home, a 4-hour fasting is necessary before the examination, and a bowel preparation applying a glycerin suppository is recommended 2 to 8 hours before the examination.

Before the examination at the radiology department, patients are asked to urinate. A full bladder prolapse may block the descent of a rectocele or uterus prolapse and prevent its identification.

Routinely, to prevent intestinal peristalsis and uterine contractions, 10 mg of butylescopolamine is injected intravenously.

The preparation at the radiology department consists of 10 mL of intravaginal ultrasound gel (to distend the vaginal fornix) and 4 syringes of 60 mL of contrast gel, using a rectal probe n° 30 for the application.

The intrarectal contrast gel is introduced until patients report a sensation of fullness and voiding urge or until complete (250 mL).

Patient Instruction

Before imaging, patients are instructed about the maneuvers they will perform as part of the MR examination (Valsalva, squeeze, and defecation). It is important to use easy-to-understand directions (eg, bear down as hard as you can, squeeze your anal muscle and pull your pelvic floor up, relax).[10]

During the dynamic examination itself, patients are instructed to initiate the dynamic movement when they hear the technologist's command, so that image acquisition will begin at rest and proceed through the desired motion. The instructions should be heard above the noise of the magnet. Confirming that patients have performed the right maneuver at the time of the scan is important to assure a diagnostic examination.[10]

Patient Positioning and MR Technique

Patients lie in the supine position. A pillow is accommodated under the gluteus, simulating a sanitary toilet (**Fig. 13**).

Patients are positioned such that the symphysis pubis is located in the middle of the phased-array coil.

The 3 compartments of the pelvic floor should be identified before and after the administration of rectal contrast medium with no need for further opacification of the bladder because the soft tissues provide an excellent contrast during MR imaging acquisition.[11]

The MR examination is divided into 3 steps:

1. *Analysis of the pelvic floor structures at rest*: Images are acquired without endorectal contrast in T2-weighted high-resolution sequences in the axial, sagittal, and coronal planes. In these images, it is possible to analyze the components of the levator ani muscle, the levator hiatus, urethral and anal anatomy and lesions, as well as the position of the pelvic organs. Another important contribution of pelvic floor MR imaging is to identify the presence of other lesions out of the pelvic floor, such as the uterine leiomyoma, which can accentuate symptoms, and the solitary rectal ulcer, which can be associated with intussusception.[11]
2. *Dynamic video evaluation during the Valsalva maneuver*: The examination is performed in the sagittal plane during the Valsalva maneuver to determine the severity of the pelvic floor injury and to identify lesions related to urethral

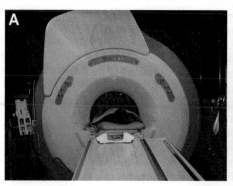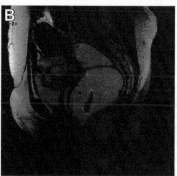

Fig. 13. Positioning in the MR unit. (*A*) Patients lie in the supine position, with legs bent. (*B*) A pillow is accommodated under the gluteus, simulating a sanitary toilet.

incontinence. In the coronal plane, the mobility of iliococcygeal component of the levator ani muscle is assessed as a reflex of unilateral or bilateral muscle bulging during increased intra-abdominal pressure (hernia).

3. *Dynamic study after the introduction of endorectal contrast medium (gel)*: The dynamic study is performed while patients are lying down with bent knees during sphincter contraction and evacuation. Images are acquired in video mode in the sagittal plane.

The high-resolution protocol at rest includes the following conventional sequences:

- Sagittal T2-weighted fast spin echo (FOV 26; thickness 4.0 × 0.2; matrix 384 × 224; NEX 4; repetition time [TR] 4400 and echo time [TE] 102; 24 slices)
- Axial T2-weighted fast spin echo (FOV 26; thickness 4.0 × 0.5; matrix 256 × 192; NEX 3; TR 4400 and TE 90; 30 slices)
- Coronal T2-weighted fast spin echo (FOV 24; thickness 4.0 × 0.2; matrix 384 × 224; NEX 4; TR 4200 and TE 101; 20 slices)

The dynamic protocol includes the following conventional sequences:

- Sagittal FIESTA sequence at rest (FOV 30; thickness 10.0 × 5.0; matrix 320 × 320; NEX 1; TE minimum; 1 slices) (to make sure the image includes the anorectal angle, bladder, urethra, and vagina)
- Sagittal Valsalva (same protocol as earlier with 20 repeats)
- Sagittal squeeze (same protocol as earlier with 50 repeats)
- Sagittal defecation (same protocol as earlier with 170 repeats) (**Fig. 14**)

The defecation dynamic study should be repeated until the endorectal gel is eliminated. The radiologist must evaluate images because a large rectocele may prevent the descent of an enterocele or identification of intussusception and rectal prolapse. Moreover, the diagnosis of spastic pelvic floor is based on the difficulty to eliminate the endorectal gel; it is necessary to make sure patients understand the radiologist's directions.

EXAMINATION INTERPRETATION

Patients referred for dynamic imaging of the pelvic floor generally possess multiple abnormalities involving the anterior (bladder and urethra), middle (vagina and uterus), and posterior pelvic compartments (rectum).

Abnormal descendant and associated findings are described later.

The examination interpretation is divided in 2 steps. The first one is to analyze the high-resolution T2-weighted images, identifying lesions in the fasciae, ligaments, and pelvic support muscles. The second part of the interpretation is to evaluate the dynamic images.

1. Levator ani muscle

The radiologist should focus on muscle morphology, thickness, and signal strength. In the T2-weighted axial images, the healthy levator ani sling should be evenly thick throughout, and the signal should be low and homogenous.

Levator ani muscle injury is characterized by asymmetric or diffuse reduction in thickness with or without fat infiltration of the muscle fibers. Fat infiltration appears as high signal intensity in the muscle fibers on T1- and T2-weighted sequences (**Fig. 15**).

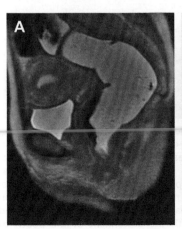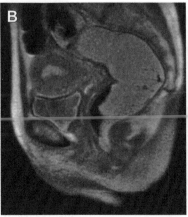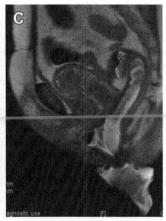

Fig. 14. Dynamic study after introduction of endorectal contrast medium (gel). (*A*) Valsalva. (*B*) Squeeze. (*C*) Defecation.

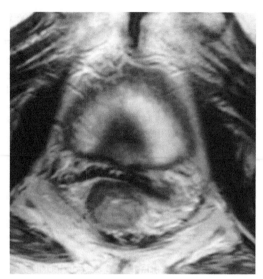

Fig. 15. Increase the levator hiatus and reduction in thickness with fat infiltration of the puborectalis muscle.

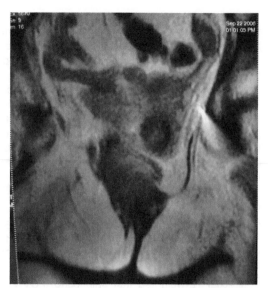

Fig. 16. Coronal imaging during Valsalva maneuver at dynamic MR showing herniation of the left levator ani muscle in a patient with muscle lesion.

In very severe lesions, the distance between the puborectalis fibers, the levator hiatus, increases in the axial plane. In women with an intact pelvic floor, the length should be at most 4.5 cm.

The puborectalis muscle may have become detached from the pubis, and the proximal extremity appears retracted and irregular. As a consequence, a paravaginal defect appears; the vagina retracts toward the injury and the urethra rotates.

Coronal imaging during Valsalva at dynamic MR can detect herniations and eventrations of the levator ani muscle in patients with muscle lesions, which cannot be seen at traditional fluoroscopy (Fig. 16).

2. Pubococcygeal line

The level of the pelvic floor on dynamic MR can be demarcated radiologically on the midsagittal image using the pubococcygeal line as described by Yang and colleagues.[12] There are other lines proposed for the radiological measuring of pelvic organ prolapse, like the H and M lines, but the pubococcygeal line is the best accepted.

This line extends from the most inferior portion of the pubic symphysis to the last horizontal coccygeal joint. This line is easily drawn and highly reproducible on MR imaging in all patients.

By convention, the descent of pelvic organs and structures is measured from the pubococcygeal line. The descent of any particular structure/organ is measured along a perpendicular line from the pubococcygeal line to the structure (Fig. 17).

The distance between the pubococcygeal line and the bladder, cervix, and anorectal junction should be measured on images obtained during rest, Valsalva maneuver, and evacuation.[11,13]

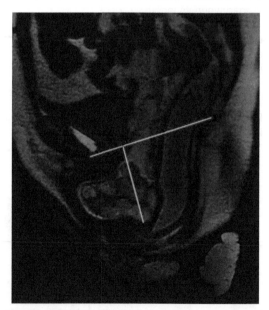

Fig. 17. Pubococcygeal line, extending from the most inferior portion of the pubic symphysis to the last horizontal coccygeal joint. Descent of any particular structure/organ is measured along a perpendicular line from the pubococcygeal line to the structure. This case is of a peritoneocele showing the protrusion of the peritoneal fat alone between the rectum and the vagina, with the descendant of the pouch of Douglas into the rectovaginal space caused by disruption of the rectovaginal fascia.

In women with normal continence, the bladder, the uterus, and the vaginal vault remain above the pubococcygeal line.[11,14]

The anorectal junction is below this line, and the distance should not be greater than 2 cm.

During the Valsalva maneuver, the pelvic organs may move very slightly; but if the organ descends from 1 to 2 cm below the pubococcygeal line, the pelvic floor has likely been weakened. If the prolapsed exceeds 2 cm, then surgery may be indicated. This sequence is very important to access lesions related to urethral incontinence.[11,14]

The puborectal hiatus line (H line) allows grading of the maximal widening of the pelvic sling in the anteroposterior dimension during straining and is the linear distance between the symphysis pubis and the rectum. The H line represents the most caudal part of the levator ani group (the puborectalis muscle). The abnormal widening of the pelvic floor, measured with the H line, is graded progressively when it exceeds 6 cm in length. The other component of pelvic floor relaxation is the M line, which is the measure of muscular pelvic floor descent.

The M lines extends perpendicularly from the pubococcygeal line to the posterior end of the H line. Abnormal descent (M line) is progressively graded when its length exceeds 2 cm.

With significant pelvic floor relaxation, variable degrees of pelvic floor widening (H line) and descent (M line) are present at dynamic MR imaging (**Fig. 18**).

Anterior Compartment

Patients with anterior prolapse may have coexisting or occult incontinence. For this reason, the imaging interpretation should include the study of urinary incontinence. Stress urinary incontinence (involuntary loss of urine during increased abdominal pressure) is related to intrinsic urethral sphincter deficiency and urethral hypermobility.

In sagittal images acquired during pelvic floor contraction, the healthy urethra remains slightly vertical and anterior to the base of the bladder. The loss of urethral integrity related to the sphincter and the anterior fascia support of the bladder leads to urethral hypermobility, as observed when comparing the organ's position during rest, Valsalva maneuver, and evacuation.[11]

The urethra and supporting ligaments are best visualized at rest MR images and the urethral hypermobility during dynamic imaging with Valsalva.

In continent patients, the normal position of the urethra is retropubic, above or at the inferior pubic level. When there is a defect of the urethral support ligaments or paravaginal fascia, we observe an inferior translation of the urethra under the pubic bone (**Fig. 19**).

Urethral hypermobility is demonstrated when the urethra rotates excessively, more than 30°, from its rest axis, from the vertical to horizontal axis (the rotational urethral descend).[4]

Funneling of the proximal urethra or the opening of the urethrovesical junction is visualized as a widening and filling of the proximal urethra. It can be seen during rest or Valsalva and it is associated with urinary incontinence; however, it can also be seen in some continent patients.

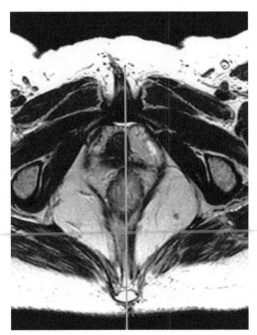

Fig. 19. Injury to the pubocervical fascia and ligaments, with consequent rotation urethra.

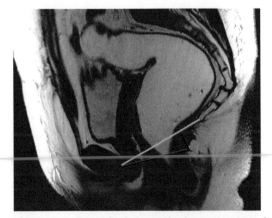

Fig. 18. Line H (*red line*): From the lower portion of the pubic symphysis to the posterior wall of the rectum. Line M (*blue line*): From the pubococcygeal line to the H line. It represents the longitudinal extent of the levator ani.

In cystocele and stress-induced incontinence, the levator ani muscle and the pubocervical fascia are injured, making the posterior bladder wall descend below the pubococcygeal line, thereby displacing the anterior vaginal wall. Depending on its severity, the injury may be identified at rest, during the Valsalva maneuver, or evacuation (**Fig. 20**).[11,15]

Many investigators consider the descent of the bladder base below the pubococcygeal line to be abnormal, defined as anterior descent or cystocele. However, some normal, continent patients demonstrate a slight descent of the bladder base below the pubococcygeal line. Consequently, we graduate the anterior prolapse as small, medium, and large.

To graduate the prolapse, the distance between the pubococcygeal line and the bladder base is measured on the MR image. It can be performed at images acquired with the Valsalva maneuver or evacuation. In the authors' institution, they considered anterior prolapse (cystocele) as small (<3 cm), medium (3–6 cm), and large (>6 cm).

Middle Compartment

The normal vagina is H shaped, indicating adequate lateral fascia support. When normal support is lost, the vagina becomes longer and sometimes asymmetrical, depending on which side of the levator ani muscle has been most severely injured.[11,12]

The vaginal vault (in patients with hysterectomies) and cervix vaginal junction can be readily seen on midsagittal dynamic MR images. It should be recognized that although many published series define vaginal vault or uterine prolapsed as occurring when the vaginal vault or cervicovaginal junction descends below the pubococcygeal line, many asymptomatic patients will have a mild descent of the vaginal vault to a point 3 cm or less below the pubococcygeal line; such descent should be considered small (**Fig. 21**).

When the uterus descends more than 3 cm below the pubococcygeal line, it can impede rectal evacuation, especially with leiomyoma.

In the authors' institution, they consider a downward displacement (uterine prolapse) as mild (<3 cm), moderate (3–6 cm), or severe (>6 cm).

Mild compartment disorders include peritoneocele. The anterior rectum is normally opposed to the posterior vaginal wall through pelvic floor maneuvers. Peritoneocele is the protrusion of the peritoneal fat alone between the rectum and the vagina, with the descendant of the pouch of Douglas into the rectovaginal space caused by disruption of the rectovaginal fascia (see **Fig. 17**).

The pouch of Douglas is considered the most inferior portion of the peritoneal cavity and is usually located at the level of the posterior vaginal fornix. However, the depth of the cul-de-sac may vary a lot, more than 5 cm. To diagnose a peritoneocele, it is necessary to identify the inferior

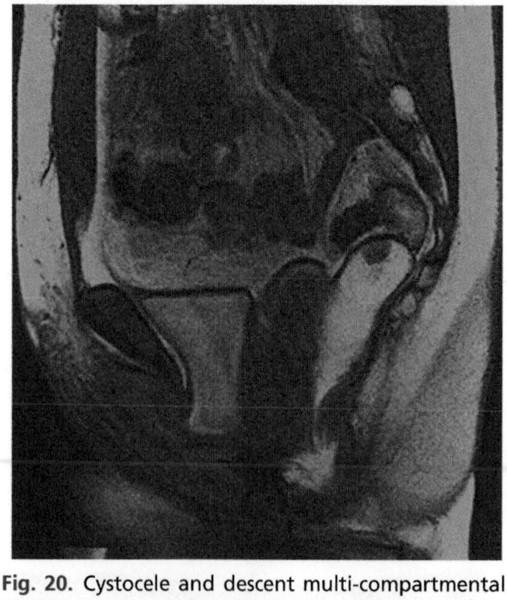

Fig. 20. Cystocele and descent multi-compartmental. Bladder, uterus, and posterior descend below the pubococcygeal line. The uterus compresses the inferior rectum wall, causing defecation obstruction.

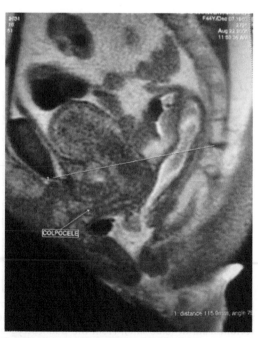

Fig. 21. Colpocele. Cervicovaginal junction descends below the pubococcygeal line.

herniation of the lower peritoneal pouch along the anterior rectal wall, forming a wide rectovaginal fossa with an increased distance between the vagina and the rectum.

The peritoneocele pouch may contain only peritoneal fat or it can be accompanied by the small bowel loops (enterocele) and the large bowel, like sigmoid or ceco (sigmoidocele or cecocele). This condition can be identified at rest and by accentuating the dynamic images acquired in the sagittal plane during Valsalva or evacuation, when the sigmoid or small bowel loops may be seen invading the space between the rectum and vagina.[2,11]

Several studies as well as the authors' experience suggest that dynamic MR imaging is more sensitive than fluoroscopic proctography for detecting enteroceles.

Sometimes it is necessary to repeat the evacuation sequence to empty the rectum or a rectocele to identify the peritoneocele. Also, its detection can be improved by undertaking a repeat posttoilet straining image.[16]

Enterocele is classified into 3 degrees: (1) herniation as far as the distal third of the vagina, (2) herniation as far as the perineum, and (3) herniation extending beyond the anal canal.

It can be asymptomatic, and sometimes it is not detected before a pelvic floor corrective surgery. However, it may evolve with increasingly visible symptoms after the procedure and eventually require another surgical correction.

Posterior Compartment

The evaluation of the posterior compartment includes some observations at rest and during the evacuation sequence, such as the following:

Rest: (1) the outline of the anterior wall to identify small rectoceles; (2) the position of the anorectal junction in relation to the pubococcygeal line; and (3) the evaluation of the levator plate.

Measurements during evacuation: (1) the anorectal angle; (2) the length and degree of the anal canal opening; (3) the position of the anorectal junction in relation to the pubococcygeal line (perineal descent); (4) the degree of rectal voiding; and (5) the duration and number of contractions required to eliminate the rectal contrast should be quantified.

The existence of voluntary loss of endorectal gel during rest, Valsalva sequence, and sphincter contraction should also be observed.

Anorectal angle

Changes in the anorectal angle during squeeze and defecation allow estimation of the puborectalis muscle function.

During squeeze, the anorectal junction should move superiorly and generally anteriorly, thus, the anorectal angle normally decreases, reflecting normal puborectalis contraction (**Fig. 22B**).

During evacuation, the anorectal junction should move downward, increasing in this angle, reflecting puborectalis relaxation (see **Fig. 22C**).

The anorectal angle is the angle between the midline of the anal canal and a line tangent to the posterior rectal wall (see **Fig. 22A**).[11]

At rest, the angle is 95° on average (range 70°–134°), although it rarely exceeds 120° in healthy individuals. The anorectal angle normally decreases during sphincter contraction and increases during sphincter evacuation because of the contraction and relaxation, respectively, of the puborectalis muscle.[11,17,18] In healthy individuals, this variation should be more than 20°.

Anal canal length

Anal canal length at rest is 16 mm (range 6–26 mm) in women and 22 mm (range 10–38 mm) in young

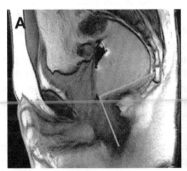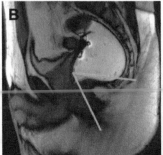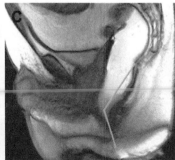

Fig. 22. Anorectal angle. (*A*) Rest. This angle is measured from the midline of the anal canal to a tangent to the posterior rectal wall. (*B*) Squeeze. The anorectal junction should move superiorly and generally moves anteriorly, thus this angle normally decreases, reflecting normal puborectalis contraction. (*C*) Evacuation. The anorectal junction moves downwards, increasing this angle, reflecting puborectalis relaxation.

men. During sphincter contraction, the length of the anal canal is slightly reduced to an average 14 mm (range 6–20 mm) in young women and 17 mm (range 9–27 mm) in young men.[11]

Perineal descent

The perineum is considered to have prolapsed or descended when it extends more than 2 cm below the pubococcygeal line during evacuation. This condition is commonly observed in patients with chronic intestinal constipation and in multiparous women (**Fig. 23**).[11,19]

The difference in the distance from the anorectum junction and pubococcygeal line at rest and during the evacuation sequence should be quantified and reported (**Box 6**).

Perineal descent may be mild (<3 cm), moderate (3–6 cm), or severe (>6 cm).[11,13]

TYPES OF DISORDERS
Rectocele

Rectocele is an anterior protrusion in the rectal wall, related to the rectovaginal fascia defect. Rectoceles reflect "give-way" of the anterior rectal, often in the context of deficient support mechanisms, such as after a hysterectomy or vaginal delivery fascia lesion (**Fig. 24**).

They are relatively common, especially in women. Rectoceles less than 2 cm are common in asymptomatic women, particularly in older women, and

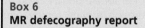

Box 6
MR defecography report
High-resolution images
Pelvic organs' position related to the pubococcygeal line
Urethral length and position
Vaginal aspect and position
Levator ani signal intensity and thickness
Levator hiatus
Anal sphincter thickness and signal intensity
Anorectal angle at rest
Dynamic images
Anorectal angle at strain (squeeze and evacuation)
Pelvic organs' position related to the pubococcygeal line
Perineal descent
Voluntary loss of endorectal gel during rest and Valsalva sequence
Degree of rectal voiding
Duration and number of contractions required to eliminate the rectal contrast
Peritoneocele (enterocele)
Rectocele (complete or partial voiding)
Intussusception and rectal prolapse

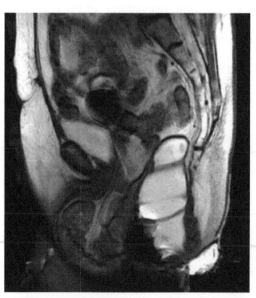

Fig. 23. Descending pelvic floor secondary to chronic constipation. History of hysterectomy and cystocele corrective surgery. Also note the presence of enterocele.

can be considered clinically insignificant. However, rectocele is an important cause of evacuation obstruction, and it may occur with a small anterior rectum wall bulge.

It is defined on image as an anterior rectal protrusion in relation to a line drawn upward from the anterior wall. Anterior rectoceles are classified according to the size of the protrusion in 3 degrees: (1) small: rectocele less than 2 cm; (2) moderate: rectocele between 2 cm and 4 cm; and (3) severe: rectocele more than 4 cm.

It is importance to describe the complete or partial voiding of the rectocele, with contrast retention, at the end of the evacuation sequence and the need for manual voiding (digital vaginal manipulation) to empty it. It is functional information to the surgeon.

Rectoceles may be secondary to excessive straining in patients with impaired pelvic floor relaxation. Impaired emptying of a rectocele may contribute not only to symptoms of disordered defecation but also to passive leakage (after defecation) in fecal incontinence.

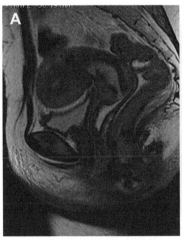
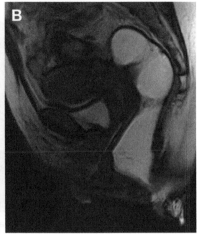

Fig. 24. Rectocele. Note the anterior protrusion in the rectal wall, related to rectovaginal fascia defect, during evacuation. (*A*) Rest. (*B*) Evacuation.

Descending Pelvic Floor Syndrome

In this syndrome, pelvic floor muscle tone is highly reduced. The diagnosis is usually based on clinical symptoms, electrophysiological test, and image findings, especially MR imaging.[11,13,20]

The descent of the rectum, bladder, and vagina in relation to the pubococcygeal line, covering 1, 2, or all 3 compartments, is defined as pathologic. The examination is performed at rest, during the Valsalva maneuver, and evacuation. The pelvic floor is likely to be more severely compromised when abnormalities are observed both at rest and during evacuation effort (see **Fig. 20**).

Pelvic floor descent may be mild (<3 cm), moderate (3–6 cm), or severe (>6 cm) in relation to the pubococcygeal line.

Spastic Pelvic Floor Syndrome

The spastic pelvic floor syndrome includes a large group of constipated patients who complain of the inability to evacuate but in whom no significant underlying structural abnormality is found. The clinical symptoms are a difficulty in initiating evacuation and incomplete rectal evacuation. It is also named as anismus and paradoxic puborectalis syndrome.

The emptying phase of the MR defecography gives important information about rectal structure and function. At rest, the puborectalis muscle drives the rectum anteriorly to maintain the anorectal angle (the angle between the posterior border of the distal rectum and the center of the anal canal); during evacuation, the anorectal junction should move downwards, increasing this angle, reflecting puborectalis relaxation.

In the spastic pelvic floor syndrome, the puborectalis muscle is not relaxed during defecation and can remain hypertonic throughout the evacuation (**Fig. 25**).[11,19,21]

Dynamic MR sagittal images reveal a smaller change in the anorectal angle, reflecting the fact that the puborectalis muscle fails to relax during the evacuation process, requiring more sequences (each of them with 150 seconds) to eliminate a small amount of the rectal contrast or even do not eliminate it. In healthy individuals, the rectum emptying process will not last more than 30 seconds.

Moreover, a prominent puborectal impression related to the paradoxic contraction of the muscle may be identified, reducing the angle during evacuation. As the result, patients make a considerable effort to evacuate.

Intussusception and Rectal Prolapse

Invaginations of the rectal wall and mucous membrane toward the rectal or the anal lumen are referred to as *intussusceptions*.[11] The invagination includes the mucous membrane and may be accompanied by parietal components, promoting wider invaginating rectal folds measuring more than 3 mm.

It can be classified as internal (intrarectal and intra-anal) and external, forming the rectal prolapse. This classification is of doubtful utility because the invagination starts in the rectal wall and extends toward the anorectal junction.

It is relatively commonly observed in asymptomatic patients. If the intussusceptions reach the anal canal, patients experience a sensation of incomplete voiding caused by obstruction.

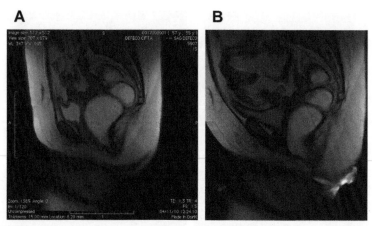

Fig. 25. Dynamic MR sagittal images reveals a smaller change in the anorectal angle, reflecting the fact that the puborectalis muscle fails to relax during evacuation process. (*A*) Rest. (*B*) Evacuation.

Intussusception is classified according to the degree of rectal exteriorization at the end of evacuation in 3 degrees: (1) intussusception is intrarectal, with minimal involvement of the rectal wall or circumferential involvement restricted to the rectum; (2) intussusception is restricted to the inside anal canal; and (3) intussusception reaches beyond the anal canal and prolapses through the anus.

Other Pathologic Conditions and Incidental Findings

MR imaging can display pelvic pathologies beyond the rectum and pelvic organ prolapsed, most typically ovarian and uterine and urethral masses, such as leiomyoma and diverticula.

SUMMARY

Dynamic MR imaging of the pelvic floor has become a recognized adjunct, problem-solving test in the evaluation of patients with defecatory disorders and pelvic floor prolapse and is increasingly used in the day-to-day practice, affecting management decisions.

Defecography with MR provides accurate evaluation of the morphology and function of the anorectal and pelvic muscles and organs involved in pelvic floor dynamics. Imaging in the sagittal plane makes it possible to completely evaluate the anal canal and the position of anorectal junction, vaginal vault, and bladder base in relation to the pubococcygeal line and thereby detect any pelvic organ descent. With high-resolution imaging, it is also possible to define the anatomy and functioning of the levator ani muscle, one of the most important components of the pelvic floor.

The spatial and temporal resolution is high enough to allow evaluation of the relevant morphologic structures and dynamics of the pelvic floor, demonstrating the major pathologies affecting the defecation mechanism. Classification of findings into mild, moderate, and severe degrees is a direct and reproducible method of describing, staging, and quantifying visceral pelvic prolapse.[11]

REFERENCES

1. Flusberg M, Sahni VA, Erturk SM, et al. Dynamic MR defecography: assessment of the usefulness of defecation phase. AJR Am J Roentgenol 2011;196: W394–9.
2. Roos JE, Weishaupt D, Wildermuth S, et al. Experience of 4 years with open MR defecography: pictorial review of anorectal anatomy and disease. Radiographics 2002;22:817–32.
3. Stoker J, Halligan S, Bartram CI. Pelvic floor imaging. Radiology 2001;218:621–41.
4. Woodfield AC, Krishnamoorthy S, Hampton BS, et al. Imaging pelvic floor disorders: trend toward comprehensive MRI. AJR Am J Roentgenol 2010; 194:1640–9.
5. Macura JK, Genadry RR, Bluemke DA. MR imaging of the female urethra and supporting ligaments in assessment of urinary incontinence: spectrum of abnormalities. Radiographics 2006;26:1135–49.
6. Tunn R, DeLance J, Quint EE. Visibility of pelvic organ support system structures in magnetic resonance images without an endovaginal coil. Am J Obstet Gynecol 2001;184(6):1156–63.
7. Handa VL, Harris TA, Ostergard DR. Protecting the pelvic floor: obstetric management to prevent incontinence and pelvic organ prolapse. Obstet Gynecol 1996;88:470.
8. Houshmand G. Imaging of the female perineum in adults. Radiographics 2012;32:E129–68.
9. DeLancey JO. Anatomic aspects of vaginal eversion after hysterectomy. Am J Obstet Gynecol 1992;166: 1717–24.

10. Baert AL, Knauth M. Imaging pelvic floor disorders. Chapter 4 (4.2). 2008;75–88.

11. Bartram CI, Madoff RD (2008). Imaging atlas of the pelvic floor and anorectal diseases. Chapter 23;219–36.

12. Yang A, Mostwin JL, Rosenshein NB, et al. Pelvic Floor descent in women: dynamic evaluation with fast MR imaging and cinematic display. Radiology 1991;179:25–33.

13. Hetez F, Andreisek G, Tsagari C, et al. MR defecography in patients with fecal incontinence: imaging findings and their effect on surgical management. Radiology 2006;240:449–57.

14. Fielding JR. Practical MR imaging of female pelvic floor weakness. Radiographics 2002;22:295–304.

15. Rodrigues CJ, Fagundes Neto HO, Lucon M, et al. Alterações no sistema de fibras elásticas da fáscia endopélvica de paciente jovem com prolapso uterino. Rev Bras Ginec Obstet 2001;23(1):234–9.

16. Kelvin FM, Maglinte DD, Hale DS, et al. Female pelvic organ prolapse: a comparison of triphasic dynamic MR imaging and triphasic fluoroscopic cystocolpoproctography. AJR Am J Roentgenol 2000;174:81–8.

17. Stoker J, Rociu E, Zwarborn AW, et al. Endoluminal MR imaging of the rectum and anus: technique, applications and pitfalls. Radiographics 1999;22:817–32.

18. Ferrante SL, Perry RE, Schreiman JS, et al. The reproducibility of measuring the anorectal angle in defecography. Dis Colon Rectum 1991;34:51–5.

19. Karasick S, Karasick D, Karasick SR. Functional disorders of the anus and rectum: findings on defecography. AJR Am J Roentgenol 1993;160:777–82.

20. Itringer WE, Saclarides TJ, Dominguez JM, et al. Four contrast defecography: pelvic "floor-oscopy". Dis Colon Rectum 1995;38:969–73.

21. Shorvon PJ, McHung S, Diamant NE, et al. Defecography in normal volunteers: results and implications. Gut 1989;30:1737–49.

Diseases of the Female Pelvis
Advances in Imaging Evaluation

Alice C. Brandão, MD[a,b,]*, Anelise Oliveira Silva, MD[a,b,c]

KEYWORDS

- MRI • Female pelvic MRI • Diffusion • Perfusion • Functional pelvic MRI

KEY POINTS

- Magnetic resonance (MR) has been widely accepted as a powerful imaging modality for the evaluation of the pelvis because of its intrinsic superior soft tissue contrast compared with other imaging modalities.
- MR imaging is mainly used for staging of uterine cancers and as a problem-solving modality in patients with ultrasonographically indeterminate masses.
- MR imaging provides multiplanar imaging of the zonal pelvic anatomy, mainly through high-resolution T2-weighted images.
- Functional study with perfusion and diffusion allows the evaluation of microvascular characteristics and cellularity of the lesions.
- Functional evaluation favors the differentiation of benign from malignant lesions.

INTRODUCTION

Magnetic resonance (MR) has been widely accepted as a powerful imaging modality for the evaluation of the pelvis because of its intrinsic superior soft tissue contrast compared with that of computed tomography (CT).[1]

At this moment, MR imaging is mainly used for staging of uterine cancers, and as a problem-solving modality in patients with ultrasonographically indeterminate masses.

At our site, characterization of congenital female pelvic anomalies, diagnosis of adenomyosis, planning of appropriate treatment for benign myometrium diseases, and endometriosis staging are other common clinical applications for MR imaging of the pelvis.

CT is applied for staging purposes in patients with ovarian, bladder, and prostate cancer, whereas MR imaging is the method of choice for local staging of uterine cancer, allowing detection of infiltration of neighboring structures.[1]

MR imaging does not use ionizing radiation, which is particularly important in the evaluation of young women and represents another advantage over CT.

The main goals of female pelvic MR imaging include (1) multiplanar display of the zonal pelvic anatomy, mainly with high-resolution T2-weighted images; (2) detection and characterization of diffuse and focal lesions; (3) detection and characterization of congenital female pelvic anomalies; and (4) follow-up of disease processes.[2]

Despite the high sensitivity of conventional MR imaging for the assessment of most pelvic lesions, in certain cases, such as peritoneal lesions, lymph node staging, and assessment of therapeutic response of some tumors, the morphologic information provided by MR imaging may be insufficient. The functional evaluation provided by perfusion

Disclosures: None.
Funding Sources: None.
a IRM, Ressonância Magnética, Rio de Janeiro, Brazil; b Department of Radiology, Clínica Felippe Mattoso, Avenida das Americas 700, 319, Rio de Janeiro 30112011, Brazil; c Department of Radiology, Hospital Federal da Lagoa, Rio de Janeiro, Brazil
* Corresponding author.
E-mail address: brandaosalomao@gmail.com

Magn Reson Imaging Clin N Am 21 (2013) 447–469
http://dx.doi.org/10.1016/j.mric.2013.01.003

and diffusion studies, which allow estimation of the microvascular characteristics and cellularity of the lesions, favors the differentiation of benign from malignant lesions.[3]

IMAGING TECHNIQUE
Standard MR Protocol

Our standard MR protocol includes axial, sagittal, and coronal T2-weighted fast spin-echo images, axial T1-weighted gradient-echo images with and without fat suppression, and sagittal T1-weighted gradient-echo with fat suppression. Sagittal and axial images are acquired before and after the intravenous injection of a gadolinium-based contrast material.

MR imaging is performed in a 1.5-T unit (Signa; GE Medical Systems, Milwaukee, WI), with a phased-array coil, which is used to improve signal-to-noise ratio.

Four to 6 hours of fasting before the examination is recommended.

It is also important to empty the bladder before the examination.

Routinely, to reduce intestinal peristalsis and uterine contractions, 10 mg of butyl scopolamine (Buscopan; Boehringer Ingelheim, Ingelheim, Germany) is injected intravenously.

For congenital female pelvic anomalies, endometriosis, and uterine carcinoma staging, to distend the vaginal fornix, 20 mL of gel is infused into the vagina.

For endometriosis, additional bowel preparation is recommended, using glycerin suppository 2 hours before the examination and 80 mL of saline solution rectally (Fig. 1).

Functional Sequences

Diffusion-weighted imaging

Diffusion-weighted imaging (DWI) is an MR technique that depicts molecular diffusion, which is the Brownian motion of water protons in biologic tissues.[1]

In the pelvis, DWI is most commonly acquired in the axial plane, as the magnetic field strength is more homogeneous close to the isocenter of the magnet, especially along the cranio-caudal direction, which leads to less susceptibility-induced signal loss and distortions in the axial images, compared with single-oblique and double-oblique acquisitions (Fig. 2).[1]

However, for endometrial carcinoma staging, we acquire the coronal oblique plane perpendicular to the uterine cavity. This sequence improves the accuracy of myometrium invasion identification (Fig. 3).

To obtain good-quality multiplanar reconstructions, the section thickness should be reduced to about 3 mm or less. If necessary, additional signal averaging might be indicated to ensure an adequate signal- to-noise ratio (SNR).

Diffusion-weighted images (DWIs) are usually acquired before contrast agent administration, although it has not yet been proved that this is required in all situations (Table 1).[1]

Choosing the b values for the DWI acquisition is not always straightforward. The largest b value used in the sequence defines the echo time of the sequence, and higher maximal b values (and subsequently longer echo times) yield greatly reduced SNR in the resulting images.

Because the b value is the strength of the diffusion sensitizing gradient, at a b value of 0 s/mm^2 (no diffusion sensitizing gradient), free water molecules have high signal intensity (SI), the SI being based on T2 weighting.

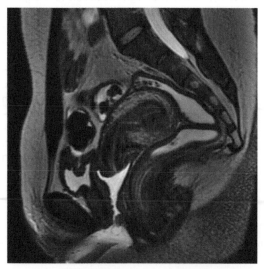

Fig. 1. T2-weighted image. Sagittal plane. Vaginal fornix distended by gel and rectum distended by saline solution.

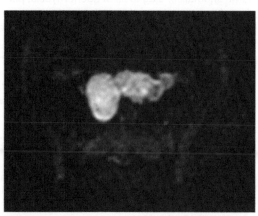

Fig. 2. DWI. Axial plane. Endometrium carcinoma staging. Note adnexal bilateral invasion presenting with high SI.

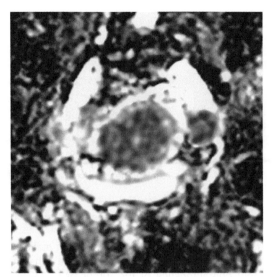

Fig. 3. DWI. Coronal oblique plane, perpendicular to the uterine cavity. Endometrium carcinoma staging. Note diffuse myometrium invasion.

By using mainly low b values, the apparent diffusion coefficient (ADC) that is calculated will be higher and reflects a combination of both perfusion and diffusion effects, whereas by using only higher b values (0.100 s/mm²), the resulting ADC values will be much lower and better approximate the true diffusion of the tissue.[1,4,5]

Studies in the literature report different choices of maximal b values, usually of 500 to 1000 s/mm². Currently used clinical MR systems should, in most cases, be capable of obtaining good-quality DWIs with a maximal b values of 1000 s/mm². A range of intermediate b values can be selected depending on the type of quantitative analysis anticipated. Minimally, only 2 b values (most often b = 0 and 1000 s/mm²) are required to calculate the ADC, expressed in square millimeters per second, if a monoexponential fit is used, by using the following equation: $S = S0 \exp (2b \, ADC)$, where S is the SI after application of the diffusion gradient, S0 is the estimated SI at b value of 0 s/mm², and b is strength of the applied diffusion-sensitizing gradients. However, application of more b values is usually recommended.[1]

The radiologist should be aware of the choice of b values to correctly interpret the resulting ADC values. We obtain DWIs with maximal b values of 1000 s/mm² with adequate SNR.

Qualitative analysis DWI is performed with at least 2 b values, including a b value of 0 s/mm² and a higher b value of 500 to 1000 s/mm².

The signal decay in tissues at different b values is generally biexponential.[6] The initial component of signal decay is signal loss caused by flowing blood (fast-moving water molecules will dephase but will not readily rephase and will loose signal even with small b values). The second component is due to the movement of water in the intracellular and extracellular spaces. A region of high signal intensity at high b-value DWI suggests restricted diffusion consistent with highly cellular tissue (tightly packed water molecules may readily be rephased by the rephasing gradient). The signal loss in water molecules at different b values can be used for lesion detection or characterization (**Fig. 4**).[6]

Quantitative analysis: ADC value The ADC represents the slope (gradient) of a line that is produced when the logarithm of relative signal intensity of tissue is plotted along the y-axis versus b values along the x-axis, thereby linearizing the exponential decay function. Quantitative analysis of DWI findings can be performed only if at least 2 b values are used for imaging. The optimal b values for tissue characterization depend on the tissue (organ) being evaluated.[6]

ADC values are related to the proportion of extracellular and intracellular components within the tissue. Increased tissue cellularity or cell density decreases the ADC measurement. Thus, high ADCs suggest benign processes with low cellularity, whereas low ADCs might indicate malignancy with large cell diameter and higher cell density, which restricts water diffusion. Therefore, ADC measurements can be valuable in differentiating benign from malignant lesions (**Fig. 5**).[4]

Dynamic Contrast-Enhanced–MR Imaging

Angiogenesis plays a vital role in the growth and spread of tumors. It means the sprouting of new capillaries from existing blood vessels, and, along with the vasculogenesis, the generation of new

							Direction	Diffusion		Pulse
TE	TR	FOV	Slice	Space	Matrix	NEX	Frequency	Direction	b Value	Sequence
Minimum	5675	40	3.0 mm	0.5	128 × 192	16	R-L	Slice	1000 mm²/s	Spin-echo

Table 1
Transverse diffusion-weighted imaging parameters in our institution

Abbreviations: FOV, field of view; R-L, right to left; TE, echo time; TR, repetition time.

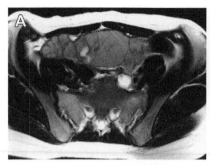
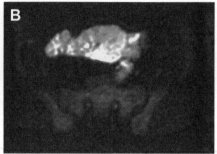

Fig. 4. Bilateral ovary mucinous adenocarcinoma. (*A*) T2-weighted image. Axial plane. (*B*) Axial plane DWI. High-SI ovaries and peritoneal lesions suggest restricted diffusion.

blood vessels, are the 2 primary methods of vascular expansion by which nutrient supply to tumor tissue is adjusted to match physiologic needs.[7]

Dynamic contrast-enhanced (DCE)-MR imaging is a noninvasive method that allows evaluation tumor angiogenesis. The findings are related to differences in microvascular characteristics observed in normal and malignant tissues. There are some features considered characteristic of malignant vasculature, which can be evaluated by DCE-MR imaging, such as poorly formed fragile vessels with high permeability to macromolecules, arteriovenous shunt, and extreme heterogeneity of vascular density.[8]

DCE-MR enables qualitative and quantitative assessment of tumor status. Insights into these physiologic processes are obtained qualitatively by characterizing kinetic enhancement curves or quantitatively by applying complex compartmental modeling techniques (**Fig. 6**).

DCE-MR imaging includes a DCE T1-weighted gradient-echo sequence, acquired before, during, and after a bolus injection of a low-molecular-weight contrast agent, gadolinium. As the agent enters into a tissue, it changes the MR signal intensity of the tissue. As the contrast agent flows out of the tissue, the MR signal intensity returns to its baseline value.

Serial images must be acquired with sufficient temporal resolution to demonstrate the enhancement characteristics of the tumor being investigated, but at the same time with enough spatial resolution so that the inherent heterogeneity of the lesion can be adequately probed. Most studies use temporal resolution in the 10-second to 30-second range. High spatial resolution is typically selected if a "semiquantitative" analysis is planned, whereas the high temporal resolution approach is selected if a full quantitative analysis is planned.[9]

Semiqualitative analysis

Semiquantitative evaluation of the DCE-MR images is based on SI changes that can be evaluated using (1) the SI curve, (2) the slope and height of the enhancement curve (time-to-peak), (3) maximum SI (peak enhancement), and (4) wash-in/washout gradient.

The technique used is a multiphase DCE T1-weighted fat-suppressed sequence obtained before intravenous administration of gadolinium-based contrast material and 0, 30, 60, 90, and

A
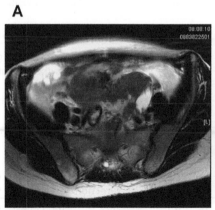

B
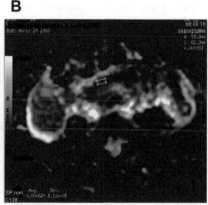

Fig. 5. Peritoneal implants. (*A*) T2-weighted image. Axial plane. (*B*) ADC map. Axial plane. Low-SI peritoneal lesions (ADC value – 0,6), suggest restricted diffusion.

automatically calculated and displayed as both numerals and SI versus time curves. These parameters include tissue SI on unenhanced T1-weighted images (SI0); SI at maximum absolute contrast enhancement (SImax); maximum relative SI (SIrel), which is relative to SI0 (SIrel = [SImax− SI0]/[SI0 × 100]); and wash-in rate (WIR), the difference between SI0 and SImax divided by time (in seconds).[10]

Another semiquantitative DCE-MR imaging technique involves rapid acquisition of DCE-MR images every 5 seconds for 2 to 4 minutes after injection of contrast material with a limited (1.5-cm) section that covers the solid portion of the mass, usually an adnexal lesion, which will be compared with the adjacent myometrium. The high temporal resolution of this DCE-MR imaging technique allows derivation of accurate time-intensity curves and other early enhancement parameters with an MR imaging workstation and additional computer software; however, the spatial resolution is lower (**Fig. 7**).[11]

This evaluation has the obvious advantage of being very straightforward to implement and can be performed in near real-time. The limitation is that the parameters do not necessarily have clear physical correlates because they are "mixed" measures. This approach has been particularly successful for breast and adnexal lesions.[9]

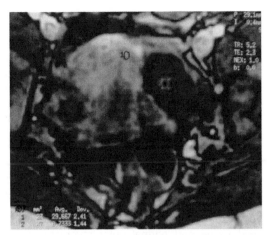

Fig. 6. Left adnexal mass. Fibrotecoma. DCE-MR imaging. DCE T1-weighted gradient-echo sequence acquired before, during, and after the bolus injection of gadolinium. As the agent enters into a tissue, it changes the MR SI of the tissue.

120 seconds after injection. The entire mass is included in the 5-point dynamic run acquisition. With standard breast MR software on a commercially available MR imaging workstation, a region of interest (ROI) is manually drawn over the most avidly enhancing solid component of the lesion, and the SI at each time point is recorded. For each ROI, enhancement parameters are

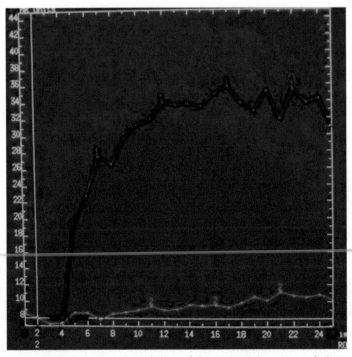

Fig. 7. Same case as Fig. 6. The high temporal resolution of this DCE-MR imaging technique allows derivation of accurate time-intensity curves.

Quantitative analysis

DCE-MR imaging is a noninvasive technique that allows measurement of the density, integrity, and leakiness of tissue vasculature. By analyzing the associated SI time course using an appropriate mathematical model, physiologic parameters related to blood flow, vessel permeability, and tissue volume fractions can be extracted for each voxel or ROI.

In the quantitative approach, a pharmacokinetic model is applied to changes in the contrast agent concentrations in tissue, and quantitative kinetic parameters are derived. They include (1) transfer constant of the contrast agent (Ktrans), (2) rate constant (Kep), and (3) interstitial extravascular extracellular space (Ve). The quantitative approach can be quite complex to implement.[12]

DCE-MR imaging related to pelvic organs

To design a DCE-MR imaging protocol, it is important to consider the goals of the study and carefully select the appropriate parameters balancing the needs of the study with resolution issues.

Uterus For uterus lesion characterization, the DCE-MR imaging consists of a sequentially ordered 3-dimensional T1-weighted fast-spoiled gradient-recalled echo of 4 contiguous sagittal sections. The bolus injection of gadopentetate dimeglumine (0.1 mmol/kg at a rate of 2 mL/s) is given 30 seconds after the beginning of acquisition and is immediately followed by a flush of 10 mL of normal saline at the same rate. The arterial phase is found at 18 seconds, based on the enhancement curves. The other 2 time points for the subtraction study are chosen by adding 60 seconds (portal venous phase) and 120 seconds (equilibrium phase) to the arterial phase (**Fig. 8, Table 2**).[13–17]

Adnexa For adnexal lesion characterization, DCE-MR imaging is acquired as a free-breathing axial

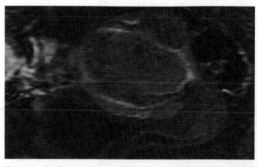

Fig. 8. Endometrial carcinoma with outer half myometrium invasion. DCE-MR imaging. Three-dimensional T1-weighted fast-spoiled gradient-recalled sagittal section.

DCE non–fat-suppressed T1-weighted gradient-echo 3-dimensional sequence. Images are obtained at 2.4-second intervals, beginning 5 seconds before the bolus injection and continuing for 320 seconds after the injection. The study must include the solid components of the ovarian tumor seen on the T2-weighted images as well as the uterus. Using a power injector at a rate of 2 mL/s, 0.1-mmol/kg of gadolinium contrast is given intravenously followed by 10 mL of normal saline to flush the tubing (**Table 3**).

A 3-dimensional FIESTA (fast imaging employing steady-state acquisition) sequence is acquired with similar parameters, being useful for the imaging analysis. The ROIs are placed within the solid tissue and normal outer myometrium selected on precontrast FIESTA images (**Fig. 9**).

ADVANCES IN UTERUS IMAGING
Endometrium

Endometrial carcinoma

The most common gynecologic malignancy, endometrial carcinoma, typically occurs in postmenopausal women, and presents with abnormal bleeding. Most endometrial malignancies are adenocarcinomas, which account for 90% of endometrial neoplasms.

Adenocarcinoma with squamous differentiation, adenosquamous carcinoma, clear-cell carcinoma, and papillary serous carcinoma represent less common histologic types. Clear-cell carcinoma and papillary serous carcinoma carry a worse prognosis.[18,19]

Depth of myometrial invasion is the most important morphologic prognostic factor, correlating with tumor grade, presence of lymph node metastases, and overall patient survival. The prevalence of lymph node metastases increases from 3% with superficial myometrial invasion to 46% with deep myometrial invasion.[20–22]

Endometrial cancer is staged based on the International Federation of Gynecology and Obstetrics (FIGO) system, which underwent an updated major revision in 2009.[20,23]

Based on the 2009-revised FIGO staging system, tumors confined to the endometrium, as well as those invading the inner half of the myometrium, are designated as stage IA tumors.[24]

Tumors invading the outer half of the myometrium are designated as stage IB tumors. MR imaging is highly accurate in distinguishing stages IA and IB tumors.[25] With the old staging system, differentiating between stages IA and IB tumors could be challenging in patients with loss of junctional zone definition or in lesions with poor tumor-to-myometrium contrast, both of which

Table 2
Parameters of dynamic contrast-enhanced magnetic resonance imaging for uterus lesion characterization in our institution

TE	TR	FOV	Slice	Space	Matrix	NEX	Direction Frequency	Fat Saturation	Pulse Sequence
Minimum	5675	40	3.0 mm	0.5	128 × 192	16	R-L	Chemical suppression	T1W 3DFSRG

Abbreviations: FOV, field of view; R-L, right to left; TE, echo time; TR, repetition time; T1W, T1-weighted.

are common pitfalls in endometrial cancer staging. The fusion of stage IA and IB tumors into a new stage IA should alleviate this problem.

Stage II tumors are those with cervical stromal invasion. In the new staging system, subsets IIA and IIB no longer exist, and tumors with endocervical glandular invasion are now considered stage I tumors.[25]

Stage III is still composed of 3 subdivisions: IIIA, IIIB, and IIIC. Stage IIIA tumors invade the serosa or adnexa, and stage IIIB tumors invade the vagina or parametrium. Previously, stage IIIC referred to any lymphadenopathy (pelvic or retroperitoneal); in the new FIGO system, however, stage IIIC is divided into stage IIIC1, which is characterized by pelvic lymph node involvement, and stage IIIC2, which is characterized by para-aortic lymph node involvement.[25]

These changes reflect prognostic data that suggest a worse outcome in patients with involvement of para-aortic nodes than in those with involvement of pelvic nodes only.[26]

Stage IV remains unchanged: stage IVA tumors extend into adjacent bladder or bowel, and stage IVB tumors have distant metastases (**Table 4**).

After administration of contrast media, endometrial tumors enhance earlier than normal endometrium, which aids in the detection of small tumors.

Normal myometrium enhances intensely compared with hypointense endometrial tumor. Maximum contrast between hyperintense myometrium and hypointense endometrial tumor occurs 50 to 120 seconds after contrast media administration. Therefore, evaluation of the depth of myometrium

invasion should be done at this stage (FIGO stage I).[25,27] Delayed-phase images obtained 3 to 4 minutes after contrast media administration are useful in detecting cervical stromal invasion (FIGO stage II). The presence of an intact enhancing cervical mucosa excludes stromal invasion (**Fig. 10**).[25]

DCE images, when evaluated along with T2-weighted images, have a diagnostic accuracy of up to 98% for assessing myometrium invasion.[25,28,29]

There is some controversy in the literature regarding the added value of DCE-MR imaging for overall FIGO staging, however. Although most published studies have shown an improvement in staging accuracy with DCE-MR imaging, some investigators have found no benefit.[25]

In the authors'opinion, the DCE images have advantages over the T2-weighted images and both should be used to better stage the lesion.

DWI DWI is a functional imaging technique that displays information about water mobility, tissue cellularity, and the integrity of the cell membranes.[29]

On DWI, endometrial cancer manifests as a high-SI mass, hypointense on the corresponding ADC map, in comparison with normal endometrium.[1,30,31]

The combination of conventional MR images and DWI seems particularly useful in assessing the depth of myometrial invasion by endometrial cancer, when there is thinning of the myometrium, or in differentiating cancer from coexisting leiomyomas or adenomyosis (**Fig. 11**).

Table 3
Parameters of dynamic contrast-enhanced magnetic resonance imaging for adnexal lesion characterization in our institution

TE	TR	FOV	Slice	Space	Matrix	NEX	Direction Frequency	Fat Saturation	Pulse Sequence
Minimum	5675	40	3.0 mm	0.5	128 × 192	16	R-L	No	T1W 3DFSRG

Abbreviations: FOV, field of view; R-L, right to left; TE, echo time; TR, repetition time; T1W, T1-weighted.

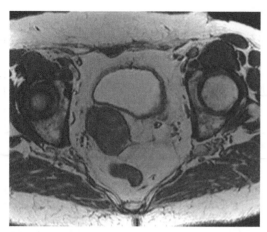

Fig. 9. Adnexal right adenocarcinoma. Three-dimensional FIESTA sequence is acquired with similar parameters.

In one study,[32] all staging errors at contrast-enhanced MR imaging were overcome by incorporating DWI.

Rechichi and colleagues[33] found that ADC values may provide useful and reliable information in differentiating normal endometrium and myometrium from malignant endometrial tissue. In this study, the mean ADC value of endometrial cancer was $0.77 \pm 0.12 \ 10^{-3} \ mm^2/s$ (average size of ROIs, 35 pixels; first–third quartiles, 29–39 pixels), which was significantly lower ($P<.0001$) than that of normal endometrium in the control group ($1.31 \pm 0.11 \ 10^{-3} \ mm^2/s$; average size of ROIs, 36 pixels; first–third quartiles, 29–40 pixels) and that of normal myometrium ($1.52 \pm 0.21 \ 10^{-3} \ mm^2/s$; average size of ROIs, 33 pixels; first–third quartiles, 29–37 pixels). There was no overlap between the 2 former distributions; therefore, it was possible to define a clear cutoff ADC

value of $1.05 \ 10^{-3} \ mm^2/s$ to distinguish between endometrial cancer and normal endometrial tissue.

Although T2-weighted imaging provides usually reliable contrast for tumor depiction, DWI may be clinically relevant in the following 2 scenarios: (1) isointense tumors, as seen in diffusely infiltrative adenocarcinomas in young women, and (2) early cervical cancer extension for exact delineation of tumor margins, if fertility-preserving surgery is planned.[1]

In a recent prospective study by Rechichi and colleagues,[34] the staging accuracy of diffusion-weighted MR imaging was superior to that of DCE-MR imaging and had a higher level of interobserver agreement.

Beddy and colleagues[29] also found a higher level of interobserver agreement of DWI when compared with DCE-MR imaging.

DWI and DCE-MR imaging are useful adjuncts to standard morphologic imaging and may improve overall staging accuracy of the endometrial carcinoma. Also, DWI can play an important role in patients who cannot accept contrast agent, such as those with renal failure.

Miometrium

Miometrial focal lesions

Leiomyomas are common benign tumors that usually are asymptomatic and may have different imaging appearances. Most leiomiomas tend to contain hyalinized collagen. Therefore, on MR imaging, uterine leiomyomas are well circumscribed, isointense to the muscle on T1-weighted images, and hypointense on T2-weighted images.[35]

These tumors are well circumscribed and surrounded by a pseudocapsule, and some of them present with a thin hyperintense rim of dilated

Table 4				
Endometrial cancer International Federation of Gynecology and Obstetrics system, 2009 revision				
Endometrial Cancer	**Stage A**	**Stage B**	**Stage C**	
Stage I	Confined to the endometrium <50% of the myometrium	Invading >50% of the myometrium	—	
Stage II	Endocervical glandular invasion			
Stage III	Invades the serosa or adnexa	Invades the vagina or parametrium	C1. pelvic lymph node	C2. Para-aortic lymph node
Stage IV	Invades bladder or bowel	Distant metastases	—	

Dynamic contrast imaging.

Data from Sala E, Wakely S, Senior E, et al. MRI of malignant neoplasms of the uterine corpus and cervix. AJR Am J Roentgenol 2007;188:1577–87; and Creasman W. Revised FIGO staging for carcinoma of the endometrium. Int J Gynaecol Obstet 2009;105(2):109.

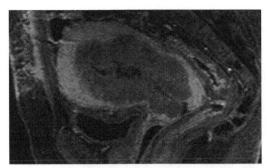

Fig. 10. Endometrial carcinoma with myometrial and cervical invasion. DCE-MR imaging. Three-dimensional T1-weighted fast-spoiled gradient-recalled sagittal section.

lymphatic clefts and dilated veins; edema may be seen on T2-weighted images and helps differentiate leiomyomas from focal adenomyosis.[9]

Degenerated leiomyomas have variable appearances on T1-weighted, T2-weighted, and contrast-enhanced images, such as (1) cellular leiomyomas, composed of compact smooth muscle cells with little or no collagen, can have relatively higher SI on T2-weighted images and marked enhancement on the contrast-enhanced images; (2) cystic degeneration shows high SI areas on T2-weighted images that do not enhance; (3) myxoid degeneration shows very high SI on T2-weighted images and enhances minimally on contrast-enhanced images; and (4) red degeneration exhibits peripheral or diffuse high SI on T1-weighted images and variable SI with or without a low-SI rim on T2-weighted images, and no enhancing areas (**Fig. 12**).

These imaging aspects can affect the aspects of uterine leiomyomas in functional images.

On MR imaging, uterine sarcomas often manifest as a large, infiltrating myometrial mass of intermediate to high SI on T2-weighted images. Differentiation between benign degenerated leiomyoma and malignant tumors may be difficult if based only on SI of nonenhanced and postcontrast MR sequences.

DWI Most leiomyomas tend to contain hyalinized collagen, so their signal is hypointense on T2-weighted images. The DWI appearance of these leiomyomas can be explained by a "T2 blackout effect" (ie, hypointensity on DWI due to hypointensity on T2-weighted images), which causes a decrease in the ADC of ordinary leiomyomas. As a consequence, all of the ordinary leiomyomas have low SI on DWI (**Fig. 13**).

Although MR imaging usually allows specific diagnosis of the much more common benign leiomyomas, degenerated leiomyomas may occasionally be associated with various types of cellular histologic subtypes, which can cause increased signal on T2-weighted images. Cellular leiomyomas can exhibit high SI on DWIs, simulating uterine sarcomas (**Fig. 14**).[36]

Bakir and colleagues[37] suggested that DWI is not useful in the differential diagnosis of degenerated benign and malignant myometrial lesions. Degenerated leiomyomas and leiomyosarcomas displayed varied signal intensities. The ADC value of leiomyosarcomas was lower than those of degenerated leiomyomas with no overlap, but this difference was not statistically significant. Furthermore, the ADC values of ordinary leiomyomas

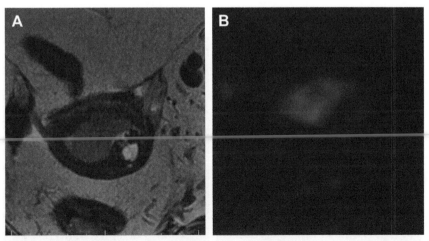

Fig. 11. Endometrial cancer confined to the endometrium and coexisting posterior adenomyosis. (A) Coronal oblique T2-weighted image. (B) DWI was useful in assessing absence of myometrial invasion.

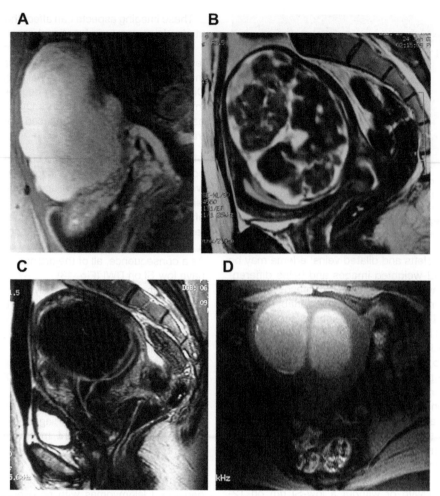

Fig. 12. Leiomyomas. (*A*) Cellular leiomyoma with marked enhancement on contrast-enhanced images. (*B*) Myxoid degeneration with high SI focus on T2-weighted images. (*C*) Hyalinized leiomyoma. Well-circumscribed mass, hypointense on T2-weighted images. (*D*) Red degeneration exhibits diffuse high SI on T1-weighted image.

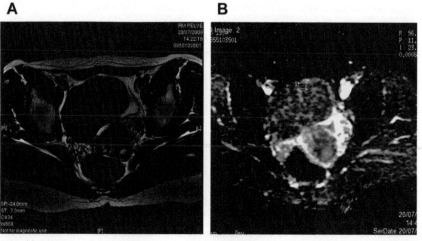

Fig. 13. Hyalinized leiomyoma. (*A*) Hypointense on T2-weighted image. (*B*) Hypointense signal on the ADC map.

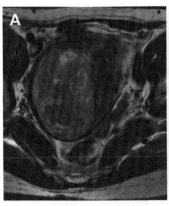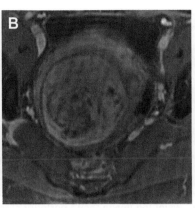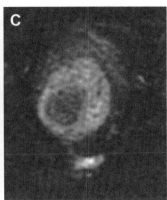

Fig. 14. Cellular leiomyomas. Well-circumscribed mass with higher SI on T2-weighted images, marked enhancement on contrast-enhanced images, and high SI on DWIs. (*A*) T2-weighted image. (*B*) Postcontrast image. (*C*) DWI.

overlapped with those of both degenerated leiomyomas and leiomyosarcomas.[37]

However, Tamai and colleagues[36] and Takeuchi and colleagues[38] reported that DWI could be useful in differentiating hyperintensity on T2-weighted images of leiomyomas from malignant lesions. All malignant tumors showed high SI on DWI with low ADC, which was significantly lower ($P<.01$) than that in benign leiomyomas. The ADC in cellular leiomyoma (1.18) was significantly lower than that in degenerated leiomyoma (1.60) and higher than that in malignant tumors. They concluded that the ADC measurement might be helpful in distinguishing benign from malignant tumors.

Recent studies have demonstrated the use of DWI to obtain "functional parameters" in both untreated and treated uterine lesions. MR imaging–guided focused ultrasound-treated leiomyoma demonstrated restricted diffusion. The heat obtained from this procedure changes the motion of water and disrupts the bound and unbound proteins within the tissue. Release of these proteins maybe the reason for the decreased water movement after this treatment. The ADC value exhibited a high similarity index and good correlation between the volumes of treated tissue. DWI could be useful as an adjunct for assessing response to treatment in uterine fibroids by MR imaging–guided focused ultrasound.[39]

Adenomyosis Adenomyosis is a common non-neoplastic gynecologic disease characterized by the presence of ectopic endometrium within the myometrium.

Adenomyosis is detected on T2-weighted images as thickening of the junctional zone to 12 mm or more, often associated with punctuate foci of high SI. Although the thickness of the junctional zone

has been reported to vary from 2 to 8 mm, the use of a lower threshold may result in false-positive diagnosis of adenomyosis because of sustained myometrial contractions, uterine peristalsis, and diffuse physiologic thickening of the junctional zone during menstruation.[9]

Typical adenomyosis appears as an ill-demarcated low-SI area on T2-weighted images owing to abundant smooth muscle proliferation. Because adenomyotic endometrium looks like the basalis endometrium, which seldom responds to hormonal stimuli, cyclic changes, including degeneration, bleeding, and regeneration, are less common in adenomyosis than in endometriosis. On T2-weighted MR images, ectopic endometrium appears as small high-SI areas similar to normal endometrium. Small cysts may also appear as high-SI spots on T2-weighted images. Sometimes, hemorrhagic foci appear as high-SI foci on T1-weighted images owing to the T1-shortening effects of methemoglobin.[40,41]

Small hemorrhagic foci (hemosiderin deposition), which are barely detectable on T2-weighted images, can be demonstrated as signal voids on susceptibility-weighted images.[41]

Susceptibility-weighted MRI is a relatively new MR technique that maximizes sensitivity to susceptibility effects and has exquisite sensitivity to blood products, such as hemosiderin and deoxyhemoglobin, and can depict discrete adenomyotic changes in the myometrium (**Fig. 15**).[41,42]

Cervix

Cervical cancer

Uterine cervical cancer is one of the most common malignancies seen by gynecologic radiologists.[43] In spite of advances in treatment enabling women to live longer, there remains a substantial associated mortality.[43]

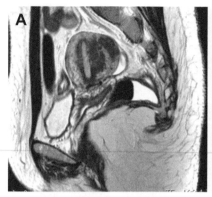
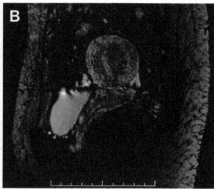

Fig. 15. Adenomyosis. (*A*) Sagittal T2-weighted image shows posterior corporal thickened junctional zone with a hyperintense foci of heterotopic endometrial tissue. (*B*) Sagittal susceptibility-weighted MRI depicted discrete hypointense foci within the adenomyotic changes in the myometrium.

Most cervical squamous cell carcinomas grow at the squamocolumnar junction (SCJ). In younger women, the SCJ is located outside the external uterine os, and the tumor tends to grow outward (exophytic growth pattern). In contrast, in older patients, the SCJ is located within the cervical canal. In these patients, cervical cancer tends to grow inward along the cervical canal (endophytic growth pattern).[43]

MR imaging can provide highly accurate information on the exact extent of cervical tumors because of its fine contrast resolution. Cervical cancers appear as hyperintense masses on T2-weighted images regardless of its histopathologic type.[43]

DWI The applications of DWI in the assessment of cervical cancer are differentiating normal from cancerous tissues and evaluating response to chemo-radiotherapy. Cervical cancer shows restricted diffusion related to an increase in cellular density, tissue disorganization, intact cellular membranes, and increased extracellular space tortuosity, features that collectively restrict the diffusibility of water molecules (**Fig. 16**).

The ADC value of cervical cancer lesions has been reported to be lower than that of normal cervical tissues, and ADC increases after chemotherapy or irradiation.[44,45]

McVeigh and colleagues[46] found that the median ADC of cervical cancers was significantly lower than the median ADC of normal cervix stroma, with very little overlap between the 2 cases. The average mean ADC for cancerous tissue was $1.09 \pm 0.20 \times 10^{-3}$ mm^2/s, whereas that of the control cervical tissue was $2.09 \pm 0.46 \times 10^{-3}$ mm^2/s (see **Fig. 16**).

Furthermore, Somoye and colleagues[47] investigated whether DWI performed early in the treatment of locally advanced cervical cancer could

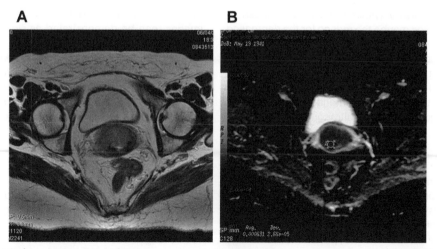

Fig. 16. Cervical carcinoma. Cervical isointense mass presenting with hypointense signal on the ADC map.

predict survival. Their study revealed an ADC difference between pretherapy ADC and ADC values at 2 weeks after treatment, indicative of tumor response; however, there was no evidence that pretreatment or post-therapy ADC variables and baseline tumor volumes were related to response.

DCE-MR imaging Although DCE-MR imaging does not significantly improve staging accuracy compared with standard T2-weighted images, it may be additionally applied for detection of early-stage cervical cancer. Moreover, some investigators have suggested that the functional assessment of the microcirculation using DCE-MR imaging would predict therapy outcome in cervical cancer, in addition to traditional factors, such as stage, extent of disease, histologic type, lymphatic spread, and vascular invasion.[44]

In a pre–radiation therapy study, a favorable outcome was demonstrated in patients with strong tumor enhancement, suggesting good tumor oxygenation. Tumors with baseline higher permeability (Ktrans) tend to show a better response to radiotherapy. After radiotherapy, tumor enhancement has been delayed compared with that before therapy.[48]

Yamashita and colleagues[49] also found that the pattern of enhancement or increased permeability in the region of the tumor correlated with the incidence of durability or local recurrence. Tumors with a homogeneous enhancement pattern showed significantly better treatment results than those with a peripheral enhancement pattern or those with predominantly poor enhancement. Tumors with increased permeability also had a higher incidence of good response to treatment.

Manelli and colleagues[50] found an inverse correlation between the percentages of nonenhancing tumor tissue evaluated using pretreatment DCE-MR imaging subtracted images and percentages of tumor regression after chemoradiotherapy in patients with advanced cervical cancer. The presence of hypoxic cells is one of the most important factors affecting tumor resistance to radiotherapy and overall prognosis in patients with advanced cervical cancer. Minimally necrotic tumors show a more homogeneous enhancement, and they have a better prognosis. These tumors are more likely to be well oxygenated and therefore more sensitive to radiation and have a better perfusion, which will also result in a higher concentration of chemotherapeutic agent within the tumor. The nonenhancing tumor areas can be necrotic, can have less biologic activity than the tumor cells, and are likely hypoxic and more resistant to therapy. Patients presenting with these tumors have a worse prognosis.[13,49]

ADNEXA
Advances in Adnexal Imaging

MR evaluation of adnexal lesions should be based on 2 features: morphology and SI. Reported morphologic signs of malignancy include bilaterality, diameter larger than 4 cm, predominantly solid mass, and cystic tumor with vegetation or intramural nodule, as well as secondary malignant features, such as ascites, peritoneal involvement, and enlarged lymph nodes (**Box 1**).[51]

The other criteria are related to the T1 and T2 contrast. The low signal of solid components on T2-weighted imaging is suggestive of benign fibrous tissue (observed in cystadenofibroma, ovarian fibroma, and Brenner tumor), with an overall accuracy of about 68% according to Sohaib and colleagues.[52] High SI on T1-weighted images is highly suggestive of benign disease, observed in lesions presenting with fat (such as benign teratoma) or blood products (endometrioma) (**Fig. 17**).[53]

For hyperintense lesions, there is no need for further characterization; however, the other reported criteria are not specific predictors of malignancy, because an overlap between benign and malignant tumors may be seen, especially in the diameter and bilaterality.

Umemoto and colleagues[53,54] reported that a solid component in an ovarian mass was the most statistically significant predictor of malignancy on MR imaging, but the accuracy of this feature is less than 50%.

Functional sequences are promising emerging techniques for better characterization of ovarian masses, based on diffusion and perfusion characteristics. Another useful technique is the susceptibility-weighted sequence, which maximizes sensitivity to susceptibility effects related to the presence of blood products, allowing

---

Box 1
Morphologic signs of malignancy on MR imaging
Solid and cystic areas within a lesion
Necrosis within a solid lesion
Irregular multiple thickened septum or irregular thickened wall
Papillary projections
Large size (>6 cm)
Bilateral lesions
Ascites, peritoneal disease, or lymphadenopathy

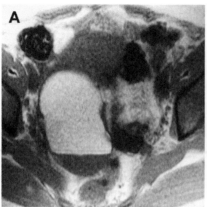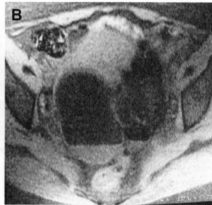

Fig. 17. Right adnexal teratoma. Lesion shows high SI on T1-weighted image, and low SI on T1-weighted image with fat suppression. (*A*) T1-weighted image. (*B*) T1-weighted image with fat suppression.

distinction between an old endometrioma and a fibrotic solid lesion.[40]

Susceptibility-weighted MRI

Endometrioma

Endometriomas are the most common manifestation of pelvic endometriosis. They are cysts with hematic content of different ages, composed of endometrial glands and stroma, which promote cyclic bleeding, resulting in hemosiderin deposition.[54]

Multiple hyperintense cysts on T1-weighted images and a hyperintense cyst on T1-weighted images that also has hypointense signal on T2-weighted images (shading) are considered definite MR imaging signs of endometrioma and have 90% sensitivity, 98% specificity, and 96% accuracy for the diagnosis.[40,42,55]

Some endometriomas, however, are filled with watery fluid on gross cut sections and may not exhibit typical MR imaging findings.[42] In such cases, visualization of hemosiderin deposition in the cyst wall may be helpful.[40]

Susceptibility-weighted MR imaging is a relatively new MR imaging technique that maximizes sensitivity to susceptibility effects and has exquisite sensitivity to blood products, such as hemosiderin and deoxyhemoglobin.[40,42]

The magnetic susceptibility effects generated by local inhomogeneity of the magnetic field caused by hemosiderin or deoxyhemoglobin is visualized as signal voids.[40]

Takeuchi and colleagues[40] found signal voids following magnetic susceptibility in 39 (92.9%) of 42 endometriomas, demonstrating the usefulness of this sequence.

It is important to note that the content of nonendometrial hematic cysts had no signal voids along the cyst walls on susceptibility-weighted images, which was attributed to the fact that these cysts do not repeatedly bleed. Thus, the finding of a thick capsule containing a cluster of hemosiderin-laden macrophages is specific for the diagnosis of endometrioma and susceptibility-weighted imaging is especially sensitive to this finding (**Fig. 18**).[40]

DWI

Tubo-ovarian abscess

Tubo-ovarian abscess (TOA) is a late complication of pelvic inflammatory disease (PID) and involves a frank abscess or an inflammatory mass resulting from breakdown of the normal structure of fallopian tubes and ovaries by inflammation. The clinical features of TOA and uncomplicated PID are similar, and differentiation is usually achieved with imaging examination.[56]

DWI is a well-established method for studying infectious diseases, especially intracranially, as well as in the breasts and abdomen.[57]

TOAs may produce complex masses with wall thickening and pseudosolid areas, thereby mimicking malignancy. The pseudosolid areas can demonstrate different SI on T1-weighted and T2-weighted images, and marked enhancement, related to high inflammatory cellularity, a matrix of proteins, cellular debris, and bacteria in high-viscosity purulent fluids, as well as large molecules playing a key role in restricting the diffusion of protons in pus. Moreover, the clinical features are not specific, and can mimic malignancy.[58]

Li and colleagues[57] found an increase of 22.5% in the diagnostic confidence of conventional MR imaging in the diagnosis of TOA using DWI. The improvement in diagnostic confidence was related to the addition of DWI to conventional MR imaging, which can differentiate pseudosolid

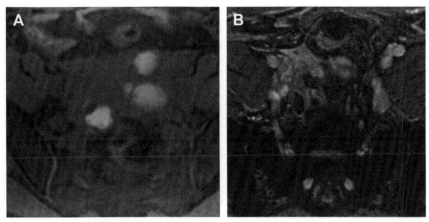

Fig. 18. Endometrioma. Hyperintense cyst on axial T1-weighted image with fat suppression and signal voids along the cyst walls on the susceptibility-weighted image. (*A*) T1-weighted image. (*B*) Susceptibility-weighted image.

(pus) from other conditions, such as the mucinous components of adnexal tumor, based on signal characteristics.[57]

Li and colleagues[57] considered that the best criteria for predicting an abscess, was the finding of a mass presenting with high or intermediate SI on T2-weighted images, no enhancement, and high SI on DWI, along with low ADC values. In this publication, DWI could also characterize and differentiate pyosalpinx from hydrosalpinx. Both of those demonstrated dilated, fluid-filled tubal structures, with variable SI on T1-weighted and T2-weighted images, but only pyosalpinx demonstrated low SI on the ADC map, related to the viscosity and high protein concentrations of the fluid contained in the pus in a pyosalpinx.[57]

Takeshita and colleagues[58] suggested that TOA presented with restricted diffusion similar to brain abscess. Thus, DWI can be an alternative for the diagnosis of TOA when the contrast study cannot be performed. The SI on the ADC map, along with the ADC measurements, may allow the correct diagnosis of TOA (**Fig. 19**).

Adnexial torsion
Ovarian torsion is the twisting of an ovary on its ligamentous supports and can result in a compromised blood supply. Adnexal torsion is a loose term that may refer to torsion of the ovary, the fallopian tube, or both. Concomitant ovarian and tubal torsion has been shown to occur in up to 67% of cases of adnexal torsion (**Fig. 20**).[59,60]

Large, heavy cysts and cystic neoplasms, such as benign mature cystic teratomas, hemorrhagic cysts, and cystadenomas, commonly predispose the ovary to swing on its vascular pedicle.[61] The

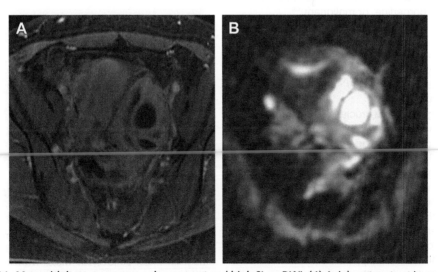

Fig. 19. TOA. Mass with heterogeneous enhancement and high SI on DWI. (*A*) Axial postcontrast image. (*B*) DWI.

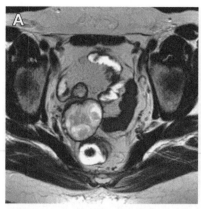
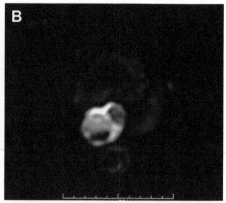

Fig. 20. Ovary edema. Axial T2-weighted image shows enlarged edematous right ovary with peripheral follicles. DWI shows restricted diffusion. (*A*) Axial T2-weighted image. (*B*) DWI.

large cystic ovaries seen in ovarian hyperstimulation syndrome are another predisposing factor for torsion. Conversely, it is rare to see ovarian torsion from cysts smaller than 5 cm.[62]

The SI of the tubal fluid is related to the presence of hemorrhage from fallopian tubal torsion and hematosalpinx and may have a similar appearance on T1-weighted and T2-weighted sequence as well as on the DWI, generally presenting with high SI on conventional images, with restricted diffusion and low ADC values.

DW imaging alone is not useful for differentiating tubal torsion and hematosalpinx from TOA and ovarian abscesses.[57]

Adnexal neoplasms

Ovarian cancer accounts for 3.7% of all cases of cancer in women.[63] Primary ovarian neoplasms are broadly categorized as surface epithelial, germ cell, or sex cord–stromal tumors and may be benign, borderline, or malignant.[64]

Surface epithelial tumors account for most ovarian neoplasms; the most common types being serous, mucinous, and endometrioid. Less common types include clear cell, transitional cell (Brenner and non-Brenner variants), and mixed epithelial tumors.[65]

MR imaging plays a crucial role in characterizing adnexal masses that are indeterminate at ultrasound and determining the origins of pelvic masses. Both MR imaging and ultrasonography have high sensitivity (97% and 100%, respectively) for depicting malignant adnexal masses. However, MR imaging has much higher specificity (84%) and accuracy (89%) for depicting malignant characteristics when compared with Doppler ultrasound (40% specificity and 64% accuracy). Therefore, an adnexal mass that appears suspicious at ultrasound may be correctly diagnosed as a benign

lesion at MR imaging, preventing inappropriate radical surgery.[66]

MR imaging characteristics that are indicative of benignity include high SI on T1-weighted images (indicative of fat or blood), loss of SI on fat-suppressed images (indicative of fat), high SI on T1-weighted fat-suppressed images (indicative of blood), and low SI on T2-weighted images (indicative of fibrous tissue or hemosiderin). In particular, solid adnexal tissue that demonstrates low SI on T2-weighted images has been shown to be highly indicative of a benign or noninvasive lesion.[11,57]

On MR imaging performed with conventional protocols, morphologic features that are indicative of a malignant adnexal mass include the presence of both solid and cystic areas within a lesion; necrosis within a solid lesion; papillary projections from the wall or septum in a cystic lesion; an irregular septum or wall; multiple thickened (>3 mm)

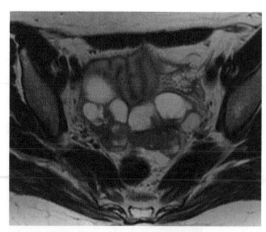

Fig. 21. Bilateral cystic adenocarcinoma showing morphologic features indicative of a malignant adnexal mass. Solid cystic mass, with irregular and thickened septations. Axial T2-weighted image.

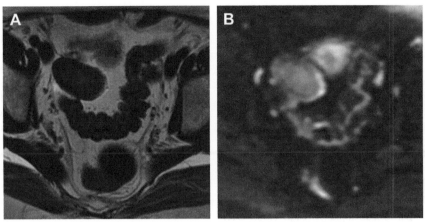

Fig. 22. Fibrotecoma. Solid adnexial lesion showing low SI on the T2-weighted and DW images. (*A*) Axial T2-weighted image. (*B*) DWI.

septations; a large size (>6 cm); bilateral lesions; and ascites, peritoneal disease, or lymphadenopathy (**Fig. 21**).[52,56]

Functional sequences are promising emerging techniques for better characterization of ovarian tumors. According to Takeuchi and colleagues, the mean ADC values of benign and malignant ovarian tumors differed significantly. Using a cutoff value of 1.15×10^{-3} mm^2/s for the ADC, differentiation of benign from malignant/borderline lesions could be done with 74% sensitivity, 80% specificity 94% positive predictive value (PPV) and 44% negative predictive value (NPV).

A cutoff ADC value of 1.0×10^{-3} mm^2/s had a sensitivity of 46%, specificity of 100%, PPV of 100%, and NPV of 32%.[67]

Thomassin-Naggara and colleagues[68] evaluated 77 solid adnexial lesions, and demonstrated that all solid lesions that presented with low SI on DWI acquired at a b value of 1000 s/mm^2 were benign (**Fig. 22**)[56]; however, there were some overlaps between the mean ADC values of the malignant and benign ovarian lesions. Thomassin-Naggara and colleagues[68] considered that their results may reflect the increased mean ADC values in some malignant lesions owing to the existence of small necrotic or cystic areas in solid tumoral components, or fluid collection intervening papillary projections, and the decreased mean ADC values in some benign lesions owing to relative hypercellularity in functioning ovarian tumors, such as thecomas, or restriction of the water diffusion by dense stromal proliferation in fibroma without edematous changes (**Fig. 23**).[69]

Katayama and colleagues[69] reported that ADC values may provide limited information in the

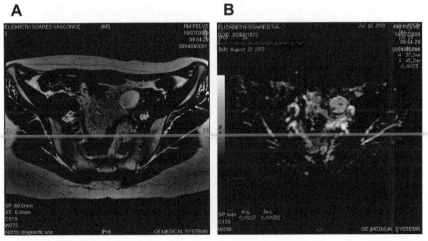

Fig. 23. Limitation of diffusion in the evaluation of cystic ovary lesions. Left ovary malignant lesion showing increased ADC owing to cystic areas within the solid tumoral component.

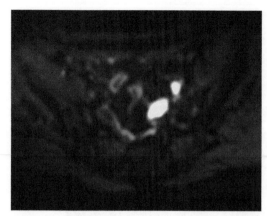

Fig. 24. Left peritoneal implants. High SI on DWI related to restricted diffusion.

differential diagnosis of cystic ovarian tumor, but most of them agree that most solid components of malignant ovarian tumors demonstrated high SI on DWI.[70,71]

When T2-weighted images and DWIs are combined, the most useful findings for predicting malignancy in adnexal masses include the presence of papillary projections (positive likelihood ratio [PLR] = 4.5), high SI on DWIs at b value of 1000 s/mm^2 within the solid component (PLR = 3.1), intermediate SI on T2-weighted images of the solid component (PLR = 2.2), ascites and peritoneal implants (PLR = 2), and a solid portion (PLR = 1.8).[1]

In contrast, the absence of high b value (1000 mm^2/s) signal was highly predictive of benignity (PLR = 10.1). A tumor displaying both low T2 and low b1000 signal was never malignant in this study. The addition of DWI increased the diagnostic confidence in 15% (see **Fig. 22**).[1,52,56]

A few studies have investigated the value of DWI in the assessment of peritoneal spread in gynecologic cancers. Compared with CT and conventional MR imaging, qualitative DWI has been shown to improve staging accuracy by enhancing

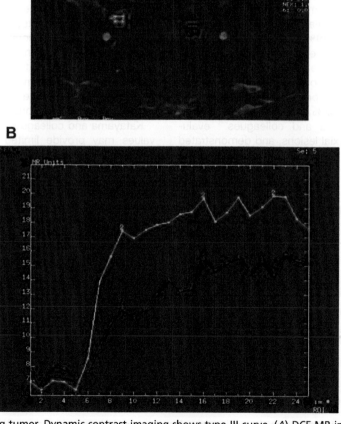

Fig. 25. Sertoli-Leydig tumor. Dynamic contrast imaging shows type III curve. (A) DCE-MR imaging. (B) Dynamic curve.

the detectability of peritoneal implants and also the detection of small peritoneal implants at sites difficult to assess with routine imaging. An early study reported that fusion of DWI with T2-weighted imaging yielded excellent sensitivity (90%) and specificity (95.5%) for assessing peritoneal spread in ovarian cancer.[1,70]

The highest incremental value of DWI was for metastases in the mesentery and for small bowel and colonic serosal surface implants (**Fig. 24**).[11]

Kyriazi and colleagues[72] demonstrated that, in patients with peritoneal ovarian cancer, DWI was potentially useful for monitoring treatment efficacy. Changes on ADC values correlated with and often preceded size and tumor-marker evidence of response, with a predictive value in assessing chemotherapy response. Response was associated with an early and sustained increase of ADCs and lack of response with stability of all histogram parameters. This is supported by the established inverse correlation between ADC and cell density.[72]

DCE-MR imaging has been used for the characterization of ovarian tumors, and it has been proven useful for distinguishing malignant from

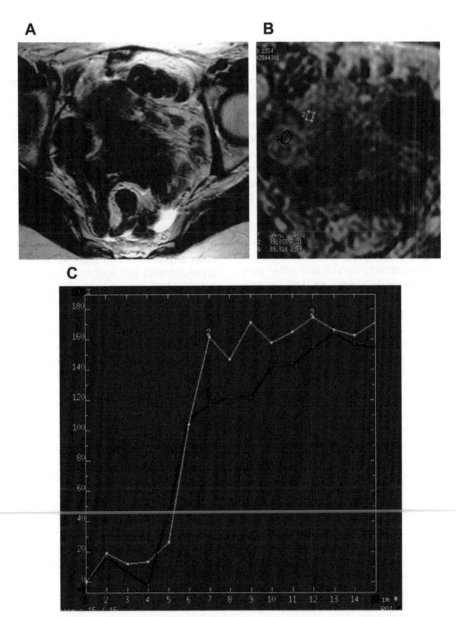

Fig. 26. Ligament right leiomyoma. DCE-MR imaging shows stronger enhancement in the leiomyoma compared with myometrium, with type III curve. (*A*) Axial T2-weighted image. (*B*) DCE-MR imaging. (*C*) Dynamic curve.

benign tumors, enabling noninvasive in vivo assessment of angiogenesis.[68]

Several studies have suggested that contrast-enhanced MR sequences are superior to noncontrast MR imaging for ovarian tumor characterization.[52,68,73] The overall accuracy of this sequence for distinguishing benign from malignant ovarian lesions reaches 90% in some series.[68,73]

Sohaib and colleagues[52] confirmed that malignant tumors exhibited stronger early enhancement (<60 seconds) than benign tumors.

Bernardin and colleagues[10] evaluated 70 complex adnexal masses (solid or mixed solid and cystic) on conventional MR images and DCE images. The parameters used were the tissue SI on unenhanced T1-weighted images (SI0); SI at maximum absolute contrast enhancement (SImax); maximum relative SI (SIrel); and wash-in rate (WIR), the difference between SI0 and SImax divided by time (in seconds). At DCE-MR imaging with semiquantitative analysis, the solid enhancing portion of malignant (borderline or invasive) tumors had significantly higher SImax, SIrel, and WIR values than did benign masses. The WIR proved to be the most significant predictive parameter, with a mean WIR of 11.8 L/s for malignant (borderline or invasive) tumors compared with 6.6 L/s for benign masses (P<.0001).

Thomassin-Naggara and colleagues[11] evaluated ovarian tumors with a high temporal resolution DCE-MR imaging technique that allows derivation of accurate time-intensity curves and other early enhancement parameters with an MR imaging workstation and additional computer software. They defined 3 patterns of enhancement of ovarian epithelial tumors, using myometrial enhancement as the internal reference, which correlated with histopathologic findings. This classification of the time-intensity curves of tumor enhancement includes types 1, 2, and 3 curves. Type 1 is a curve showing a gradual increase in the signal of solid tissue, without a well-defined shoulder. Type 2 is a curve with moderate initial rise in the signal of solid tissue relative to that of myometrium, followed by a plateau. Type 3 is a curve with intense initial rise in the signal of solid tissue steeper than that of myometrium. Thomassin-Naggara and colleagues[11] demonstrated that only invasive tumors displayed time intensity curve type 3 (specificity 100%). Enhancement curve types 1 and 2 corresponded to benign and borderline ovarian tumors, respectively. In addition, semiquantitative parameters, like enhancement amplitude, maximal slope, and initial area under the curve within the first 60 seconds ratios were significantly higher for invasive lesions than they were for benign and borderline masses (Fig. 25).[11]

Box 2
Adnexial lesions: functional features of malignancy

High SI on DWIs (low on ADC map) in the solid component of a solid/cystic lesion or in the papillary projection

Stronger early enhancement

Type 3 curve on DCE-MR imaging (intense initial rise in the signal of solid tissue, steeper than that of myometrium)

Peritoneal nodes with high signal on DWI and low signal on ADC map

---

The mechanisms explaining the different enhancement curves are dependent on tissue-specific factors, such as the number and maturity of microvessels, interstitial space, and the interstitial pressure. Malignant tumors demonstrate poorly formed and highly permeable fragile neoangiogenic vessels, explaining a type 3 curve, with intense initial rise in the signal of solid tissue.[74]

Thomassin-Naggara and colleagues[56] identified a correlation between semiquantitative parameters and vascular endothelial growth factor receptor 2 (VEGFR-2) expression. Enhancement amplitude correlated with VEGFR-2 expression on endothelial and epithelial cells, and maximal slope was associated with low smooth muscle actin expression and high VEGFR-2 expression on endothelial and epithelial cells.

DCE-MR imaging has also proved to be useful for distinguishing solid pelvic masses, especially ovarian fibromas and uterine leiomyomas. With normal myometrium used as the reference, enhancement of ovarian fibromas was weaker and slower than that of uterine leiomyomas (Fig. 26).[75]

Limitations of this technique include partial coverage of the adnexal mass, the need for the uterus to be present, the requirement that the solid portion of the tumor be at the same level as the myometrium to allow comparisons, and potential variations in myometrial perfusion.[65,76]

Despite their high specificity for depicting invasive lesions, DCE-MR technique is also prone to pitfalls. False-negative results may occur with poorly vascularized malignant tumors, and false-positive enhancement characteristics may be seen in benign lesions with a high blood supply, such as TOA, which may appear complex and indeterminate with all imaging modalities (Box 2).[65,76]

SUMMARY

Conventional MR imaging has been widely accepted as a powerful imaging modality for the evaluation of the pelvis because of its intrinsic superior soft tissue contrast. Functional study with perfusion and diffusion allows the evaluation of microvascular characteristics and cellularity of the lesions. These sequences improve the differentiation of benign from malignant lesions. Moreover, the functional study allows the characterization of lesions, both benign and malignant, thus increasing the specificity of resonance imaging.

REFERENCES

1. Thoeny HC. Genitourinary applications of diffusion-weighted MR imaging in the pelvis. Radiology 2012;263(2):326–42.
2. Hussain SM. MR Imaging of the female pelvis at 3T. Magn Reson Imaging Clin N Am 2007;14:537–44.
3. Thomassin-Nagara I. Characterization of complex adnexal masses: value of adding perfusion- and diffusion-weighted MR imaging to conventional MR imaging. Radiology 2011;258(3):793–803.
4. Le Bihan D, Breton E, Lallemand D, et al. Separation of diffusion and perfusion in intravoxel incoherent motion MR imaging. Radiology 1988;168(2):497–505.
5. Thoeny HC, De Keyzer F, Boesch C, et al. Diffusion-weighted imaging of the parotid gland: influence of the choice of b-values on the apparent diffusion coefficient value. J Magn Reson Imaging 2004; 20(5):786–90.
6. Qayyum A. Diffusion-weighted imaging in the abdomen and pelvis: concepts and applications. Radiographics 2009;29:1797–810.
7. Padhani AR, Harvey CJ, Cosgrove DO. Angiogenesis imaging in the management of prostate cancer. Nat Clin Pract Urol 2005;2:596–607.
8. Alonzi R, Padhani A, Allen C. Dynamic contrast enhanced MRI in prostate cancer. Eur J Radiol 2007;63:335–50.
9. Yankeelov TE, Gore JC. Dynamic contrast enhanced magnetic resonance imaging in oncology: theory, data acquisition, analysis, and examples. Curr Med Imaging Rev 2009;3(2):91–107.
10. Bernardin L. Effectiveness of semi-quantitative multiphase dynamic contrast-enhanced MRI as a predictor of malignancy in complex adnexal masses: radiological and pathological correlation. Eur Radiol 2012;22(4):880–90.
11. Thomassin-Naggara I. Dynamic contrast-enhanced magnetic resonance imaging: a useful tool for characterizing ovarian epithelial tumors. J Magn Reson Imaging 2008;28(1):111–20.
12. Tofts PS, Brix G, Buckley DL, et al. Estimating kinetic parameters from dynamic contrast-enhanced T(1) weighted MRI of a diffusable tracer: standardized quantities and symbols. J Magn Reson Imaging 1999;10:223–32.
13. Manelli L. Evaluation of nonenhancing tumor fraction assessed by dynamic contrast-enhanced MRI subtraction as a predictor of decrease in tumor volume in response to chemoradiotherapy in advanced cervical cancer. AJR Am J Roentgenol 2010;195(2):524–7.
14. Brown MA. MRI of benign uterine disease. Magn Reson Imaging Clin N Am 2007;14:439–53.
15. Lee JK, Gersell DJ, Balfe DM, et al. The uterus: in vitro MR-anatomic correlation of normal and abnormal specimens. Radiology 1985;157:175–89.
16. Gull B, Karlsson B, Milsom I, et al. Transvaginal sonography of the endometrium in a representative sample of postmenopausal women. Ultrasound Obstet Gynecol 1996;7:322–7.
17. Levine D, Gosink BB, Johnson LA. Change in endometrial thickness in postmenopausal women undergoing hormone replacement therapy. Radiology 1995;197:603–8.
18. Togashi K, Nakai A, Sugimura K. Anatomy and physiology of the female pelvis: MR imaging revisited. J Magn Reson Imaging 2001;13:842–9.
19. Brown MA. MRI of malignant uterine disease. Magn Reson Imaging Clin N Am 2007;455–69.
20. Creasman W. Revised FIGO staging for carcinoma of the endometrium. Int J Gynaecol Obstet 2009; 105(2):109.
21. Larson DM, Connor GP, Broste SK, et al. Prognostic significance of gross myometrial invasion with endometrial cancer. Obstet Gynecol 1996;88(3):394–8.
22. Berman ML. Prognosis and treatment of endometrial cancer. Am J Obstet Gynecol 1980;136(5):679–88.
23. Sala E, Wakely S, Senior E, et al. MRI of malignant neoplasms of the uterine corpus and cervix. AJR Am J Roentgenol 2007;188:1577–87.
24. Odicino F. History of the FIGO cancer staging system. Int J Gynaecol Obstet 2008;101(2):205–10.
25. Beddy P. FIGO staging system for endometrial cancer: added benefits of MR imaging. Radiographics 2012;32:241–54.
26. Morrow CP. Relationship between surgical-pathological risk factors and outcome in clinical stage I and II carcinoma of the endometrium: a Gynecologic Oncology Group study. Gynecol Oncol 1991;40(1):55–65.
27. Yamashita Y. Normal uterus and FIGO stage I endometrial carcinoma: dynamic gadolinium-enhanced MR imaging. Radiology 1993;186(2):495–501.
28. Manfredi R. Local-regional staging of endometrial carcinoma: role of MR imaging in surgical planning. Radiology 2004;231(2):372–8.
29. Beddy P. Evaluation of depth of myometrial invasion and overall staging in endometrial cancer: comparison of diffusion-weighted and dynamic contrast-enhanced MR imaging. Radiology 2012;262:530–7.
30. Koh DM. Diffusion-weighted MRI in the body: applications and challenges in oncology. AJR Am J Roentgenol 2007;188(6):1622–35.

31. Whittaker CS. Diffusion-weighted MR imaging of female pelvic tumors: a pictorial review. Radiographics 2009;29(3):759–74 [discussion: 774–8].

32. Takeuchi M. Diffusion-weighted magnetic resonance imaging of endometrial cancer: differentiation from benign endometrial lesions and preoperative assessment of myometrial invasion. Acta Radiol 2009;50(8):947–53.

33. Rechichi G. Endometrial cancer: correlation of apparent diffusion coefficient with tumor grade, depth of myometrial invasion, and presence of lymph node metastases. AJR Am J Roentgenol 2011;197(1):256–62.

34. Rechichi G. Myometrial invasion in endometrial cancer: diagnostic performance of diffusion-weighted MR imaging at 1.5 T. Eur Radiol 2010;20(3):754–62.

35. Murase E, Outwater EK, Tureck RW. Uterine leiomyomas: histopathologic features, MR imaging findings, differential diagnosis, and treatment. Radiographics 1999;19:1179–97.

36. Tamai K, Koyama T, Saga T, et al. The utility of diffusion-weighted MR imaging for differentiating uterine sarcomas from benign leiomyomas. Eur Radiol 2008;18(4):723–30.

37. Bakir B, Bakan S, Tunaci M, et al. Diffusion-weighted imaging of solid or predominantly solid gynaecological adnexial masses: is it useful in the differential diagnosis? Br J Radiol 2011;84:600–11.

38. Takeuchi M. Hyperintense uterine myometrial masses on T2-weighted magnetic resonance imaging: differentiation with diffusion-weighted magnetic resonance imaging. J Comput Assist Tomogr 2009;33(6):834–7.

39. Jacobs MA. Comparison between diffusion-weighted imaging, T2-weighted, and postcontrast T1-weighted imaging after MR-guided, high intensity, focused ultrasound treatment of uterine leiomyomata: preliminary results. Med Phys 2010;37(9):4768–76.

40. Takeuchi M. Susceptibility-weighted MRI of endometrioma: preliminary results. AJR Am J Roentgenol 2008;191:1366–70.

41. Takeuchi M. Adenomyosis usual and unusual manifestations, pitfalls and problem solving imaging technique. Radiographics 2011;31:99–115.

42. Haacke EM, Xu Y, Cheng YC, et al. Susceptibility weighted imaging (SWI). Magn Reson Med 2004;52:612–8.

43. Okamoto Y. MR imaging of the uterine cervix: imaging-pathologic correlation. Radiographics 2003;23:425–45.

44. Nakai A. Functional MR imaging of the uterus. Magn Reson Imaging Clin N Am 2008;16:673–84.

45. Naganawa S, Sato C, Kumada H, et al. Apparent diffusion coefficient in cervical cancer of the uterus: comparison with the normal uterine cervix. Eur Radiol 2005;15:71–8.

46. McVeigh PZ. Diffusion weighted MRI in cervical cancer. Eur Radiol 2008;18:1058–64.

47. Somoye G, Vanessa H, Semple S, et al. Early diffusion weighted magnetic resonance imaging can predict survival in women with locally advanced cancer of the cervix treated with combined chemoradiation. Eur Radiol 2012;22(11):2319–27.

48. Boss EA. Post-radiotherapy contrast enhancement changes in fast dynamic MRI of cervical carcinoma. J Magn Reson Imaging 2001;13:600–6.

49. Yamashita Y. Dynamic-contrast enhanced MR imaging of uterine cervical cancer: pharmokocinetic analysis with histopathologic correlation and its importance in predicting the outcome of radiation therapy. Radiology 2000;216:803–9.

50. Balleyguier C. Staging of uterine cervical cancer with MRI: guidelines of the European Society of Urogenital Radiology. Eur Radiol 2011;21(5):1102–10.

51. Umemoto M, Shiota M, Shimono T, et al. Preoperative diagnosis of ovarian tumors, focusing on the solid area based on diagnostic imaging. J Obstet Gynaecol Res 2006;32(2):195–201.

52. Sohaib SA, Sahdev A, Van Trappen P, et al. Characterization of adnexal mass lesions on MR imaging. AJR Am J Roentgenol 2003;180(5):1297–304.

53. Rosai J. Female reproductive system. Ackerman's surgical pathology. 8th edition. St. Louis (MO): 1996.

54. Togashi K, Nishimura K, Kimura I, et al. Endometrial cysts: diagnosis with MR imaging. Radiology 1991;180:73–8.

55. Kim SH. Unusual causes of tubo-ovarian abscess: CT and MR imaging findings. Radiographics 2004;24:1575–89.

56. Thomassin-Naggara I, Daraï E, Cuenod CA, et al. Contribution of diffusion-weighted MR imaging for predicting benignity of complex adnexal masses. Eur Radiol 2009;19(6):1544–52.

57. Li W, Zhang W, Wu X. Pelvic inflammatory disease: evaluation of diagnostic accuracy with conventional MR with added diffusion-weighted imaging. Abdom Imaging 2012. DOI:10.1007.

58. Takeshita T. Diffusion-weighted magnetic resonance imaging in tubo-ovarian abscess: a case report. Osaka City Med J 2009;55:109–14.

59. Chang HC. Pearl and pitfalls in diagnosis of ovarian torsion. Radiographics 2008;28:1355–68.

60. Lee EJ, Kwon HC, Joo HJ, et al. Diagnosis of ovarian torsion with color Doppler sonography: depiction of twisted vascular pedicle. J Ultrasound Med 1998;17(2):83–8.

61. Graif M, Shalev J, Strauss S, et al. Torsion of the ovary: sonographic features. AJR Am J Roentgenol 1984;6:1331–4.

62. Warner BW, Kuhn JC, Barr LL. Conservative management of large ovarian cysts in children: the value of serial pelvic ultrasonography. Surgery 1992;112(4):749–55.

63. Ferlay J, Shin HR, Bray F, et al. GLOBOCAN Cancer incidence and mortality worldwide: IARC CancerBase no. 10. International Agency for Research on Cancer, Lyon. 2008. Available at: http://www.globocan.iarc.fr. Accessed January 11, 2011.

64. Ellenson. Female genital tract. In: Kumar V, Abbas AK, Aster J, et al, editors. Robbins and Cotran pathologic basis of disease. Philadelphia: Elsevier Saunders; 2010. p. 1005–64.

65. Mohagegh P. Imaging strategy for early ovarian cancer: characterization of adnexal masses with conventional and advanced imaging techniques. Radiographics 2012;32:1751–73.

66. Sohaib SA. The role of magnetic resonance imaging and ultrasound in patients with adnexal masses. Clin Radiol 2005;60(3):340–8.

67. Takeuchi M, Matsuzaki K, Nishitani H. Diffusion-weighted magnetic resonance imaging of ovarian tumors: differentiation of benign and malignant solid components of ovarian masses. J Comput Assist Tomogr 2010;34(2):173–6.

68. Thomassin-Naggara I, Marsault C, Bazot M. Dynamic contrast-enhanced MR imaging of ovarian neoplasms: current status and future perspectives. Magn Reson Imaging Clin N Am 2008;16:661–72.

69. Katayama M, Masui T, Kobayashi S, et al. Diffusion-weighted echo planar imaging of ovarian tumors: is it useful to measure apparent diffusion coefficients? J Comput Assist Tomogr 2002;26:250–6.

70. Fujii S, Kakite S, Nishihara K, et al. Diagnostic accuracy of diffusion-weighted imaging in differentiating benign from malignant ovarian lesions. J Magn Reson Imaging 2008;28:1149–56.

71. Low RN, Sebrechts CP, Barone RM, et al. Diffusion-weighted MRI of peritoneal tumors: comparison with conventional MRI and surgical and histopathologic findings— a feasibility study. AJR Am J Roentgenol 2009;193(2):461–70.

72. Kyriazi S, Collins DJ, Messiou C, et al. Metastatic ovarian and primary peritoneal cancer: assessing chemotherapy response with diffusion-weighted MR imaging—value of histogram analysis of apparent diffusion coefficients. Radiology 2011;261:182–92.

73. Hricak H, Chen M, Coakley FV, et al. Complex adnexal masses: detection and characterization with MR imaging—multivariate analysis. Radiology 2000;214(1):39–46.

74. Jain RK. Determinants of tumor blood flow: a review. Cancer Res 1988;48(10):2641–58.

75. Thomassin-Naggara I, Darai E, Nassar-Slaba J, et al. Value of dynamic enhanced magnetic resonance imaging for distinguishing between ovarian fibroma and subserous uterine leiomyoma. J Comput Assist Tomogr 2007;31(2):236–42.

76. Thomassin-Naggara I. Dynamic-contrast enhanced MR imaging to assess physiologic variations of myometrial perfusion. Eur Radiol 2010;20(4):984–94.

Index

Note: Page numbers of article titles are in **boldface** type.

Magn Reson Imaging Clin N Am 21 (2013) 471–474
http://dx.doi.org/10.1016/S1064-9689(13)00025-1
1064-9689/13/$ – see front matter © 2013 Elsevier Inc. All rights reserved.

Moving?

Make sure your subscription moves with you!

To notify us of your new address, find your **Clinics Account Number** (located on your mailing label above your name), and contact customer service at:

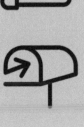

Email: journalscustomerservice-usa@elsevier.com

800-654-2452 (subscribers in the U.S. & Canada)
314-447-8871 (subscribers outside of the U.S. & Canada)

Fax number: 314-447-8029

Elsevier Health Sciences Division
Subscription Customer Service
3251 Riverport Lane
Maryland Heights, MO 63043

Printed and bound by CPI Group (UK) Ltd, Croydon, CR0 4YY

03/10/2024

01040347-0003